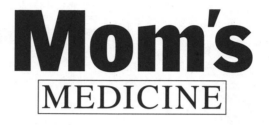

Mom's
MEDICINE

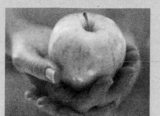

Mom's

MEDICINE

HOW TO PROTECT YOUR

KIDS, HUSBAND, AND PARENTS

AGAINST MORE THAN

100 HEALTH CONDITIONS

AND MEDICAL EMERGENCIES

BY THE EDITORS OF *PREVENTION* Health Books. *for* Women

EDITED BY SHARON FAELTEN

RODALE

Mom's Medicine is a trademark and *Prevention* Health Books is a registered trademark of Rodale Inc.

Printed in the United States of America
Rodale Inc. makes every effort to use acid-free ∞, recycled paper ♺.

Cover photograph © 2000 by Amy Neunsinger/Stone

Interior photographs © 2000 by Arthur Tilley/FPG International LLC on page 21; © 2000 G & M David de Lossy/The Image Bank on page 159; Digital Stock on page 269; Kurt Wilson/Rodale Images on page 377; and Rodale Images on page 479

Illustrations © 1999 by Melanie Powell on pages 324–27; © 1999 Michael Gellatly on pages 483–86, 502, 504, 506, 507; and © 2001 Judy Newhouse on pages 490–92

Library of Congress Cataloging-in-Publication Data

Medicina de mamá. English
  Mom's medicine : how to protect your kids, husband, and parents against more than 100 health conditions and medical emergencies / by the editors of Prevention Health Books for Women ; edited by Sharon Faelten.
      p.   cm.
  Includes index.
  ISBN 1–57954–469–X hardcover
  ISBN 1–57954–490–8 paperback
  1. Family—Health and hygiene.   2. Children—Health and hygiene.
  3. Medicine, Popular.   4. Self-care, Health.   I. Prevention Health Books for Women.   II. Title.
  RA777.7 .M4313   2001
  616.02'4—dc21   2001019873

Distributed to the book trade by St. Martin's Press

2   4   6   8   10   9   7   5   3   1   hardcover
2   4   6   8   10   9   7   5   3   1   paperback

Visit us on the Web at www.rodalestore.com, or call us toll-free at (800) 848-4735.

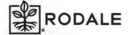

WE **INSPIRE** AND **ENABLE** PEOPLE TO IMPROVE
THEIR LIVES AND THE WORLD AROUND THEM

About *Prevention* Health Books

The editors of *Prevention* Health Books are dedicated to providing you with authoritative, trustworthy, and innovative advice for a healthy, active lifestyle. In all of our books, our goal is to keep you thoroughly informed about the latest breakthroughs in natural healing, medical research, alternative health, herbs, nutrition, fitness, and weight loss. We cut through the confusion of today's conflicting health reports to deliver clear, concise, and definitive health information that you can trust. And we explain in practical terms what each new breakthrough means to you, so you can take immediate, practical steps to improve your health and well-being.

Every recommendation in *Prevention* Health Books is based upon reliable sources, including interviews with qualified health authorities. In addition, we retain top-level health practitioners who serve on the Rodale Books Board of Advisors to ensure that all of the health information is safe, practical, and up-to-date. *Prevention* Health Books are thoroughly fact-checked for accuracy, and we make every effort to verify recommendations, dosages, and cautions.

The advice in this book will help keep you well-informed about your personal choices in health care—to help you lead a happier, healthier, and longer life.

Notice

MOM'S MEDICINE STAFF

EDITOR: Abel Delgado
MANAGING EDITOR: Sharon Faelten
WRITERS: Laura Catalano, Betsy Bates Freed, Matthew Hoffman, Jana Murphy
COVER AND INTERIOR DESIGNER: Lynn N. Gano
PHOTO EDITOR: Robin Hepler
EDITORIAL RESEARCHERS: Jennifer Goldsmith Cerra, Joanne D. Policelli, Paula Rasich
SENIOR COPY EDITOR: Karen Neely
COPY EDITOR: Jennifer Strouse
EDITORIAL PRODUCTION MANAGER: Marilyn Hauptly
LAYOUT DESIGNER: Jennifer H. Giandomenico
MANUFACTURING COORDINATORS: Brenda Miller, Jodi Schaffer, Patrick T. Smith

RODALE WOMEN'S HEALTH BOOKS

VICE PRESIDENT, EDITORIAL DIRECTOR: Elizabeth Crow

EDITOR-IN-CHIEF: Tammerly Booth

VICE PRESIDENT OF MARKETING: Karen Arbegast

PRODUCT MARKETING MANAGER: Stephanie Hamerstone

PRODUCT MANAGER: Dan Shields

BOOK MANUFACTURING MANAGER: Eileen Bauder

WRITING DIRECTOR: Jack Croft

RESEARCH DIRECTOR: Ann Gossy Yermish

ART DIRECTOR: Darlene Schneck

MANAGER OF CONTENT ASSEMBLY: Robert V. Anderson Jr.

DIGITAL PROCESSING GROUP MANAGERS: Leslie M. Keefe, Thomas P. Aczel

OFFICE STAFF: Julie Kehs Minnix, Catherine E. Strouse

BOARD OF ADVISORS

Contents

INTRODUCTION xv

PART ONE
The Basics of Mom's Medicine

Here you'll learn what equipment you need to take care of your "patients." And since many of the remedies recommended in this book are herbal, we include a basic guide to herbal medicine and how to use it to better take care of your family.

WHAT TO KEEP ON HAND 3

HERBAL MEDICINE FOR MOMS 11

PART TWO
Mom's Medicine for Kids and Teens

Kids and teens are the main "patients" for the majority of moms. In this section, we go beyond covering simple problems such as pulling out splinters, which you probably already can do, to tackle various problems—both physical and emotional—that require more complicated approaches.

ACNE 23

ASTHMA 28

BAD GRADES 34

BULLIES 41

CAVITIES 47

COLDS 53

CONSTIPATION 59

DATING 64

DRUGS 71

EATING DISORDERS 80

FEVER 85

GANGS 91

HAY FEVER AND ALLERGIES 99

LONELINESS 105

NIGHT TERRORS AND NIGHTMARES 113

OVERWEIGHT 118

SEX 123

SIBLING RIVALRY 131

STOMACHACHE 134

STUTTERING 140

TEEN REBELLION 144

TV ADDICTION 150

VOMITING 154

PART THREE
Mom's Medicine for Men

Some women claim that the hardest "children" to take care of are their husbands. In this part, our experts offer you not only remedies to take better care of your husband when he's sick but also support tactics to teach him to take better care of himself.

ABDOMINAL FAT 161

BACK PAIN 165

BALDNESS 170

BURSITIS AND TENDINITIS 173

DIABETES 178

FLATULENCE 184

GOUT 188

HEART DISEASE 193

HEMORRHOIDS 198

HIGH BLOOD PRESSURE 202

HIGH CHOLESTEROL 207

IMPOTENCE 213

INHIBITED SEXUAL DESIRE 216

KIDNEY STONES 220

PREMATURE EJACULATION 225

PROSTATE PROBLEMS 229

SMOKING 236

SNORING 243

SPORTS ADDICTION 249

SPRAINS 253

STRESS 257

ULCERS 262

PART FOUR
Mom's Medicine for Older Folks

When you were little, your parents cared for you with the love and wisdom they had learned from their parents. Now it's your turn to take care of them. Learn how to handle the most common problems that affect older people.

ARTHRITIS 271

DEMENTIA 276

HEART PALPITATIONS 285

HIP PAIN 288

INCONTINENCE 292

INSOMNIA 297

INTERMITTENT CLAUDICATION 303

MACULAR DEGENERATION 308

MEMORY PROBLEMS 313

MOBILITY PROBLEMS 320

MUSCLE SORENESS 328

NECK PAIN 333

NIGHT VISION PROBLEMS 337

NUTRITION 342

OSTEOPOROSIS 348

PARKINSON'S DISEASE 354

PHLEBITIS 360

PNEUMONIA 365

POOR CONCENTRATION 370

PART FIVE
Mom's Medicine for Mom Herself

Even the best doctors have to take care of themselves. If they don't, then what good are they to their patients? The same applies to you. In this part, our experts tell you how to combat the ills that most affect women so that you can stay in tip-top shape.

ANEMIA 379

BREAST DISCOMFORT 384

CANCER PREVENTION 390

CAREGIVER STRESS 395

CHRONIC FATIGUE 400

COLDS AND FLU 408

CONSTIPATION 413

DEPRESSION 418

INACTIVITY 424

INFERTILITY 428

MENOPAUSE 434

MENSTRUAL DISCOMFORTS 440

OVERWEIGHT 445

TENSION HEADACHES AND MIGRAINES 451

URINARY TRACT INFECTIONS 457

VAGINITIS 462

VARICOSE VEINS 467

YEAST INFECTIONS 473

FIRST AID

BASIC LIFESAVING TECHNIQUES 481
Here we present some of the basic first-aid techniques you should know in case of an emergency.

FIRST AID FOR CHILDREN 487
Step by step, you'll learn what you should do if the unexpected—and dreaded—happens and your child is hurt.

Bleeding 487
Breathing Problems and Suffocation 488
Minor Burns 488
Severe Burns 489
Choking 490
Convulsions without Fever 492
Drowning 493
Electric Shock Injuries 494
Eye Injuries 494
Falls 496
Finger or Toe Injuries 496
Frostbite 497
Head Injuries 498
Poisoning 500

FIRST AID FOR ADULTS 501
When it's an adult in a dangerous situation, the steps you take vary only a little, but we've included these specific directions to prepare you just in case.

Broken Bones 501
Broken Nose 503
Burns 504

Choking 505
Drowning 508
Electric Shock 509
Falling 511
Open Wounds 512
Poisoning 513
Seizures 514
Severed Appendages 515

Index 517

Introduction

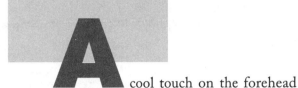cool touch on the forehead when we have a fever, an adhesive bandage and a kiss to heal a skinned knee, tea to soothe an upset stomach—these are the things we think of when we hear the term *Mom's medicine*. Sure, our dads took care of us, but mostly it seemed that their job was to make sure we didn't do anything too dangerous, like running into traffic or jumping off a rooftop using an umbrella as a parachute. But when we had splinters in our fingers, bee stings, or any other kind of ache or pain—even a bad day at school—we didn't go to Dad. We went to Mom. Why? Because we knew she'd find a way to make it better. As kids, we never really thought about it. But today, as a mother yourself, you now realize how important you are to your kids' health.

And not just to their health. What about your husband's bad back? Or your mother's high blood pressure? Sure, the doctor will examine them and prescribe treatments, but who keeps your husband from throwing his back out trying to be Hercules while moving furniture? And who makes sure that your mother takes her medication and avoids fatty foods? You do this, usually amid lots of other motherly and wifely duties.

So the fact is, Mom's Medicine goes way beyond kissing a boo-boo or two. It's about making sure everybody in the family is healthy and stays that way. And not just physically. You see problems all the time that a kiss won't make better. For one thing, drugs and gangs threaten our children. How can we stop those scourges of society from entering our homes? Between shows like *The Jerry Springer Show* and racy videos on MTV, how do we talk to our kids about sex? And on a lighter note, how do you unglue your husband from the couch and get him actually to do something with the family during football season?

You'll find these answers and more in this book. We interviewed a wide range of health experts—from doctors, scientists, and nutritionists to psychologists, herbalists, and naturopathic physicians—to get solutions to the problems that most affect families. But there's no medical jargon here. We translated it all into momspeak, so you can keep your kids drug-free forever, stop your husband's gout, or improve your dad's memory. And we didn't forget about you: We devoted a whole section to women's health problems, ranging from anemia to varicose veins. After all, if you're sick, you won't be able to practice Mom's Medicine very well.

Some of us here at *Prevention* are moms too, and we tried to keep it simple so you can get what you need right away. The first chapter tells you what you should have in the house to take care of your patients, and the second gives you a quick primer on herbal healing, since a lot of the best remedies in this book are simple herbal preparations. Then we divide your family up, going from kids and teens to men to older folks to yourself, covering the most common problems with the simplest solutions. And in the back, we added first-aid information for both kids and adults.

So does your husband need to lose weight? Are your kids bringing home bad grades? Is arthritis pain making your mom miserable? Are you looking to boost your energy and combat fatigue? Well, don't worry. It's nothing that you—and *Mom's Medicine*—can't handle. Grab this book and look it up. It's time to make things all better.

—The editors of *Prevention* Health Books for Women

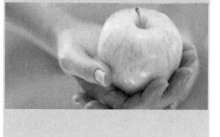

PART ONE

The Basics of Mom's Medicine

What to Keep on Hand

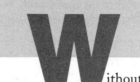**W**ithout instruments, a doctor (male or female) can only help so much. Certain equipment is necessary for diagnosis and treatment. The same applies to you as the doctor of the house. In this chapter, medical experts will let you know some of the basic things you'll need in your home to keep your family members healthy and to treat them for minor problems if they come up.

Medicines

The following items are worth keeping in your medicine cabinet.

Acetic acid. For athlete's foot and poison ivy. Example: Domeboro.

Alpha hydroxy products. To relieve dry skin and to prevent acne, use a moisturizer with alpha hydroxy acids. To make wrinkles less apparent, to help eliminate a double chin, and to prevent scarring, use an alpha hydroxy cream. Example: Alpha Hydrox.

Antacid. To relieve heartburn. A good choice is Mylanta, which contains a combination of magnesium and aluminum.

Antibacterial soap. To prevent burns and open wounds from becoming infected; to treat chafing, jock itch, and boils; and to prevent body odor. Example: Lever 2000.

Antihistamine. For eczema, poison ivy, and motion sickness. Example: Benadryl.

Baby powder. To relieve rectal itching and to prevent various skin problems such as blisters, boils, and chafing. Generic brands are readily available.

Calamine lotion. For itchy skin caused by poison ivy or sunburn. Generic brands are readily available.

Colloidal oatmeal bath. To relieve itching caused by sunburn, rashes, shingles, and psoriasis. Example: Aveeno Bath Treatment.

Cotton swabs and cotton balls. For applying medicines topically. Generic brands are readily available.

Cough medicine. For a productive cough (one that gets rid of phlegm), use a brand containing guaifenesin, such as Robitussin. For an unproductive cough (a dry cough that keeps you up at night), use a brand that contains dextromethorphan, such as Robitussin DM.

Decongestant. To relieve a stuffy head caused by allergies, a sinus infection, or a cold. Our experts recommend brands that contain pseudoephedrine, such as Sudafed.

Elastic bandages. For treating knee pain, sprains, tendinitis, and bursitis. Example: Ace bandage.

Fiber supplement. For occasional use, when eating foods high in fiber doesn't relieve constipation. Metamucil, which contains psyllium fiber, is a good choice. Taken with meals, a fiber supplement can also prevent overeating.

Hydrocortisone cream. For itching and inflammation caused by rashes, poison ivy, or razor burn. Generic brands are readily available.

Nasal spray. For a stuffy nose, use one containing oxymetazoline, such as Afrin.

Pain medicine. For headaches and minor pain. Because certain pain medications are better for certain conditions, you should keep three different kinds on hand: acetaminophen, aspirin, and ibuprofen. For example, you should give acetaminophen rather than aspirin or ibuprofen if your *adult* "patient" has an ulcer, an earache, or pain associated with a bruise or open wound. You should also avoid giving aspirin if your loved one has a fever or gout. But if your loved one is having chest pains that may be from a heart attack, having him chew one aspirin may help save his life.

To know what pain relievers to give to children, ask your pediatrician or see the specific instructions in the chapters that recommend them.

Pepto-Bismol. For a stomachache, diarrhea, or nausea. The pink stuff's active ingredient, bismuth, is also available in generic brands.

Petroleum jelly. To treat chapped lips and psoriasis and to prevent scarring, chafing, saddle sores, and hangnails. Generic brands are readily available.

Thermometer. To take a temperature to determine whether your loved one is running a fever.

First-Aid Kit

You should also keep a well-stocked first-aid kit on hand so that you're prepared for any emergency. Here's a list of items to get your kit started.

Antibiotic ointment. To prevent blisters, burns, cuts, and other open wounds from becoming infected. Example: Polysporin.

Butterfly bandages. To keep the edges of a wound together.

Disposable latex gloves. To wear whenever administering first aid to another person to protect yourself from picking up diseases such as hepatitis and HIV.

Face mask. To wear when doing cardiopulmonary resuscitation or when giving mouth-to-mouth resuscitation.

Hydrogen peroxide. To clean an open wound or to use as a mouthwash to disinfect irritated gums.

Ipecac syrup and activated charcoal. For treatment after swallowing certain poisons.

Reusable, instant-activating ice bags. For icing injuries.

Rubbing alcohol. To sterilize tweezers before using them.

Saline solution for contact lenses. To moisten sterile gauze used to bandage a broken bone that breaks through the skin or to wrap up a severed appendage so that you can take it to the hospital and possibly have it reattached.

Sterile gauze. To bandage open wounds, burns, blisters, and corns.

Tweezers. To remove dirt or debris from an open wound, a tick that is attached to someone's skin, or a splinter.

Vitamins and Minerals

For adults, a multivitamin serves as an insurance policy, says Cathy Kapica, R.D., Ph.D., professor of nutrition and dietetics at Finch University of Health Sciences/Chicago Medical School. "It doesn't excuse one, however, from eating a well-balanced diet."

One caution: Make sure that the multivitamin you choose for your man does not contain extra iron, says David Meyers, M.D., professor of internal medicine and preventive medicine at University of Kansas School of Medicine in Kansas City. Most men get too much iron in their diets already, and excess iron has been linked to higher risk of heart disease and cancer in men.

For each nutrient that follows, listed as well is the Daily Value established by the Food and Nutrition Board, which is the minimum amount one needs of each nutrient every day to stay healthy at the most basic level. Throughout this book, our experts recommend getting more than the Daily Value for many of these nutrients to help in healing, to combat fatigue, and to prevent illnesses such as heart disease.

In addition to a multivitamin, you might want to consider making sure your family eats foods that are good sources of these vitamins and minerals to help them reach the optimal amounts recommended by our experts.

Calcium. Builds strong bones and teeth. Daily Value: 1,000 milligrams for people younger than 65 and 1,500 milligrams for people older than 65. Food sources: milk, yogurt, and cheese.

Magnesium. Involved in metabolism and nerve functions. Daily Value: 400 milligrams. Food sources: meats, poultry, dairy products, cereal, and dark green leafy vegetables.

Vitamin C. Strengthens resistance against infection and helps form collagen, which fortifies blood vessel walls and forms scar tissue. Daily Value: 60 milligrams. Food sources: oranges, cranberry juice, cantaloupe, broccoli, red and green peppers, pink grapefruit, and kiwifruit.

Vitamin E. Combats heart disease and certain cancers. Daily Value: 30 IU. Food sources: vegetable and nut oils, sunflower seeds, whole grains, wheat germ, and spinach.

Zinc. Strengthens immune system, helps in the healing of wounds and sperm production. Essential for brain function. Daily Value: 15 milligrams. Food sources: red meats, poultry, eggs, and oysters.

Herbs

Among the healing herbs that our experts recommend throughout this book are the following:

Aloe. For burns, including sunburn, and to relieve rectal itching. An aloe poultice can draw a splinter to the surface of the skin. Aloe vera juice can also help relieve constipation.

Arnica. For sprains and muscle soreness, and to speed the healing of bruises as well as other injuries due to trauma.

Calendula. Also known as garden or pot marigold, this herb is effective in treating blisters, canker sores, chafing, and razor burn.

Chamomile. To help settle an upset stomach and to relieve gas.

Echinacea. Also known as coneflower, echinacea strengthens the immune system and helps fight off colds, ear infections, flu, pneumonia, and perhaps even Lyme disease.

Ginger. Contains anti-inflammatory properties that make it useful for people with arthritis, bursitis, or tendinitis. It can also help relieve gas, diarrhea, nausea, motion sickness, allergies, bad breath, and hiccups.

Ginkgo. Improves bloodflow to the brain, keeps you mentally sharp, and elevates your mood. May help relieve impotence, depression, back pain, and absentmindedness.

Ginseng. May boost energy and libido. Can help relieve stress, burnout, and impotence.

Goldenseal. To help fight ear infections, pneumonia, and a cough associated with a cold. It can also ease the pain and speed the healing of canker sores and gum ailments.

Kava. To relieve muscle cramps, muscle soreness, and restless legs that keep you up at night.

St. John's wort. For moderate depression, seasonal affective disorder, and fatigue associated with mild depression.

Saw palmetto. For frequent urination or incontinence caused by an enlarged prostate.

Foods

Keeping the right stuff in your kitchen can keep your family healthier. Here are a few foods that our experts suggest keeping in your refrigerator and pantry.

Bananas. To help relieve diarrhea and muscle cramps. Eating potassium-packed bananas as part of a regular diet can also help relieve the pain associated with sciatica and can even help bring down high blood pressure.

Cayenne pepper. To help relieve congestion, a stubborn cough, a sore throat, and bad breath. Cooking with cayenne on a regular basis can help lower cholesterol.

Chewing gum. To help relieve bad breath, dry mouth, heartburn, and even an in-flight earache.

Chicken soup. To unclog a stuffy nose and to slow the body's phlegm production. Homemade chicken soup would be better, but condensed, canned chicken soup does work.

Fish. The omega-3 fatty acids in fish such as salmon, mackerel, tuna, herring, and sardines may relieve depression, skin rashes, and eczema. They can reduce the pain and stiffness of rheumatoid arthritis and may prevent and even reverse heart disease.

Flaxseed oil. To help relieve constipation, dry skin, eczema, and rashes. Also available in seed and supplement form.

Garlic. Can help fight off colds and flu as well as athlete's foot, relieves a nagging cough and diarrhea, and helps lower cholesterol, making your blood less likely to form dangerous clots. Of course, fresh garlic is best, but if you're worried about repelling your friends and coworkers as well as vampires because of garlic's notorious odor, fear not. Odor-free garlic capsules are readily available.

Hard candy. For a sore throat or hiccups.

Honey. To help relieve constipation, heartburn, a sore throat, bad breath, and even a hangover.

Horseradish. To relieve congestion.

Lemon. To soothe wasp stings or to get rid of body odor. It is also an ingredient in remedies recommended by our experts to relieve a cough, a sore throat, bad breath, and hiccups.

Milk. To relieve and prevent muscle cramps, to prevent kidney stones from forming, and to soothe sunburn. Just make sure that your family members are drinking fat-free or low-fat milk so that they're not clogging their arteries or putting on extra pounds.

Olive oil. Use as your regular cooking oil for a healthy heart.

Orange juice. To help curb nicotine cravings, prevent kidney stones from forming, and help soften the stools of those with diverticular disease of the colon.

Sports drinks. To prevent muscle cramps, replenish fluids lost during a bout of diarrhea, or prevent symptoms caused by inflammatory bowel disease. Gatorade is one brand to try.

Vinegar. White vinegar as a remedy to soothe wasp stings, as eardrops to help dry up moisture and stop any itching, and as a soak to get rid of foot odor. Apple cider vinegar as a digestive aid to ease heartburn and as a rinse to fight dandruff and dry hair.

Wheat germ. To help restore coenzyme Q_{10} levels in the hearts of people with angina and to relieve restless legs that wake you up in the middle of the night.

Yogurt. For an energy boost to relieve that early-afternoon slump. Eating yogurt is also a good way for those who are lactose intolerant to get their calcium. They generally can tolerate yogurt because the lactose is digested by the live bacteria found in most yogurt.

Other Helpful Items

The following items don't fall under the other categories but are recommended by experts elsewhere in this book for problems that your family is likely to face. So add these to your in-house doctor's medicine cabinet.

Art supplies. To work through emotional and psychological problems such as bad dreams, a midlife crisis, and envious feelings. All you or your loved one needs to give art therapy a try is an unlined pad of paper and some colored pencils or markers.

Date book. Keeping better track of one's appointments and scheduling weekly chores can help change bad habits such as sloppiness, chronic lateness, and absentmindedness. It can also help when one is trying to kick an addiction. And if sexual desire is down, you can try setting a date for sex. Maybe you and your husband will discover that it's a real libido lifter . . . and the one appointment that you're most likely to keep.

Heating pad. To speed the healing of bruises and to relieve back or neck pain, arthritis pain, heartburn, or an earache.

Humidifier. To keep skin and nasal passages moist, especially during the winter months. It will help relieve dry mouth, dry skin, eczema, bronchitis, laryngitis, and nosebleeds.

Herbal Medicine for Moms

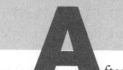

After learning about the basic herbs that you need in your home's medicine cabinet in the last chapter, you may be wondering why this chapter is taking the trouble to address herbs in greater detail. The answer is that herbs are a big part of Mom's Medicine, at least in this book. Many of the experts interviewed offered herbal remedies in addition to standard tips for solving the health problems of your family because they're generally very safe, effective, and easy to obtain. In some cases, herbs also can be a nice alternative to prescription drugs and their harsh side effects.

The fact that these are not prescription drugs doesn't mean that they can't be dangerous, however. Herbs can interact with drugs and with each other. Also, taking them is not always as easy as popping a pill. Sometimes you need to make special preparations or buy certain kinds of herbal products. What follows is a brief overview of herbal healing. Read it, and you'll be able to take maximum advantage of the herbal remedies included in this book.

Teas. There are two kinds of tea remedies most often called for in herbal medicine. If you're using the soft parts of a plant (the leaves or flowers), you steep the herb by pouring boiling water over it and letting it stand, or steep, for a set amount of time, usually between 5 and 20 minutes. That's called an infusion.

The plant's harder parts (the root, rhizome, or bark) yield their healing properties more reluctantly, so to use them, you have to decoct rather than infuse. With a decoction, you usually place the herb in the water before you bring it to a boil, then let the mixture simmer (rather than steep) for 10 to 30 minutes.

For both infusions and decoctions, you need to strain out the plant material before drinking the tea. Of course, there are variations on these instructions; those are explained with the individual remedies in this book.

Tinctures. Alcohol is nature's great extractor of an herb's healing properties. Thus, one of the best ways to take your herbal medicine is in an alcohol-based liquid extract called a tincture. Modern technology has improved the process considerably, but tinctures are essentially the result of soaking an herb in alcohol for several weeks. Sold in little dark bottles capped with droppers, tinctures are widely available, easy to take, and often recommended.

Alcohol is such an efficient extractor that tinctures are usually more potent than teas. Virtually all of the properties of the plant itself are in the liquid, including the taste. Also, the absorption rate is swift—meaning that the healing constituents get into your bloodstream faster than with, say, capsules. There are also nonalcohol tinctures, which are glycerin-based (often called glycerites).

Tincture doses are often given in drops, droppers, teaspoons, or milliliters. Most tinctures come in bottles with droppers that allow you to measure drops and sometimes milliliters. To ensure that you achieve the proper dosage when measuring in teaspoons, use a standard liquid measuring spoon, not a teaspoon from your silverware drawer. Drugstores sell measuring spoons and dosing syringes marked with both teaspoons and milliliters. These may be easiest to find near the children's medicine section.

If you want to make your own tinctures, here are some basic instructions: Put the finely cut herb and a 40 percent clear alcohol solution (vodka works fine) in a glass jar with a tight-fitting lid. You should use 1 part herb to 5 parts liquid, which roughly translates into putting in enough vodka to cover the herb with ¼ inch to spare. Store it in a dark place for 6 weeks, shaking the bottle once or twice a day. Then strain out the herb, squeezing as much of the liquid from it as you can, and behold, you have a tincture.

As you may have guessed, it gets more detailed than that. For one thing, different herbs require different alcohol strengths, so vodka isn't always best. Each herb's specific requirements can be found in herbal compendiums. Or you could take a class, which many herb stores or herbalists offer. Having somebody show you how to do it at least once may help you get comfortable. Then you can make tinctures forever, using books.

Capsules and tablets. One of the most convenient ways to get an herb dosage is with capsules or tablets. These days, herbal supplements are as easy to find in stores as vitamins. And taking them is as simple as reading the instructions on the package label to determine the dosage and then swallowing the recommended number of capsules. As an added bonus, herbs that taste or smell bad are easier to take in capsule or tablet form, as opposed to a tincture or a tea. You also avoid the alcohol that's in the majority of tinctures, which can be an issue for some people.

The average capsule is filled with a dried herb that's been ground up. This isn't exactly the most effective herb form, though, since the process of grinding exposes more of the herb to air and makes it oxidize quickly. There's a good chance that it could lose most of its healing power by the time you buy it.

Technology has stepped in to build a better herb capsule. Processes such as freeze-drying yield a dry herbal extract that makes a more potent and stable capsule. These are called, not surprisingly, freeze-dried extracts. The one downside that capsules have is that it's harder for your body to absorb the herb's healing properties than it is when you drink a tea or tincture.

Essential oils. An essential oil is distilled from an herb via a complicated evaporation and condensation process that yields an extremely concentrated liquid. These oils are used as part of two forms of natural medicine called aromatherapy and hydrotherapy. As its name implies, aromatherapy taps into the sense of smell to soothe and promote healing. Hydrotherapy uses water for healing. Some of the remedies in this book may combine herbs with aromatherapy and hydrotherapy. For instance, one of the experts may recommend inhaling the steam from a mixture of boiling water and a few drops of oil. This kind of treatment can be useful if you have a cold.

Solid extracts. A favorite with naturopathic physicians, a solid extract is actually a gooey syrup that's a concentrated source of herbal medicine.

Salves. It's often better to put herbs on your body than in it. Relief from muscle pain is a case in point. An herbal salve, usually prepared with olive oil, beeswax, or both for good consistency and penetration, is a good way to do that. Salves let you take advantage of herbs that are dangerous if taken internally, such as arnica, as do similar topical herbal products (those that are applied to the skin), such as ointments, balms, creams, and lotions.

Poultices. A poultice is little more than mashed or ground herbs in the form of a soft, semiliquid, pulplike mass that is usually spread over wounds, bites, or sores and held in place with a bandage or cloth.

Compresses. Another simple and effective way to apply herbs is with a compress—a cloth or pad that you press onto your skin. Since this is an herbal remedy, you will probably soak the material in a tea or a water-diluted tincture and then hold it near the source of inflammation or muscle pain. If the compress is hot, it may be called a fomentation.

Shopping for Herbs

Unless you're ready to dedicate half your life to growing herbs in your garden and the other half to studying botany so that you can safely harvest them in the wild, you should get most of your herbal medicines by buying them.

Thanks to the herbal renaissance and the market it created, you can find just about any herb from alfalfa to yellow dock with no problem. If you live near a city of any size, buying herbal remedies is as simple as taking a trip to any of the well-stocked health food stores or sometimes to one of the larger drugstores or grocery stores. If you live in an area that's not as well-supplied, mail-order companies will deliver herbs to you quickly, as a glance at the Internet or health-oriented magazines will confirm.

That same herbal renaissance has also complicated herbal shopping, however. Growing interest in herbal medicine has stimulated the proliferation of both high-quality herb suppliers and marginal ones. In other words, there's a lot of junk out there.

How do you avoid the junk? Mainly by being a wary shopper. If you need aspirin, you're probably not averse to simply running into any store that's open, grabbing a bottle of whatever says "aspirin" on the label, and trusting that the FDA has determined that it's perfectly good aspirin. Unfortunately, you can't take the same lackadaisical approach to the wide-open and still mostly unregulated herb market.

Here are some tips to help you make the best buys possible.

Buy by reputation. A basic ground rule is always to buy from a reputable herb supplier. Check a store or mail-order company's reputation by asking questions, talking to friends, reading up on the store or company, and using common sense. There's no set way to judge, but in the end, you should feel confident that you can trust the supplier.

Grill the store owner. Talk to the health food store owner and ask a lot of questions. Where is he getting the herbs? How is he ensuring quality? How does he keep track of how long the herbs have been in stock? The owner of a good store will know these things. And insist on answers before you buy. If a shopkeeper doesn't have this information or won't provide it, that tells you something.

Buy what you need, not what they sell you. The commercial herb business tends to dream up a lot of herbal combinations that have more to do with sales than with healing. It's not necessarily that they're bad, but they can distract you from your particular herbal remedy. Stick to your guns and buy exactly what you need.

How to Buy Herbs in Bulk

There are two basic ways to buy herbs. One lets the suppliers do the preparing and packaging of the tinctures, capsules, oils, salves, and other herbal medicines. Your job is to check for quality, buy the product, take it home, use it, and feel better. The other way is to purchase the actual loose plant in bulk. You can buy it fresh or dried. You can buy the whole herb or certain parts, such as the leaves, root, bark, flowers, or fruit. You can buy it intact or cut up. Whatever way you buy it, you'll take it home and make it into medicine yourself.

You're surely going to be doing both kinds of shopping. The higher-tech products such as extracts in capsules and essential oils aren't the kinds of things that you're likely to whip up in your garage. On the other hand, you need loose herbs to make some teas as well as to prepare certain poultices, baths, compresses, and the like. You even have the option of extracting your own tinctures.

Even bulk herbs can be packaged so that you can buy fixed, weighed amounts, such as 1 ounce, 4 ounces, or even 1 pound, in some kind of sealed bag—a must if you're ordering by mail. Frequently, though, you'll help yourself to what you need, just like buying coffee beans at the co-op. Herb stores will have big containers of herbs—leaves, roots, flowers,

(continued on page 18)

How to Find a Well-Informed Professional

There are times when no one but a pro will do—someone who's well-versed in herbal remedies and can not only assist you in becoming a better home herbalist but also help you heal when home remedies aren't enough. Herb-savvy health care practitioners can tailor herbal remedies to meet your special needs and can put together complex formulas for complex problems.

The professional that you seek may be an herbalist, a naturopathic physician (N.D.), a medical doctor (M.D.) or osteopathic doctor (D.O.) who uses herbs, or some other qualified healer such as a chiropractor, a licensed acupuncturist (L.Ac.), or a practitioner of Traditional Chinese Medicine. That's a lot of options. But even with the booming interest in herbal medicine, finding someone who's qualified to practice it is still no cinch. Here are some tips for a successful search.

Ask your doctor. Sometimes, you find what you're looking for where you least expect it. "The first thing to try is to ask your doctor if he'll work with herbal medicine," says Robert Rountree, M.D., a holistic physician at the Helios Health Center in Boulder, Colorado. "You may be surprised." Even if your doctor won't deal with herbal remedies, he may be able to refer you to someone who does.

Go where the action is. "Ask the people at your local health food store if they're aware of any doctors who are sending their patients over," Dr. Rountree suggests. "That's a great way to find out." Don't forget to ask your fellow customers, too.

Contact the guild. Most herbalists aren't licensed to practice medicine, but the good ones are well-trained in herbal healing methods. The best way to find a qualified practitioner is to contact the American Herbalists Guild (AHG) to see if any of their professional members are located in your area. "They keep a register of all the professional members—herbalists who have passed an extensive peer-review process," says Chanchal Cabrera, a professional member of the AHG, a member of Britain's National Institute of Medical Herbalists, and an herbalist in Vancouver. The address is American Herbalists Guild, 1931 Gaddis Road, Canton, GA 30115. The organization also includes a referral list of professional members on its Web site. If you have access to the Internet, use your Web search engine to find the guild's site.

Nab a naturopath. Naturopathic doctors with degrees from accredited natural medical schools such as Bastyr University in Kenmore, Washington, are often highly qualified physicians who practice a broad range of natural modalities, including herbal medicine. Their principal professional organization, the American Association of Naturopathic Physicians, offers a referral service that may put you in touch with an herbal practitioner near you. Write to 8201 Greensboro Drive, Suite 300, McLean, VA 22102, or search for their Web site and physician database on the Internet.

Hunt for the holistic. Many medical doctors who use herbal remedies in their practices consider themselves holistic physicians and may be affiliated with the American Holistic Medical Association. The association's referral directory costs $5 and may help you locate an herb-oriented holistic M.D. who practices in your area. For more information, write to the American Holistic Medical Association, 4101 Lake Boone Trail, Suite 201, Raleigh, NC 27607. You can also locate the organization's site on the World Wide Web.

or whatever. Just measure out as many ounces as you want and put it in a bag to take home.

Such self-service shopping is cost-effective, since you buy only what you need (perhaps just the right amount to follow a remedy in this book), and there are no packaging costs. It's also kind of fun.

Again, though, you have to pay attention to what you're buying, or you can end up with a decidedly nonmedicinal pile of leaves. Here are some tips to make sure that you get what you pay for.

Trace the age. Once an herb has been unearthed, its flowers and leaves start to deteriorate, especially if they're finely chopped. A big chunk of dried root or bark might keep for a year or two, but if it has been cut and sifted, or if it is made up of the leaves or flowers, it's good for 6 months maximum. It has a finite life span. So ask the store owner or manager how long ago the herb was picked. Track down not just how long it's been in the store but also how long it was in a warehouse or with brokers before it got to the store.

Rate the display. Air and light are enemies of herb potency. A store that protects its herbs properly from those two things is more likely to be selling good ones. Make sure the herbs are in airtight containers that are either dark or stored out of the light. "If they're in those big clear plastic bins with flip-up lids, they're not protected," says Chanchal Cabrera, a professional member of the American Herbalists Guild, a member of Britain's National Institute of Medical Herbalists, and an herbalist in Vancouver.

Check the color. Fading color is a sign of age. Look for a nice bright color before you buy.

Sniff around. A stale-smelling herb is probably an impotent herb, so give it the sniff test before you buy. Check for that really fresh, herby smell.

Give your herbs a good home. Herbs are just as sensitive to light and oxygen after you buy them as they are in the store, so at home follow the same storage rules that you demand from the store. Keep your herbs stored in a tightly covered glass container and keep that container somewhere away from light exposure.

The Herbal Standard

You hear laments about declining standards in the modern world, but not in herbal medicine. Indeed, standardization is a trusty aid in your herb quest. Why? When you buy herbs in capsule or tincture form, it helps to know whether the product has a certain standard percentage of the herb's most important healing constituent (or constituents). A standardized extract has been tested and found to contain enough of the principal active constituent for the herb to do its healing.

For example, there are lots of capsules on the market for the popular immune-system–boosting herb echinacea. If the label indicates that the capsules contain an extract with at least 15 percent of the polysaccharides known as echinacosides, you can be fairly confident that this standardized product will have the desired effect. If not, you could be swallowing an ineffective substance.

Not everyone loves standardized extracts. Some natural practitioners consider standardization a contradiction of a widely adopted tenet in herbal medicine that *all* of the plant's chemicals work together to heal. Still, using a set amount of one constituent as a marker for overall plant potency is the closest thing to consumer protection that exists in herbal medicine.

The importance of standardization also depends on the severity of the illness or condition you are treating. The more serious and pervasive the problem, the more you want to start looking at standardized preparations. But if it is at the lower end of the disease spectrum, where you're looking more to prevent than to treat, then increased potency as determined by standardization isn't as important as just being sure to take the herb on a daily basis.

The Art of Home Herb Use

This book offers specific herbal remedies for specific conditions, with clear instructions on how to prepare those remedies. But there's more to herbal medicine than just following instructions. There's science in herbal medicine, but there's also an element of art. Besides the general guidelines, there are elements that you, the individual, bring into play. That's why so many people like herbs.

What you learn about herbs as you practice your home-herbalist skills expands your healing possibilities. The more you become personally involved with herbs, the healthier you can be. That's something to keep in mind as you consider these last tips for getting the maximum benefit from your herbal home remedies.

Spread out the doses. When a remedy calls for three cups of tea a day or 1 teaspoon of tincture three times a day, that almost always means a morning-noon-night schedule, not a triple shot with breakfast. Experts say that you'll absorb the herbs better if you spread the doses out over the day.

Take most herbs between meals. Almost all herbs should be taken between meals so that they don't have to compete with foods for absorption. You'll find plenty of exceptions, of course, but between-meal dosing has another advantage. Taking herbs at least 15 minutes before meals can aid your digestion, because they prime your digestive system for handling the food.

Refrigerate. Capsules or any other kind of powdered herb should be kept in the fridge. That will prolong their shelf life a little bit.

Develop a plan. Always remember that herbal remedies are just one part of natural healing. "Take your herbs in conjunction with vitamins, diet changes, and stress management," says Susan B. Kowalsky, N.D., a naturopathic physician in Norwich, Vermont. "Natural medicine isn't a matter of popping a different kind of pill. It's about lifestyle."

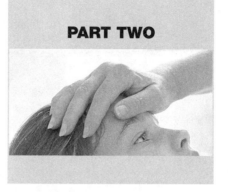

PART TWO

Mom's Medicine for Kids and Teens

Acne

If there's anything more challenging than getting through the acne years, it's watching your children go through them. Blackheads and pimples may be as inevitable among teenagers as the latest fashion trends, but these years are among the most difficult that young people go through.

Teenagers are incredibly self-conscious about physical appearance, and even mild cases of acne can shake their self-confidence to a harmful degree, says Guy Webster, M.D., Ph.D., vice chairman of the department of dermatology at Jefferson Medical College of Thomas Jefferson University in Philadelphia. "I've read that acne can even affect your future success—that unemployment is higher among those who suffered severe acne when they were teenagers."

Fortunately, most acne can be controlled or even eliminated with a combination of home remedies and simple over-the-counter medications, says Debra Jaliman, M.D., a dermatologist and clinical instructor of dermatology at Mount Sinai School of Medicine of New York University in New York City.

Blame It on Hormones

Acne is almost always triggered by the action of hormones called androgens, which stimulate the growth of the oil-producing sebaceous glands in the skin. There's a surge in androgens between the ages of 11 and 14. Boys have the most androgens, but girls have them, too.

The oils produced by sebaceous glands are essential for keeping the skin pliable and healthy. During puberty and adolescence, however, the glands produce too much oil. The surface skin doesn't shed normally, so these dead skin cells plug the pores. The oils can't get out, and oxygen can't get in. This creates a perfect environment for acne-causing bacteria called *P. acnes.*

"Everyone has plenty of oil and plenty of these bacteria," Dr. Webster says. "But some people have an immune system reaction to the organisms." That's what causes the inflammation and bumps known as pimples.

Blackheads, which doctors call comedones, are also caused by the buildup of oils in the skin. Unlike pimples, however, they aren't accompanied by inflammation or infection. Otherwise, the treatments for pimples and blackheads are the same.

It's important for parents to understand that hygiene really isn't a factor, says Dr. Webster. Skin oils are involved, but the action takes place *beneath* the surface of the skin. Sugar and fatty foods are unlikely to be factors either. "A lot of parents work hard to make their kids feel guilty about what they eat, but it probably has nothing to do with the acne," he adds.

The Secrets to Clear Skin

For most people, acne starts to disappear once the hormonal kick of adolescence loses steam. In the meantime, teenagers can usually eliminate outbreaks just by keeping the pores clear and bacteria-free. Here are some home treatments you may want to try.

Keep a lot of washcloths handy. "The most important thing is to encourage teenagers to wash their faces several times a day—not just with soap and water, but with a washcloth. As an alternative to soap, Dr. Jaliman recommends Cetaphil Oil-Free Cleanser (which comes in liquid or bar formulations) and Neutrogena Extra Gentle Cleanser. Using a washcloth helps remove dead skin cells and oils that clog the pores, a process called exfoliation.

Insist they use a fresh washcloth every time. Doing the extra laundry will be a nuisance, but it's essential for teenagers to use a fresh washcloth every time they wash their faces. Otherwise, skin bacteria that's picked up during one washing will be deposited right back on the skin, says Dr. Jaliman.

Make sure the entire face gets washed. Teenagers are always looking for shortcuts, which means they're likely to scrub pimples that have already formed while leaving the rest of the face untouched. Not

Instant Blemish Cover-Ups

A teenager's worst nightmare, apart from losing the use of the car for a month, is to have an evil-looking pimple pop up just before a big date. Even though doctors discourage using makeup to hide pimples, sometimes it's the only way to prevent a big night from turning into an emotional mess.

Makeup experts have a few simple tricks for making pimples disappear—or at least making them a little less noticeable.

"One thing they can do is dab on a little Visine, the same product that's used for red eyes," says Betsy West, instructor of cosmetology and aesthetics at Jean Madeline Education Center for Cosmetology in Philadelphia. "It contracts the blood vessels in the skin and lessens the redness a little bit."

A longer-lasting approach is to use concealer makeup. Dab a little concealer on the pimple, let it sit for a minute, then gently pat it (don't wipe it) so it blends with the skin. This works for boys as well as girls. Concealer comes in dozens of colors, so your child will have to try it out in the store to make sure it's a good match with the skin.

"It's very good camouflage," West says. "It won't make the pimple disappear entirely, but from a distance it's almost completely unnoticeable."

only can this irritate the skin, but it allows acne-causing bacteria to remain on the skin, says Dr. Jaliman. You have to make sure that your kids wash their entire faces, from their hairlines down to their necks.

Buy some cotton pads. An alternative to using dozens of washcloths every week is to pick up some simple cotton facial cleanser pads, which come in circular tubes. They have a slightly abrasive surface that's perfect for acne. "You put on some cleanser and wash the face in a circular motion," says Dr. Jaliman. "That gets rid of a lot of dead skin cells and surface bacteria."

Pick up some granular cleanser. Cleansers called skin scrubs, which are usually sold as creams or lotions, contain tiny particles that lightly scrape and abrade the surface of the skin. You don't want to use them often, but they can play an important role in unblocking pores and letting oils out. "About once a week, have your child exfoliate the skin more deeply by using a granular cleaner," says Dr. Jaliman. It's easy to get carried away when using these cleansers, she adds. Using them too often or too aggressively will irritate the skin and make it more inflamed. "You don't want to weaken the skin too much," she says. Use them as you would any other soap—to give the skin a thorough cleaning, not to rub it raw.

Take advantage of over-the-counter medicines. Pharmacy shelves are loaded with antiacne remedies, some of which are extremely effective. Look for products that contain the following ingredients:

- Benzoyl peroxide. This is an antibacterial ingredient in many acne gels, creams, and pads. "It's a wonderful drug," says Dr. Webster. "A lot of people would get better if they'd just use this one medication."

  Benzoyl peroxide comes in several strengths—the 5 percent formulation is strong enough for most people. "Don't use it as a spot treatment," Dr. Webster instructs. "It has to be applied anywhere on the face where acne tends to appear."

- Salicylic acid. Products with this ingredient are often used in combination with benzoyl peroxide. It helps remove dead skin cells from the surface of the skin and keep the pores open, says Dr. Jaliman.

- Glycolic acid. It belongs to a family of compounds called alpha hydroxy acids. It removes dead skin cells from the surface, which helps the oils beneath the skin drain, Dr. Jaliman says.

Take an inventory of shampoos and cosmetics. A lot of the products that teenage girls use, such as foundation, rouge, and other kinds of makeup, contain oil-based ingredients that clog the pores, says Dr. Jaliman. Only use products that say "non-comedogenic" on the label, she advises. You should look for this label on hair conditioners and hair mousse as well, because the oils that many of these products contain may cause acne on the scalp or below the hairline.

Remind them to keep their hands away from the skin. It's hard for teenagers to resist touching or squeezing pimples, but it's essential that they leave them alone. Otherwise, they'll cause more inflammation and spread bacteria to other parts of the face, says Dr. Jaliman.

Help from Your Doctor

Apart from the emotional turmoil, most acne doesn't cause long-term problems. In some cases, however, the pimples are so numerous or badly inflamed that they start leaving scars. That's when home treatments simply aren't enough. "If your child isn't getting better within about 4 weeks of home care, you need to see a doctor," says Dr. Webster.

Medical treatments for acne have become extremely effective, Dr. Webster adds. "I'm always nervous about using the word *cure*, but, in fact, many cases of acne can be cured with the proper treatments."

The standard medical treatments for acne include the following:

Retinoids. Derived from vitamin A, these prescription creams are designed to break apart the oily deposits that are blocking the pores. The medications are usually applied to the skin for several weeks. They're very effective at controlling flare-ups and getting "active" acne under control.

"The retinoids are extremely safe, but they're a little irritating," Dr. Webster says. "Most people feel better when they use a moisturizer at the same time. Also, the retinoids are often combined with oral tetracycline to control bacteria. The combination works a lot faster than retinoids alone."

Isotretinoin. This oral medication, sold under the brand name Accutane, is very effective at controlling acne. In some cases, it virtually eliminates the problem for a year or more. But despite the benefits, doctors are often reluctant to use this medication because it can cause birth defects. "You have to be careful when using it," says Dr. Webster. "Girls who take Accutane have to take every precaution against pregnancy. But invariably, people who take Accutane get dramatically better."

Asthma

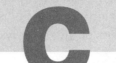

Cases of childhood asthma are increasing. Obviously, this may be worrying you. Fortunately for you and your children, increase in the incidence of asthma has been accompanied by a great deal of research on this disease, and today, many physicians are able to recognize the first symptoms of asthma and help those children experiencing it.

It is not always easy for parents to recognize when a child has asthma. "Almost half of those that experience asthma never gasp for air," says Ted Kniker, M.D., professor of pediatrics and internal medicine at the University of Texas in San Antonio.

"Coughing is the most common symptom, especially coughing at night. Your child could also complain of tightness in the chest and a general feeling of tiredness, particularly after exercise."

What happens during an asthma attack? Airflow decreases as airways inflame and swell. Muscular contractions and heavy mucus obstruct breathing. Many things can cause asthma: pollen, a viral respiratory infection, pollution, dust, animal dander, mold, or even exercise.

If you believe that your child has asthma, take her to the doctor as soon as possible. If this condition is diagnosed, your physician may prescribe medicine to prevent the inflammation of the respiratory passages and a bronchodilator, which is a medicine that must be used during the attacks to help open the respiratory passages. These medicines are given by way of inhalers and atomizers. Your doctor may also prescribe the regular use of a spirometer, a concave tube with a built-in numbered gauge that measures how much air is getting to the airways.

Here are tips from experts to help you manage your child's asthma.

Establish a routine. Daily readings with the spirometer allow you to know how well your child is breathing. Have your child use the spirom-

WHEN TO SEE THE DOCTOR

Even though asthma is a chronic condition that can generally be managed effectively at home with the help of your child's physician, some attacks may be so severe that they are life-threatening.

Unfortunately, there is no specific limit to establish when medical assistance is required, says Thomas Irons, M.D., professor of pediatrics at East Carolina University School of Medicine in Greenville, North Carolina. "But there are defined symptoms that could indicate that your child is in danger and requires medical attention from her personal physician or from an emergency room."

You should seek medical help if:

- Your child is fighting to get air. Her nose may be plugged or her skin sunken at the ribs or collarbone.

- Your child is too busy breathing to be able to talk.

- She is sitting up and leaning forward in an effort to get air.

- She grunts with each breath.

- Your child sits quietly and tries to get air (is not rising or walking).

- She refuses food or beverages.

- She does not feel better within 15 minutes after receiving asthma medicine.

Because this illness can be life-threatening, you should consult your physician immediately if you have any doubts, says Dr. Irons.

eter at a specific time every day, for instance, upon waking up in the morning. A lower-than-normal reading indicates that less air is entering the respiratory passages. If this is the case, ask your physician if you can give your child more medicine to prevent an attack, says Thomas Irons, M.D., professor of pediatrics at East Carolina University School of Medicine in Greenville, North Carolina.

Help your child practice blowing into the spirometer. To produce an accurate reading on the spirometer, your child needs to inhale deeply, close her lips around the nozzle, and exhale as strongly and rapidly as she can. This may require practice. To help your child develop the technique of exhaling, place a cotton plug on one end of a straw, suggests Nancy Sander, president and founder of the Allergy and Asthma Network–Mothers of Asthmatics in Fairfax, Virginia.

"Do it as a game. Make your child breathe in deeply, then place the other end of the straw in her mouth and tell her to blow as hard and as fast as possible. The object is to make the cotton plug shoot out from the straw to reach the other side of the room. This will give your child a sense of how much effort is needed to use the spirometer," explains Sander.

Keep an asthma log. "Keep a record of the symptoms and what caused them, the spirometer's daily readings, and the medicines," says Gary Rachelefsky, M.D., professor of pediatrics at the University of California, Los Angeles. This information can help your child avoid those things that cause the symptoms to surge, and it will help your physician adjust the medication for your child as needed.

Know the medicines your child is taking. "This includes the benefits and the side effects," says Sander. Ask your pharmacist to include the package insert that comes with any medicine you get. Ask her or your doctor any additional questions you may have about the medicines and write down the information to avoid any confusion later.

Ask for a meeting. All those involved with a child with asthma—from the parents to the child care workers to the school personnel—need to be aware of the seriousness of this condition and know the details of the treatment for your child, says Dr. Kniker. Organize where the medicines are going to be kept during school hours and what plans will be followed if symptoms should develop.

Encourage practice. Your physician may recommend a metered-dose inhaler for an older child to take asthma medications, but these devices are difficult to use and require practice. "It takes a little bit of co-ordination and time to use them well," says Dr. Kniker. "Some children can already use them correctly when they are 7 years old, but most will not do it well until they are 10 or 12." With these inhalers, one has to aim them perfectly at the throat, pressing at the same time one breathes in. Oftentimes, children do not do it well, and the medicine ends up in their mouths or on their tongues. The disagreeable taste of the medicine and the difficulty in using the inhalers are the reasons that children don't want to use them.

Fortunately, many children find that it is more convenient to utilize the inhaler by using a *spacer*. This device is a little tube connected to the inhaler that collects the medicinal mist coming out of it. That is, instead of the medicine coming out of the inhaler directly into the child's mouth, it first goes to the spacer. This gives the child more time to inhale the medicine. If your child is starting to use the inhaler, watch closely to see that she is following the doctor's instructions. Later, check every now and then to see that your child is following the appropriate procedure. If you want to get a spacer for your child, consult your physician.

Visualize for healing. Some children breathe the medicine in their inhalers very fast, or they don't do it deeply enough, so most of the med-icine is deposited in their mouths or throats. To help your child use the inhaler correctly, teach her to understand what the medicine does and have her visualize where the medicine should end up, says Sander. "Ex-plain to your child that her lungs are hurt and that the medicine should go where the problem is, which is deep in her lungs. Then, show your child how to breathe slowly while mentally saying a simple sentence or a rhyme as she inhales. After, your child should hold her breath as long as possible to allow the medicine to go as deeply as possible." This will allow your child to prolong the inhalations.

Make your home "antiallergenic." Nearly 90 percent of children younger than 16 who have had asthma also have allergies, according to the National Institute of Allergy and Infectious Diseases in Bethesda, Maryland. "This means that if your child with asthma has been diag-nosed as allergic to cats, dust, or any other thing, you will need to 'im-munize' your home against allergies," says Dr. Kniker. For instance, encase your child's mattress and pillows with plastic covers, and consider removing the carpet from your child's room. Ideally, those pets to which your child is allergic should be removed from the house. Otherwise, you should wash the pet regularly to reduce the allergen and keep the pet out of your child's bedroom. (For more tips, see Hay Fever and Allergies on page 99.)

Ward off smoke. Smoke from tobacco, fireplaces, and wood-burning stoves may trigger an asthma attack, says Dr. Kniker. No one should be allowed to smoke in a house where a child with asthma lives. If your house has a wood-burning stove, it would be better if you installed another type of heating system.

Teach your child to breathe with her abdomen. Slow breathing, twice a day, 10 times each occasion, can help your child learn to use a metered-dose inhaler. Additionally, deep breathing may help her calm down during an asthma attack, says Dr. Irons. But it is the type of breathing that makes the difference. Help your child practice diaphragmatic breathing, which means keeping the upper chest still while breathing deeply and moving the abdomen.

To do this, make your child lie on the floor and place a book on her abdomen, suggests Dr. Irons. Tell your child to make the book move up and down every time she breathes. "Your child should close her lips tightly and breathe in as deeply as possible. Then show your child how to loosen her lips and let the air out very slowly."

Do fun breathing exercises. To develop pulmonary strength and exercise the airways, your child can play a musical instrument or blow up balloons, says Sander. In both cases, you should encourage your child to do more diaphragmatic breathing rather than "chest breathing."

Keep extra inhalers handy. In case of an asthma emergency, you will want to have medication immediately available, says Sander. "Always have one inhaler more than what you estimate necessary. Keep this additional one covered in the lower drawer of the kitchen." But do not keep an inhaler near the stove or in your car's glove compartment during the summer, because the heat can break the valves of the can and allow small quantities of the medicine to escape. Extreme heat may cause the inhalers to explode. These medicines keep well for almost 2 years, so you should check the expiration dates, says Sander.

Consider giving medicine before exercise. "If your child has exercise-induced asthma, you can prevent an attack by simply giving her a dosage of the prescribed medicine in an inhaler, a few minutes before the sports activity or exercise starts," says Dr. Kniker.

Determining the correct pre-exercise dosage will require some trial and error, which should always be done in consultation with your physician.

"Many children need two inhalations from their inhaler to have the appropriate protection," says Dr. Kniker. "Sometimes, children need to repeat the dosage they used before, an hour or more later. Weather can also affect the quantity needed. Warm weather is easier on asthma than cold days."

Keep your cool during the crisis. When an attack occurs, keep calm and speak in soothing tones. "An asthma attack affects parents greatly," says Dr. Irons, "but it will help calm the child down if she sees that you are also calm." If your child gets upset, coughs, or cries, her nervousness or panic will aggravate the attack.

Talk to your child. During an asthma attack, talk calmly with your child, says Sander. "Tell your child, 'I am here, and I am going to help you. First, we are going to use your inhaler. We will use it together. Now that the medicine is inside you, you will soon feel better. So, let us relax while the medicine does its work. Weren't the vacations we took last summer great?'" Talking about fun times you have enjoyed as a family helps to divert your child's feelings of panic as the attack subsides, she explains. If the asthma attack does not respond to the medicines your doctor prescribed, seek medical attention immediately.

Search for a tape or a book. "A child that starts to panic during an asthmatic crisis can frequently be calmed with her favorite tape, be it audio or video," says Dr. Rachelefsky. "If your child concentrates on the music or the program, she will be distracted from the attack." You can also help your child by reading aloud her favorite book.

Bad Grades

Report card day—that moment of revelation when you solve the "How is my child doing in school?" mystery. You open that long, white envelope, scan the page filled with succinct marks that give cryptic shape to your child's accomplishments. And then, disheartened, you slip it back into its envelope and wish the mystery had been left unsolved. Because now you have a whole slew of new mysteries tugging at your brain, like why are your child's grades sagging? Is he on an inevitable road to failure? Can you help set him on a new course?

Children perform poorly in school for a number of reasons, says Patricia Rivell, Ph.D., an educational counselor in Princeton, New Jersey. So the first step toward improving scores is to figure out why they're low to begin with. If your son or daughter really can't keep up with the class, attention deficit disorder or a learning disability could be at fault. While such disorders often become evident in the early grades, some don't surface until later years, especially ones that impact comprehension or other complex functions. (For more information, see "Attention Deficit/Hyperactivity Disorder: What to Look For" on page 36 and "When to Suspect a Learning Disability" on page 38.)

If you've ruled out the possibility of a learning disorder, you'll probably have to do a little guesswork to determine why your child isn't up to speed. To help, we've included some common reasons that dismal report cards show up at different grade levels and ages, and some tips aimed at brightening report card day.

Grades 1 to 3

If reading, writing, and arithmetic seem like unworkable tasks to your elementary school child, the problem could stem from an environment that does not stress education, a distaste for reading, or a vision flaw. You can often improve your young child's grades by providing an enriching home environment that prepares and motivates him to perform tasks required in the early grades. Here are some ways you can help.

Enrich their environment. "Often, kids are in a barren place with nothing but TV," says Dr. Rivell. By filling your home with enriching activities, you'll help prepare and motivate young children to perform tasks required in the earliest grades. Try the following strategies:

- "Spend time seeing things with children," says Dr. Rivell. "Teach them how to ask questions and how to find the answers." Nurturing your children's natural curiosity gets them excited about learning.

- Have plenty of books at their disposal, and read to your kids to stimulate their interest in the printed word. Read newspapers and magazines in front of them, and talk about what you've read.

- Keep crayons, paints, markers, and paper on hand and encourage your children to experiment with them. That will invite them to explore writing and creativity outside the classroom.

Play games. Board games that involve patterns, counting games, and games that keep score require children to use basic math skills in a practical setting.

Do math daily. Show your children that math is something people use every day. Let them help you calculate the savings from coupons at the grocery store or the distance between their house and a friend's.

Show them how to skim and scan. Reading is key to academic success, but not every child loves doing it. If your youngster dreads reading, ask the teacher for tips on skimming and scanning the text for information. "If you make sure that your children's reading skills are really good, then they'll be reading with maximum efficiency whenever they do have to read," says Dr. Rivell.

Ask for explanations. When your child finishes his math homework, ask him to explain how he did it. That will help you pinpoint any areas where he needs help. For example, if he's adding but has trouble carrying numbers to the next column, you'll know he needs additional instruction on that concept. If you can't help him at home, call the teacher for suggestions.

Attention Deficit/ Hyperactivity Disorder: What to Look For

f your child just can't seem to get it all together and listen attentively in class, he may be suffering from attention deficit/ hyperactivity disorder, or ADHD. Here are a few telltale signs.

- Your child is easily distracted by minor stimuli, such as a leaf rustling against a window or someone walking past the classroom.

- He makes many careless mistakes, doesn't pay attention to details, and seems to drift off frequently.

- He often forgets or loses items needed for a task.

- Your child behaves impulsively, blurting out answers or inappropriate remarks.

- He has difficulty taking turns in games.

Schedule a vision check. Your child is constantly growing and changing, so vision problems can crop up suddenly. If reading and learning numbers are a problem, a pair of glasses could clear things up.

Grades 3 to 9

Poor organizational skills and sloppy homework habits can send your child's top-notch grades to the bottom of the barrel. That's often the reason low scores replace straight A's in the third, sixth, or ninth grades. "There is a completely different level of expectations at each of those grades," explains Noreen Joslyn, a psychiatric social worker with the Cleveland Clinic Westlake in Westlake, Ohio. To get your kids back on

- He is hyperactive, fidgets or talks incessantly, and gets out of his seat at times when other children can behave quietly. Hyperactivity is common but is not always present.

- The symptoms described here appeared before the age of 7, have lasted for at least 6 months, and have created a real handicap not just in school but in another setting as well, such as at home or social events. If your child exhibits any of these symptoms, see your pediatrician or a child psychologist, who can assess whether or not the problem is ADHD.

Once your child is diagnosed with ADHD, a doctor or psychiatrist may recommend a stimulant medication to reduce symptoms. This has been shown to improve the behavior and classroom performance of children with ADHD. Concerns have been raised that medication is being overprescribed for ADHD, although studies have unearthed little evidence of this. If you strongly object to putting your child on stimulant medications, ask your doctor about behavioral therapies, which can improve certain behaviors but may not reduce inattention, hyperactivity, or impulsivity, the core symptoms of ADHD.

track, coach them with some homework rules and organizational strategies. But be patient. It takes time to establish a habit.

Support them with strategies. Kids who regularly forget to bring home books and papers may need a memory boost. Teach your child to write down all assignments or to say something aloud to make sure it gets committed to memory, suggests Adrienne Gioe, Ph.D., a certified school psychologist in Philadelphia. By saying, "I'm putting my science book in my locker, but I have to bring it home after school," your child will be less likely to forget.

Stick to a set time. Your kids may do best when homework is done at a set time every day, because it helps them develop a consistent routine, says Dr. Rivell. Agree on a time that works for all of you, and require them to have everything completed before they can watch TV.

Do homework at a desk. Having a quiet spot set aside just for homework helps eliminate distractions. Another benefit of sitting at a desk is that it keeps the body in the proper posture for learning. "When you're lying on the floor or in bed or cuddling in a chair, you're not sending messages to your brain to stay alert," says Dr. Rivell.

Enforce your rules. Let your children know what they stand to lose if their homework isn't done or is done poorly. Place restrictions

When to Suspect a Learning Disability

A learning disability, such as dyslexia, a common reading disorder, can be detected through an educational evaluation performed by the school or a private psychologist. If your child has a disability, he'll need remedial reading, writing, or arithmetic programs to help him acquire techniques necessary for learning. Your child could have a disorder if he or she:

- Has difficulty spelling, sounding out words, identifying new words, or playing rhyming games.

- Is unable to compose complete, grammatical sentences or to comprehend what is read.

- Has poor fine motor skills that make it a chore to copy off the board or write a paragraph.

- Has difficulty memorizing words or facts.

- Has problems aligning numbers or recognizing numbers and symbols.

on TV, computer games, and, for adolescents, going out on weekends.

Check work. When a passing grade is at stake, check homework nightly. But if you have an adolescent who is showing improvement and who resists nightly inspections, you can limit your checks to once a week. Make it the same night, says Joslyn, preferably when you know the school sends information home.

When the Mark of Growing Up Is a D

If your child went careening off the honor roll the moment he hit adolescence, a bad attitude, negative peer pressure, and low self-confidence could be to blame. Here's how to help.

Present a positive attitude. In our culture, teens often believe it's not cool to be smart. You can offset negative peer pressure by always maintaining and voicing a positive attitude toward education, says Joslyn. To be effective, the same message should be coming from your spouse.

Put limits on part-time jobs. Teens who work long hours may have little time to study. If your child doesn't really need the money, insist that he keep hours light.

Never say can't. "Teens really get into the word *can't*," says Dr. Rivell. Make that word off-limits and insist, instead, that your child address specifics, such as "I don't know how" or "I'm overwhelmed." Then, work together to find a solution, thereby bolstering your teen's self-confidence.

Squelch social problems. If your teen is being bullied at school or feels that he is not accepted socially, it's likely he'll develop a negative attitude that affects his grades. In such a case, the parent should first talk to the child and determine the extent of the problem. Then, develop a course of action, says Dr. Rivell. If one or two kids are bullying him, go to the guidance counselor or teacher for assistance. If the issues are more wide-ranging, a counselor may need to step in to work with your child.

Unearth underlying causes. Sometimes drugs, family conflicts, and emotional problems lead teens to neglect their studies. Such problems often require the assistance of a psychologist or family therapist. Below are some reasons you should seek professional help for your teen.

- Drugs. If your adolescent's uncharacteristic Ds are accompanied by other behaviors that are strikingly out of character, suspect drugs, says Dr. Gioe. If you find evidence of drugs or are convinced that your child is taking them, ask the guidance office for a referral to an agency that can help.

- Emotional problems. If your teen loses interest in grades and seems generally distracted or unhappy, he could be suffering from depression. Since serious depression can lead to teen suicide, it is essential that you get him to a psychologist or psychiatrist for a diagnosis.

- Family conflict. "Sometimes there are problems in family dynamics, and kids are angry at the parents, and they use bad grades as a way to get back at them," explains Dr. Gioe. Since this spirals into a power struggle, professional intervention is often needed to resolve the conflict.

Don't Go It Alone

No matter what age your child is when he has trouble in the classroom, input from teachers, administrators, guidance counselors, and other parents may be warranted.

Talk to the teacher. Parent-teacher conferences provide the perfect opportunity for you to meet the teacher, find out where your child stands in relation to his peers, and ask about district-run programs that offer help with learning problems, suggests Dr. Gioe. Some high schools don't offer regular conferences, but teachers remain accessible through voice mail or e-mail. If you get no response, contact the guidance department for assistance. When you do meet with a teacher, maintain a nonadversarial attitude even if you think he has been unfair.

Request reminders. If your child constantly forgets to bring home papers or write down assignments, you might need to rally his teachers to help, says Dr. Rivell. At the elementary school level, make arrangements with the homeroom teacher for daily checks before your child heads home. In later grades, where multiple teachers are involved, an advisor or guidance counselor may supply reminders.

Be an advocate for your child. Do you think a school-related problem, such as overcrowding or inadequate programs, is affecting your child's performance? Contact other parents and see if they agree. If so, join with them to solicit the school board for smaller class sizes or other improvements.

Bullies

Jay Carter, Psy.D., remembers what it was like to be bullied. In middle school, he was the new kid. At the park one day, he met up with a group of boys from his school. They were playing ball, and when he tried to get into the game, they refused to include him and began teasing him. In school, they continued teasing and picking on him whenever they had the chance. Back then, Dr. Carter learned how to stop the bullying by taking a confident stand. Today, he is a psychologist in West Reading, Pennsylvania, and coauthor of *Taking the Bully by the Horns*.

If your child is the victim of a bully, he's hardly an anomaly. "Bullying is one of the most enduring and underrated problems in U.S. schools," says Ronald Stephens, Ed.D., executive director of the National School Safety Center in Westlake Village, California. In fact, one out of seven kids is either a bully or the victim of one, according to Dr. Stephens. Kids of all ages, from preschool through high school, can be affected. And, while most people conjure up images of bullies as adolescents, bullying is actually most prevalent in grades three through six, he says. The problem is often more pronounced in teens, though, because kids who haven't learned to curtail a tendency toward physical aggression may become more violent at that age.

Even in cases where physical violence isn't a threat, bullying can have a serious impact on the self-esteem of the victim, says Carol Watkins, M.D., a psychiatrist in Baltimore. Taunting, teasing, name calling, racial slurs, and even shunning are all forms of bullying that your child may be faced with. We've included tips to help your kids deal with both psychological and physical bullying.

When Teasing Takes Its Toll

Kids tease each other all the time; it's fairly normal. If a kid teases your child with the deliberate intention of hurting his feelings, that's bullying, says Dr. Carter. But, if your child isn't particularly sensitive to that type of teasing, he may not feel bullied, and no action may be required on your part. You should step in with advice, though, whenever the teasing begins to bother your child, and especially if you feel that it is impacting his self-esteem.

Your daughter may be verbally attacked by a classmate because of the way she looks or acts. She may be shunned from a clique because she doesn't make the grade. Or your son may be singled out and taunted because he isn't good at sports. Even on a mild level, that may be bullying, but some kids won't be as sensitive to it, says Dr. Carter. If your child starts to feel hurt, you'll need to step in with advice on how to handle bullies. In some cases, you may need to intervene by contacting the school or the bully's parents. But it's most empowering for your children to learn to effectively deal with bullies on their own. Here are some recommendations for advising them.

Recognize the signs. "Often parents don't know that their kids are being teased," says Dr. Stephens. That's because children don't always report incidents of teasing to their parents or teachers, administrators, or law enforcers. Therefore, before you can even help your child, you should be attuned to possible signs of bullying. Your daughter may suddenly become reluctant to go to school, or her grades may plummet. If she comes home famished every day, she could be handing her lunch over to bullies. A lot of bullying takes place in restrooms, so if your young son sometimes soils himself at school, he could be avoiding restrooms out of fear. One mother became suspicious when she saw the impression of a footprint on the back of her son's shirt. If you suspect bullying, ask a few questions, like "Are there any kids in your school who are making you feel uncomfortable?" or "Are there kids involved in name calling?" suggests Dr. Stephens. And caution your kids against keeping secrets.

Teach them not to be targets. Kids who are loners are most often the targets of bullies, because bullies are less likely to pick on groups of kids. One of the best pieces of advice that you can give your kids, therefore, is to avoid being alone. They should find someone to sit with on the bus, walk to school with, and play with at recess. If you have a young child who is shy and has difficulty socializing, you may need to help him make friends by contacting other mothers in your neighborhood and setting up play dates, says Muriel Savikas, Ph.D., a child psychologist in

Manhattan Beach, California, and founder of the Web site Parenting 101. Your adolescent could benefit from peer-counseling programs, which are available in many school districts. Such programs offer help with conflict resolution and social skills. For teens, Dr. Carter sometimes recommends a course that teaches communication skills, such as the Dale Carnegie course "How to Win Friends and Influence People." (For more information, see the Loneliness chapter on page 105.)

Think good thoughts. If your child occasionally complains about mild bullying, advise him to think good thoughts about himself while he's being teased. By reminding himself of something he's done well, such as a success on the soccer field or a good grade on a test, his confidence will remain elevated, and his self-esteem won't be impacted, says Dr. Watkins.

Encourage eye contact. If your son is being teased by someone on the bus or playground, suggest that he remain calm and maintain eye contact with the bully. "Just look the bully in the eye and don't look intimidated or nervous. Just see him for what he's being," advises Dr. Carter. Your son could also state the facts at this point, saying in a confident voice something like, "You're just trying to get me upset." Since bullies don't usually want to be confronted, this could squelch future incidents.

Suggest remaining unruffled. "Bullies pick on people whom they feel they can get a reaction from," cautions Dr. Watkins. A young child who cries or a teen who acts upset by taunting can invite future bullying. Tell your child to act as though the teasing doesn't bother him. Telling a joke is one of the best ways to handle mild bullying, she adds. Laughing off a hurtful comment and then changing the subject can put a quick stop to teasing. For example, if your son is teased about the way he dresses, he could make a humorous comment or give a quick laugh, then look for a sympathetic person or group nearby and begin talking to them about something else, such as something he saw on TV last night or a popular song. "Deflecting saves face for both parties," says Dr. Watkins.

Help them accept their differences. In the case of children who are overweight or otherwise different, should you suggest that they erase those differences, by losing weight, for example, or changing their manner of dress?

It is probably better to address issues of self-esteem, says Dr.

Watkins. "A strong, self-confident attitude and a friendly manner can make more difference than personal appearance," she says. You can help boost your children's self-confidence by encouraging them to use their talents socially. For example, your academically talented daughter could offer to help another student study. Your son who likes to fly model airplanes could demonstrate for his Boy Scout troop.

It's also a good idea to ask your child what he believes the problem is. If he doesn't believe his appearance is the real issue, he won't be motivated to change it, says Dr. Savikas. If, on the other hand, he is convinced that his looks are putting him at the mercy of bullies, help him to do what he feels is necessary to make a change.

Be supportive. If your child is taunted or shunned from a clique of former friends, you need to be there for him. Offer emotional support and allow him to vent, says Dr. Watkins.

When Bullies Get Physical

Bullying that involves pushing, hitting, pinching, punching, or any act of physical aggression is actually common in very young kids because they don't know how to express themselves verbally. But, in adolescence, things can get serious if a bully becomes violent enough to threaten your child with bodily harm. Here's what experts recommend you tell your child when dangerous bullies are in his school or the neighborhood.

Try to avoid fighting back. If you find out that your child is being pushed around by a peer, it's not usually a good idea to tell him to reciprocate. "We counsel young people not to fight back because generally that only escalates the problem," says Dr. Stephens. With teens, fistfights can potentially spiral out of control and transition into gun fights, he points out. Therefore, it's best to warn your son or daughter to be assertive without being aggressive. In a case where physical aggression poses a serious threat, you may want to advise your child to tell a teacher or school official. This should be done confidentially, to prevent your child from gaining a reputation for ratting.

Nevertheless, experts agree that there are times when kids may have to fight simply to defend themselves, so telling them never to fight may not be advisable. Fighting should be a last resort—only if you cannot get away. If someone is really trying to seriously harm your child and he can't escape, he will have to fight back just to defend himself. And, if a bully or a gang of kids is trying to get your child to an isolated place, he should fight back and try to get away.

Sign up for a karate class. A good martial arts class that teaches your child defensive moves can benefit him in two ways. First, it will enable your child to protect himself from bullies. Second, it can empower him with a confident air that will discourage bullies from targeting him. "If you can be lightning fast about something, like a good block and spin, that can be very impressive," says Dr. Watkins. She recommends finding a class, such as the Japanese martial art aikido, which teaches respect and confidence and emphasizes restraint, so that the skills are never used in an inappropriate manner. And remember, it's not only boys who can benefit from self-defense lessons. Girls may need them to ward off unwanted sexual advances.

Recommend running. Tell your child that if a bully or a gang is posing a serious physical threat—which can mean being threatened with weapons, being in an isolated place, or even just having a feeling that he is in serious danger—he should try to escape. "There's a lot to be said for running and screaming loudly," says Dr. Watkins. This may be especially important in circumstances where a group is attacking him.

Avoid danger. "Try to teach your child to avoid situations where he is likely to be in physical danger," says Dr. Watkins. Stress that he should steer clear of isolated places, whether he is in or away from school. If your child walks to school and is physically threatened by someone en route, consider accompanying him or getting another adult to do so.

Set up safe houses. Students who walk to school should know of homes along the way where they can go when they are in danger, says Dr. Watkins. Some schools set up safe house programs. If yours doesn't, get to know the people who live along your child's route, and approach those families that you feel you can trust. Tell your child to stop there whenever he is in fear of a bully.

Don't ask for mercy. It's not a good idea to recommend that your child appeal to a bully for mercy, says Dr. Carter. If your child says, "Stop bothering me" or "Please leave me alone," it probably won't do any good. "Bullies are capable of respect, but they're not capable of mercy," he explains. Your child can gain respect by behaving confidently or reacting with humor.

Call the cops. Physical assault is against the law, but knowing when to involve police in the case of adolescent bullying can be tricky. "I would weigh it out," says Dr. Carter. "If a kid commits a clearly antisocial act, I wouldn't hesitate at all to do it." An antisocial act is one in which a kid deliberately physically hurts another child, and the severity of the act is enough to concern you about future threats. Find out if the bully has a history of violence. You can do this by asking other parents in the neighborhood or the school. A phone call to the bully's parents or to school officials may be all that's necessary when the bully is a young child. If, however, you know of a teen who is repeatedly physically hurting other children as well as your own child, legal intervention could be warranted. If you do press charges, and the bully is found guilty, it is likely that he will be put on probation. If he continues behaving violently, he will then be sent to a juvenile detention center.

When You Can't Go It Alone

When bullying involves physical attacks, racism, or persistent, emotionally damaging verbal assaults, you'll need to work together with the school, community, and other parents to stop it. Here are some suggestions.

Counter prejudice. If your child is the victim of regular racial slurs or is teased because of his ethnicity or religious beliefs, you may need to get some support. Contact the school and talk to teachers about running programs on cultural diversity. Arrange for a speaker from a local ethnic or religious organization to come in and talk to students. Or, band together with other members of your community and form a positive awareness group that can be visibly constructive in the school and community. That way, you will be sure that your child sees his culture in a positive light, says Dr. Watkins.

Take it up with a youth group leader. If both your child and the bully are members of the same church, ask the parish youth group leader to act as a mediator. "Getting one's cultural or religious group involved in these things can be a valuable resource," says Dr. Watkins.

Call the parents. If your child is routinely tormented by another child, you should consider calling the parents. It's best to call in cases where you know the parents and you believe they will be supportive. Articulate your concerns for your child, and ask them, "Is there some way we can work together on this?" suggests Dr. Watkins.

Gather evidence. As soon as you become aware of any incident of bullying that involves your child, try to get as much information about it as possible, advises Dr. Stephens. Write down the date, time, and place of the event. Document exactly what happened and find out if there were witnesses. Collecting data is particularly important for bullying that takes place on school grounds, since details will aid school officials in handling the problem.

Call the school. Provide teachers and administrators with as much information as you can, and expect them to take action. A guidance counselor, principal, or teacher should talk to the bully about his behavior, and outline consequences for it. If it's a wide-ranging problem, the district may need to include programs on conflict resolution. Always follow up on your complaint to make sure the matter is being handled.

In cases where a bully is physically aggressive or violent, expect school officials to take the matter very seriously and consider transferring that child to an alternative school.

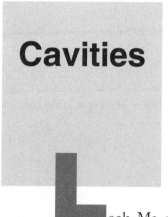

Cavities

"Look, Ma, no cavities!" yells the child with the angelic face on the TV commercial . . . precisely what all parents like to hear.

Fortunately, this is not only television advertising. It is possible for your child to show no cavities at all in her dental checkups, according to Luke Matranga, D.D.S., a dentist in Omaha, Nebraska.

Of course, nothing can substitute for good dental care, and many dentists recommend a checkup every 6 months after your child reaches age 2. But besides the attention from the dentist, there are certain habits that should be followed at home that may support cavity prevention.

This chapter gives an explanation of those habits and how to promote them in your home so that your children have strong, healthy teeth.

Tips for Tooth Care

Avoid the baby's bottle at sleep time. Allow your child to go to sleep with a baby bottle only if it contains water instead of milk or juice, says Dr. Matranga. When your baby falls asleep with milk or juice in her mouth, sugars in those drinks combine to form tartar, a film over the teeth that promotes bacterial development. This twosome of decomposition may decay the teeth. Indeed, most cases of extensive cavities in infant teeth are known as baby bottle syndrome, he says.

Clean your baby's gums. Good habits start at an early age, even before teeth come out. "You should get your baby used to mouth care, cleaning her gums with a soft and damp washcloth after each meal," says William Kuttler, D.D.S., a dentist in Dubuque, Iowa, who has been treating children for more than 20 years.

Guide the brushing. Start brushing the teeth as soon as they appear, and for babies use a soft brush with rounded edges *without* toothpaste, recommends Jed Best, D.D.S., a pediatric dentist and professor of pediatric dentistry at Columbia University School of Dentistry in New York City. Continue helping your child to brush as long as she needs it, he advises. The child will probably not be able to brush her teeth properly until she is 4 to 6 years old.

"An excellent general rule is that if your child is skillful enough to tie her shoelaces, she can probably brush her own teeth," says Dr. Best. "Until then, let your child do it the best she can, and then you should brush those parts she missed."

Allow your child to choose the toothbrush. When your child is old enough to brush her teeth, she is more likely to enjoy it if she has a brush she likes, such as one with the figure of a cartoon character. "As long as it is a toothbrush appropriate for children—with a small soft head and nylon bristles with rounded edges—your child may choose any toothbrush," says Dr. Matranga.

Look for fluoride toothpaste. When your child has six or seven teeth, it is time to start using regular toothpaste, but it should not be a tartar-control toothpaste, advises Cynthia Fong, professor of general

Avoiding Dental Phobia

You probably know what dental phobia means, that horrible sensation that makes you wish you could turn around and run instead of stepping into the dentist's office, even when you are only scheduled for a routine dental checkup.

If you do not want your child to develop that irrational fear toward the dentist, you need to start early. First, do not let your child sense that you expect her to be afraid of the dentist or that you feel uncomfortable there. Children are experts at picking up your feelings. "Don't make a big deal over the visit to the dentist," says Philip Weinstein, Ph.D., professor at University of Washington School of Dentistry in Seattle. "Act as if it were as normal as going shopping."

Be sure to take your child to the dentist before any dental problem arises, he says. That way, the first visit can be a new and exciting experience instead of an intimidating and possibly painful one. The first visit should take place sometime between the first and second birthday.

Many dentists specialize in treating children, and a pediatric dentist may be more experienced in that aspect than your own dentist. A conscientious dentist will explain to your child what he is doing and why and will give her a measure of control over the procedure. "He will suggest, for instance, that the child raise her hand when something is bothering her during the treatment," says Dr. Weinstein. "He can give her a mirror to look at herself and ask to 'help,'" which can be comforting to the child and in fact make her enjoy the experience.

dentistry at the University of Medicine and Dentistry of New Jersey in Newark. She says that some tartar-control products may be abrasive, and tartar is not frequently a problem in small children. Also, make sure that your child knows which tube of toothpaste is exclusively hers. She will feel much more important when she has her own toothpaste.

Brush twice a day. Many people, children and adults alike, brush their teeth superficially. It takes time to remove bacterial plaque and the residues from the teeth. Doing it once a day is not enough. "Your child should brush her teeth for 2 to 3 minutes at least twice a day," says Dr. Best. One of the brushings should be just before going to bed, so that food particles and tartar don't remain on her teeth during the whole night.

Introduce dental floss early. As soon as your child has premolars, it is time to use dental floss daily, a task you should carry out for a time, probably until your child is 7 or 8 years old, says Dr. Best. "It requires greater manual dexterity than brushing," he explains.

The easiest way to clean your child's teeth with dental floss is to sit behind her while she is standing or kneeling, with her head on your lap. "He is now in a position similar to being in the dentist chair," says Fong. This will allow you to reach your child's teeth more easily and see what you're doing.

Pass the dental floss in front of the TV. Flossing doesn't have to be done in the bathroom. If your child becomes impatient while you are cleaning her teeth, change locations. "Many children will grumble less if you take them to the place they like," says Dr. Matranga. "So settle yourself in front of the TV, place your child's head on your lap, and floss there."

Try an electric toothbrush or an irrigator. The buzzing of the electric device may make daily dental care more attractive for some children and will also reduce the time needed to do it. "Be it electric or battery operated, these dental brushes do an excellent job of cleaning the teeth in nearly half the time of a manual brush," says Dr. Matranga. Oral irrigators that shoot a spurt of water to the teeth help remove the particles that are stuck between them, but mothers should not assume that oral irrigation is a substitute for brushing and flossing, he says.

Points to Prevent Cavities

Eat less frequently. There is a reason why many dentists recommend limiting snacks between meals. Each time your child eats, her teeth are

Supervise the Teeth-Cleaning Routine

Let us suppose that you have already bought a toothpaste with fluoride and a toothbrush with very bright colors for your child. You have already shown her how to use the brush and the dental floss, and each evening you check that the brush is wet.

Mission accomplished, right?

Wrong. Your child may be brushing and using the dental floss daily and still not have clean teeth. To examine them, use special disclosing tablets, which you can obtain from your dentist, says John Brown, D.D.S., a dentist in Claremont, California.

Make your child chew on the tablet after she has brushed. If the brushing was not correctly done and there is still bacterial plaque, those areas will turn red temporarily. That way, you and your child will know that those teeth need to be brushed more carefully.

You should also control how much toothpaste your child squeezes on the brush, says Cynthia Fong, professor of general dentistry at the University of Medicine and Dentistry of New Jersey in Newark. An amount the size of a pea is sufficient, she says.

"If your child uses very little toothpaste, she will not obtain the sufficient anticavity protection. And if the child uses too much, she will be swallowing a good dosage of toothpaste," explains Fong. She also suggests that you keep the toothpaste out of the reach of children to avoid the temptation of eating it. Although it doesn't happen frequently, consuming too much fluoride when swallowing or eating toothpaste can cause spotted teeth.

covered with food particles and sugars that can cause cavities. "The more often food comes in contact with the teeth, the more opportunities there are for cavities," explains Dr. Matranga. If your child brushes after each snack, however, the damage is reduced.

Choose your snacks carefully. Some snacks are worse than others, Dr. Kuttler points out. Dentists say that the best options are cheese, air-popped popcorn, and raw vegetables. Fresh fruit is also acceptable, according to Dr. Kuttler, but it is not the best option since it has natural sugars. Candy, snacks high in carbohydrates such as cookies and cakes, and dried fruits are poor options because they leave a very sticky residue on the teeth that makes it easy for cavities to develop. "The worst culprits are soft drinks because of their sugar and acid content," says Dr. Kuttler. Juice can also be harmful.

This does not mean that you have to deny your child these foods and drinks. Just make sure that she eats them only if she brushes her teeth immediately afterward.

Protect your child with straws. If your child drinks soft drinks or juices, the potential damage can be minimized if she uses a straw. The straw directs the beverage past the teeth, so they don't get "bathed" with sugars. The straw reduces the time in which the drink is in contact with the teeth, says Dr. Kuttler. "And so, less damage is done."

Rinse her mouth. Once your child has eaten, make her rinse her mouth with water. "This removes some of the food and sugar particles," says Fong. Brushing is better, but if no brush is handy, rinsing with water is better than nothing.

Supply sugarless gum. Sugarless chewing gum is another anticavity option because chewing it for 20 minutes may help clean the teeth, says John Brown, D.D.S., a dentist in Claremont, California. "Chewing gum stimulates the flow of saliva, which helps remove from the teeth the residues and substances that make up the bacterial plaque."

Be a good example. If your child sees that you brush, use dental floss, and choose healthy snacks for the teeth, it is more likely that she will do the same. "Good dental care is a learned behavior," says Dr. Kuttler. "If the parents value the care of their own teeth, it is likely that their children will want to do the same."

Colds

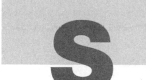

Some kids seem to have a cold brewing almost all the time, which is not surprising when you consider that approximately 200 viruses can cause the common cold. Most of these cold viruses are extremely hardy. They can survive for several hours on hands, clothing, and hard surfaces as well as in the air, giving your child ample opportunity to pick up something infectious somewhere. Small wonder, then, that most kids average about six colds every year.

Spending 7 days, more or less, soothing a child with a cold isn't most parents' idea of a good time. Before a typical cold runs its course, you'll have to deal with sniffles and sneezes, stuffiness and coughs, runny nose and scratchy throat, and maybe even a low-grade fever. But it's reassuring to know that these symptoms seldom turn out to be serious.

"The vast majority of kids—even infants—do just fine with a cold," says Michael Macknin, M.D., head of the section of general pediatrics at the Cleveland Clinic Foundation in Ohio, clinical professor at Pennsylvania State University College of Medicine in Hershey, and associate professor of pediatrics at Ohio State University College of Medicine in Columbus. "It's a very common ailment that rarely causes a problem."

That doesn't mean that you should just ignore your child's cold, however. Although there is no cure for a cold virus (antibiotics only vanquish bacterial infections, such as those that cause strep throat or ear infection), you can give your child some relief from annoying symptoms. And you may be able to prevent some colds entirely. Here's what the experts suggest.

Boost immunity by breastfeeding your baby. "To prevent colds in infants—as best we can—it pays to breastfeed," notes Naomi Grobstein, M.D., a family physician in Montclair, New Jersey. "Breastfeeding can provide extra protection against those cold viruses to which the mother has already developed an immunity," she says.

Go easy on the acetaminophen for fever. "You don't have to treat a low-grade fever," says Dr. Grobstein. "Fever mobilizes the immune system and helps fight off infection." But if you choose to treat the fever because your child is intolerably uncomfortable, use acetaminophen—Children's Tylenol or any other brand, she suggests. Check the package directions for the correct dosage for your child's age and weight. If your

WHEN TO SEE THE DOCTOR

As long as your child has no fever and is eating and sleeping well despite her cold, there is no reason to go to the doctor, says Flavia Marino, M.D., a clinical instructor in pediatrics at New York University Medical Center, Tisch Hospital, and a pediatrician in New York City. "If the symptoms worsen, if there is a low-grade fever (100° to 101°F) for a few days, or if the fever shoots higher, however, it's time for a visit to the pediatrician. Your child may have a bacterial infection rather than a cold," says Dr. Marino.

If your child's runny nose and cough haven't improved after 10 days, your child may have a sinus infection. "Sinusitis may follow a cold because the sinuses become inflamed and can't drain properly," says Michael Macknin, M.D., head of the section of general pediatrics at the Cleveland Clinic Foundation in Ohio, clinical professor at Pennsylvania State University College of Medicine in Hershey, and associate professor of pediatrics at Ohio State University College of Medicine in Columbus.

Sinus infections are particularly common among preschoolers. "For a child under age 6 who's had a runny nose with or without a cough for 10 days and isn't getting better, chances are close to 90 percent that there's a sinus infection," Dr. Macknin says. For 6- to 12-year-olds, chances are 70 percent. Unlike a cold virus, a sinus infection should be treated with doctor-prescribed antibiotics, he adds.

child is under age 2, consult a physician. "You should never give aspirin to your child with a virus," she adds, "because it has been linked to Reye's syndrome, a serious disease that affects the brain and liver."

Smooth something soothing on a sore nose. "Most children are not bothered by a runny nose, except when the skin around it becomes chapped and raw from frequent wiping," says Flavia Marino, M.D., clinical instructor in pediatrics at New York University Medical Center, Tisch Hospital, and a pediatrician in New York City. To prevent that, she recommends applying a layer of petroleum jelly just beneath your child's nose as often as necessary.

Ask for hand washing. "Cold viruses are frequently transmitted through hand contact," says Dr. Macknin. "So simple hand washing is the best way to prevent the spread of infection." And be sure your child uses soap when he washes up, he says.

Put the squeeze on excess mucus. During the first few months of life, babies have a harder time than the rest of us if they're forced to breathe through the mouth, notes Dr. Marino. "Nasal blockage caused by a cold may make it difficult for an infant to nurse or drink from a bottle," she says. "But you can make breathing easier for your baby with the help of saline (saltwater) drops and a rubber suction bulb."

You can purchase saline solution (sold under brand names such as Ayr Saline Nasal Mist and Ocean) from a drugstore. Or you can mix your own, dissolving ¼ teaspoon of salt in 1 cup of lukewarm water. "Put a couple drops into your child's nose and wait a few moments," says Dr. Marino. "Then squeeze the suction bulb and insert the tip gently into one nostril. Slowly release the bulb to suction out mucus." After you dispose of the mucus in a tissue, repeat the procedure for the other nostril, she says. Be sure to sterilize the bulb afterward in boiling water.

Serve warm liquids. Offer your child plenty of warm drinks or soup, suggests Dr. Grobstein. "Warm liquids help relieve congestion, and they can also soothe a sore throat," she says.

Mix a mild gargle. Another way to soothe a sore throat is to have your child gargle with warm water in which some salt has been dissolved, says Dr. Marino. This can be repeated several times a day, she says.

Don't squelch a daytime cough. "Coughing is a protective mechanism that keeps bacteria and debris out of the lungs," says Dr. Marino. So leave the cough alone during the day. If coughing is keeping your child up at night, though, an over-the-counter cough suppressant may help him sleep, she says. "Check with your physician for the appropriate dosage," says Dr. Marino, "and schedule an office visit if the cough lingers for more than a few days or if fever persists."

Say okay to school. "Unless he has a fever or feels really lousy, there is no reason to make your child stay indoors or keep him home from school just because he has a cold," says Dr. Grobstein.

Ditch the decongestants and antihistamines. These over-the-counter cold medicines have never been proven effective for kids under the age of 5, says Dr. Macknin. "They may work, but there's not a single article in the scientific literature for the last 40 years that supports their use," he says.

Dr. Macknin concedes that decongestants, at least, may offer some symptomatic relief, but both types of remedies have side effects. "Decongestants may make a child hyperactive, and antihistamines may make him sleepy," he says. "And in some instances, kids may have other, more unusual or severe reactions." The bottom line is that cold medications won't make the cold go away faster. So unless your child feels truly miserable, don't use them.

Check for stress. Studies have shown there is a link between stress and illness. "When your child is very fatigued, worn out, or under a lot of stress, he is more likely to become ill with a cold," Dr. Macknin says. If you discover that your child is facing a stressful situation, either at play or at school, consider what steps can be taken to relieve his concerns. Pressure at school, trouble with friends, or too many activities may be contributing factors.

Herbal Options

In the other parts of this book, which offer tips for dealing with the adults in the house, you'll notice that the general health recommendations include some herbal recipes. In this part we haven't done that because we want to give you some overall guidelines about giving herbal remedies to kids before getting into specific herbal tips.

First of all, although some herbalists believe that kids can be given medicinal herbs, we advise you to *never* give them to your children unless you consult their pediatrician first and get her approval. The tips we offer in this section are designed for kids that are at least 8 years old. If your son or daughter isn't a baby but has not yet reached that age, you should consult your pediatrician before giving them any of the following remedies. The fact is, there has been very little research done on the effect of medicinal herbs on kids. Therefore, you need to be very cautious when using these remedies. Always clear up any questions you may have with your pediatrician beforehand and stop using any herbal remedy if you notice that your little one has a negative reaction.

That said, here are some herbal healing options.

Employ echinacea. From Alaska to Australia, the herb echinacea has achieved superstar status as a cold remedy. "Almost everybody in this country has heard of echinacea," says Gill Stanard, a member of the National Herbalists Association of Australia and an herbal practitioner in Melbourne. "It's now right up there with vitamin C in the arsenal that people choose when they have a cold."

While Stanard warns that echinacea is no cure-all, it does work wonders in rallying the immune system when one has a cold. Using numerous active constituents, the herb increases production of the white blood cells in the body that go after the cold virus. It also activates the killer cells that destroy virus-infected cells. Use echinacea early, at the first hint that your child is coming down with something, because it doesn't work well once a cold is full-blown.

Use ½ to 1 teaspoon of tincture three times a day, says Mary Bove, N.D., a naturopathic physician at the Brattleboro Naturopathic Clinic in Vermont and a member of Britain's National Institute of Medical Herbalists. Echinacea is safe, but some herbalists feel that it may lose its effectiveness if given to your child regularly for more than a few days.

To make the echinacea tincture more palatable, try putting it in juice or water. Sometimes echinacea can cause a tingling or numbing sensation on the tongue. Don't worry, this is a common side effect and completely harmless.

Note: A tincture is a highly concentrated herbal liquid. It's made by soaking leaves in alcohol or glycerin—which extracts the herb's medicinal properties—for at least 6 weeks. Tinctures are sold in health food stores in small bottles with eyedroppers to give doses. Be sure to store them out of the reach of children.

Make it all better with a mix. Try a blend of herbs that have antiviral properties, recommends Kathi Keville, an herbalist in Nevada City, California, and director of the American Herb Association. Put ½ teaspoon each of Oregon grape root, licorice root, and echinacea root in a pan with 2 cups of water. Simmer for 2 minutes, then remove from heat and steep for about 20 minutes. Strain out herbs. For a 50-pound child, give one cup of tea daily. To improve the flavor, the tea can be mixed with an equal amount of juice, such as apple or grape juice.

Give some sage assistance. A few years ago, several leading herbalists were sitting around talking shop when the subject of cold remedies came up. Interestingly, neither echinacea nor goldenseal won by consensus. The winner? Sage. "Sage is antiseptic and astringent," says Cascade Anderson Geller, an herbal educator and consulting herbal practitioner in Portland, Oregon. That means that it helps fight infections while drying up problems like postnasal drip.

Steep 1 teaspoon of dried medicinal sage leaves in 1 cup of water for 15 minutes, recommends Keville. Then sweeten with $1/4$ teaspoon of honey since this tea is fairly bitter. For a 50-pound child, give at least $1/2$ cup. If he wants more, that's perfectly fine, according to Keville. You can find dried medicinal sage at the health food store.

Nip it in the bud with another herbal blend. Drinking pots and pots of hot yarrow tea is a time-honored folk remedy for colds. The classic formula is yarrow, elder flowers, and peppermint. A fourth ingredient, catnip, is recommended by Dr. Bove as a decongestant that also encourages relaxation. "Basically," she says, these are "all diaphoretic herbs, meaning that they stimulate the immune system by raising the body's temperature." Since turning up the body's temperature is one of the body's natural defense mechanisms against foreign invaders, it will help fight off the cold virus. It makes the body's environment inhospitable to germs because bacteria, parasites, and viruses replicate more slowly at high temperatures.

Combine equal parts of elder and yarrow flowers and peppermint and catnip leaves, all in dried form. You may want to skimp a bit on the bitter catnip and add a little extra peppermint to improve the flavor, Dr. Bove suggests. Make an infusion by steeping 1 heaping teaspoon of the blend in 8 ounces of water in a covered pan for 5 to 10 minutes and sweeten with a little fruit juice or honey. Offer the tea while it's nice and warm, at least three or four times a day, starting at the onset of a cold. Up to one cup can be given every 2 hours. Give the last cup with a warm bath in the evening before bedtime, Dr. Bove says.

Constipation

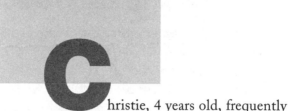

hristie, 4 years old, frequently goes 3 or 4 days without having a bowel movement. That worries her mother, who fears that Christie is constipated. But when she goes to the bathroom, Christie has never had problems. So, even though her mother is worried, Christie has no complaints. Is she constipated or not?

"Some parents believe that unless the child has a bowel movement every day, something is wrong," says Kevin Ferentz, M.D., professor of family medicine at the University of Maryland in Baltimore. "But regularity is highly variable and something very personal. Even if the girl has a bowel movement only twice a week, as long as there is no discomfort associated with this and the stool is relatively soft, then she has bowel movements regularly. She is not constipated."

For the majority of children with real constipation, the cause is their diets, says Dr. Ferentz. The digestive tract is designed to work better with a high-fiber diet, that is, with whole grains, beans, fruits, and vegetables. For many children, those are not necessarily their preferred foods.

Other children, especially those that have been trained to go to the bathroom by themselves, become constipated because of changes they are going though and not because of their food habits. As part of their resistance to the training process, these children involve themselves in what has been called the battle of the bowels with their parents. In other words, they literally refuse to go, and as a result, their stools impact.

Despite all potential roads toward irregularity, constipation in children can be easily corrected and prevented. "No child *ever* has to be constipated," says Dr. Ferentz. Here is what you can do to help your child.

WHEN TO SEE THE DOCTOR

Constipation may be a symptom of several physical or emotional conditions, warns Marjorie Hogan, M.D., instructor of pediatrics at the University of Minnesota and a pediatrician at the Hennepin County Medical Center, both in Minneapolis. When constipation appears in babies, it will *always* require a medical checkup, she says, because it could be a symptom of an intestinal blockage.

Likewise, if the baby you are nursing has not had a bowel movement in 2 or more days, you definitely should consult your physician, according to Kevin Ferentz, M.D., professor of family medicine at the University of Maryland in Baltimore. For older children, you should call the doctor if:

- Your child is in a lot of pain, her stomach is distended, and she is not eating well. (This could mean a blockage or other intestinal problem.)

- There is blood in the stool.

- Your child appears to be avoiding a bowel movement for emotional purposes, especially during toilet training.

- Your child has accidental bowel movements when she is not in the bathroom. Over time, withholding stools can cause encopresis, a condition in which the child becomes so impacted that she loses control over the sphincter and feces come out.

Tips for Babies

Try a slick solution. Small children and babies can be given glycerin suppositories. "They are very thin, bullet-shaped waxy substances that melt as soon as they are inserted in the rectum," explains Dr. Ferentz. "They relieve constipation two ways: They stimulate the rectum, and they 'grease the walls' to eliminate the waste. But use them only occasionally, because if the child becomes dependent on them, she will not be able to have a bowel movement without their help."

Glycerin suppositories for babies and children can be obtained at any drugstore, and the instructions for using them are on the package.

Try using the thermometer. Once the doctor diagnoses infant constipation, you can use a rectal thermometer approved for child use to help her defecate. "Lubricate the thermometer well with petroleum jelly," advises Dr. Ferentz. "Insert it in the baby's rectum no more than

When a Baby Grunts, Strains, and Goes, All Is Well

Tony, a baby just 3 weeks old, appeared to be making more effort than a weight lifter trying for a world record. He grunted, strained, and bent his legs as if he were in pain. His mother, worried that her child was constipated, called the pediatrician.

"I don't think I've ever had a new mother who didn't call me to say that she thought her newborn was constipated because of the baby's strain," says Kevin Ferentz, M.D., professor of family medicine at the University of Maryland in Baltimore. "Then, when I asked them if the stool was soft, the typical answer is 'Yes, soft and moist.' When that is the answer, I know that the child is not constipated."

"All newborns grunt," points out Dr. Ferentz. "It has nothing to do with difficulty in moving their bowels. Babies grumble because they don't have as much abdominal strength as adults; therefore, they have to work at straining to push the stool out. It is perfectly normal, and they don't require any help."

1½ inches and take it out. Sometimes you will get a 'little present' along with the thermometer."

Defeat your child with sweetness. "For all babies, a teaspoon of Karo syrup in a baby bottle of 6 to 8 ounces of formula or ½ teaspoon in a 4-ounce baby bottle can soften the stool very well," says pediatric nurse Shirley Menard, professor of nursing at the University of Texas in San Antonio. The syrup takes water into the intestine and keeps stools soft, she says.

Tips for Children

Give your child a mild laxative . . . but only a little of it. If a child 10 years or older is already constipated, there are several medicines that do not require a prescription and can give her temporary relief. "For an older child, it is all right to use over-the-counter laxatives, such as milk of magnesia or mineral oil," says Dr. Ferentz. "But use them only when a doctor recommends them. Mineral oil, in particular, should not be used regularly because it interferes with the absorption of oil-soluble vitamins." Other laxatives as well can cause problems if taken regularly. A child can become so dependent on them that she will lose the natural stimulus to have a bowel movement.

Keep a daily food record. Write down everything that your child eats and drinks each day, advises Marjorie Hogan, M.D., instructor of pediatrics at the University of Minnesota and a pediatrician at the Hennepin County Medical Center, both in Minneapolis. This will allow you to point out accurately what is causing the constipation in your child.

"For instance, if your child drinks a quart of milk a day, maybe that is the connection," says Dr. Hogan. Consuming too many dairy products can constipate, she says. Other foods that can constipate—and are included frequently in children's diets—are applesauce, bananas, and white rice.

Make some high-fiber muffins. "Fiber in the diet helps keep the stools soft," says Dr. Ferentz. "Unfortunately, in our society, we eat very few foods rich in fiber, such as fruits, vegetables, whole wheat breads, and bran cereal."

You can introduce your child to eating high-fiber foods with some that are tasty and fun. "For instance, there is no reason that a child cannot eat a bran muffin daily," says Dr. Ferentz. To make muffins more appetizing, add some raisins. "Many children love raisins," says Dr. Ferentz.

Serve snacks fit for a rabbit. "When your child gets hungry between meals, try giving her some raw vegetables, such as carrots or celery. Many children like them because they are crunchy," says Dr. Ferentz. To make these snacks even more appetizing, decorate them with something. "A stalk of celery spread with a little bit of peanut butter is excellent to prevent constipation."

Disguise those vegetables that your child hates so much. You may want to force your child to eat cauliflower or broccoli, vegetables that are very high in fiber and that can help her with her constipation. Instead, disguise them to make them tastier, says Dr. Hogan. "Be creative. Try cutting them in different shapes; tell your child that broccoli florets are little trees and, if you have to do it, chop the vegetables and hide them in a meat loaf where your child cannot find them."

Take advantage of fruit favoritism. Children who don't eat vegetables generally will eat fruit. There are many types of fruits available to get their intestines moving. "Offer them many apples, pears, and peaches," suggests Menard. "But avoid giving them bananas and applesauce, which tend to constipate."

Offer your child many liquids. "Make sure that your child drinks a great deal of liquids, including fruit juices, to help her prevent constipation," says Menard. This is particularly important if you are introducing bran and other high-fiber foods into your child's diet. Liquids help give the fiber volume so that the stool is soft and easy to pass.

Do not start toilet training too soon. Children who are not ready to use the toilet may hold in their stool as a way to gain control over their bodies, says Dr. Ferentz. "A 2-year-old child wants to be in control so desperately that if you tell her, 'You have to go the bathroom,' she will try not to go just to show you who is in charge."

Therefore, instead of forcing your child, have patience and watch for signs that indicate that the child is ready to go to the bathroom. "Most kids are not what you'd call very interested in learning to go to the bathroom by themselves until they are almost 3 years old. It is when they reach that age that you should start to train them," says Dr. Ferentz.

Yield a little. Children who are engaged in a stool-withholding power struggle perhaps need freedom to make some decisions by themselves, says Dr. Ferentz.

"You can focus your attention on other aspects of control over the life of your child—for instance, the clothing she uses or the type of sandwich she takes for lunch. If you allow your child to participate more in making these decisions, she will feel that *you* are budging a little, and that is important for your child," suggests Dr. Ferentz. "The child can feel more relaxed, and the stool will pass more easily."

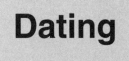

Dating

During their preadolescent years, your daughter thought that boys had cooties and your son treated girls like germs. It's clear to you now: Those were the good old days. These days, your budding teens talk for hours on the phone with members of the opposite sex, and they even meet with them in groups at the mall. You know they'll begin dating soon. It's obvious they're ready for it. The question is, are you?

If the idea of sending your teen off on a date makes you nervous, you're not alone. The early dating years are generally difficult ones for both parents and teens, says Thomas Olkowski, Ph.D., a clinical psychologist in Denver. "Most parents realize that it's sort of a normal step, but it's also another sign that their kids are growing up and becoming separate individuals."

The age at which kids begin dating differs dramatically by individual and even by community, Dr. Olkowski says. Teens raised in urban environments may be more likely to start dating earlier than those in rural areas, for example. And keep in mind that your children will each develop at their own rates. For that reason, if your 17-year-old has never been on a date, don't press the matter, unless you feel that he's socially isolated. By the same token, experts seem to agree that you shouldn't try to restrict dating before a certain age. If your 14-year-old is interested in boys, it may not be realistic to expect her to refrain from dating until she's 16, says Dr. Olkowski.

That doesn't mean that you should give her free rein to date however she chooses. "Set it up so that she can date appropriately," recommends Muriel Savikas, Ph.D., a psychologist in Manhattan Beach, California, and author of *Guilt Is Good!* Young teens shouldn't be going on dates alone, so it's best to help your child organize group outings where she can date safely.

Despite feeling uneasy about your children's dating, remember that it, like many other pastimes that occupy your teens, is really an opportunity for learning social skills and for developing new relationships, according to Dr. Savikas. Your role, then, is to guide, encourage, and support your teens as they test out the murky world of girl-boy relationships. Here's some advice from the experts to help you do this.

Set up some ground rules. "You want to teach your kids how to make responsible decisions as they grow," says Dr. Olkowski. To do that, you should give voice to your values, and let your kids know how you expect them to uphold those values. It's a good idea to begin relaying this information as early as possible. "If a parent has taught values all along, kids are more likely to uphold them as they grow up," Dr. Olkowski says. Your principles will probably differ from those of other families, but you'll undoubtedly want to draw the line at drinking and driving, attending unchaperoned parties, and breaking curfews.

Don't be a dictator, however. Place too many restrictions on your teen, and you'll risk inciting resentful and rebellious behavior, warns Dr. Savikas. Sit down and talk with your teen. Find out how he feels about a rule and, when possible, be flexible. For example, try to come up with a curfew that's agreeable to both of you.

Encourage group activities. Don't act put out when your teen asks you to drive him, his date, and a few other friends to the skating rink. Being a driver or a chaperone is a good way to offer your child support and encouragement for one of the earliest and most significant rituals of adolescence: group dating. Young teens usually aren't ready for one-on-one dates, explains Dr. Savikas. They feel safest and most comfortable dating when they learn how to do it with a group of friends. Only after they've become accomplished at functioning in a group are they ready to go out on their own.

Invite their amour over. How important is it to meet the person your child is dating? Experts agree that it's very important. For one thing, it's been shown that girls are less likely to become pregnant when their parents know their boyfriends, according to Maura Quinlan, M.D., associate professor in the department of obstetrics and gynecology at Emory University School of Medicine and medical director at Grady Teen Clinic, both in Atlanta. That's probably because parental involvement helps sanction the relationship, making it more likely that the couple will use birth control if they do have sex. On another level, knowing your child's friends is essential to maintaining an open, healthy parent-child relationship.

Speak up about sex. If you want your teen to get good information about sex, you have to supply it yourself, says Debra W. Haffner, president and chief executive officer of the Sexuality Information and Education Council of the United States in New York City and author of *From Diapers to Dating: A Parent's Guide to Raising Sexually Healthy Children*. Discuss your expectations with your children and give them solid data about health risks and contraception. What's the best way to do this? Don't limit it to one big talk, says Haffner. Look for everyday opportunities to talk about sex—sitcoms with intimate situations, news stories about AIDS, and magazine articles on contraception all can provide a springboard for conversations on sexuality.

Get them thinking. What if you meet your daughter's boyfriend, and you think he's a bad influence? Should you forbid her to see him? You could inadvertently push her more deeply into the relationship. "I think the best approach is to get the child to think on her own that this is not such a good idea," advises Dr. Savikas. Ask questions like "What do you think your best friend would tell you to do?" or "What are the best qualities about this person?" Ultimately, you want to empower your child to make her own wise choices. Nevertheless, there may be times when forbidding a relationship is appropriate. For more on this, see "When Dating Turns Dangerous" on the opposite page.

Treat siblings equally. In some families, girls face a number of constraints while their brothers are permitted to go anywhere, do anything, and stay out as late as they want with their girlfriends. If you create this kind of double standard in your family, you may also be creating trouble, says Nedda de Castro, a licensed social worker in New York City, who specializes in teen pregnancy and parenting. Your daughters will be more likely to break whatever rules you set for them, and both sexes run the risk of running into trouble.

Prepare for parties. One day your teen informs you that he and his girlfriend have been invited to a party. Your mind fills with questions: Where is this party? Who's holding it? Who's going and how will it be chaperoned? The best way to get answers is to pick up the phone and call the family. But what if you don't know the parents? "Get to know them," advises Dr. Savikas. "Invite them over for coffee." Then, you can talk to them about what the teens will be doing at the party and make certain that chaperones will be present.

If your teen wants to host a party, you'll have to walk the fine line between being respectful of his space and keeping an eye on things. You can stay in another part of the house, says Dr. Savikas, but if everyone grows too quiet, go down to see what's going on.

When Dating Turns Dangerous

For the most part, dating can be a positive experience for your teen. Unfortunately, some dating situations can turn risky. Date rape, stalking, statutory rape, and cyberstalking are all potential hazards your children could face. Here are a few measures you can take to protect them.

Warn your daughters. One study of more than 1,000 university women found that more than half had experienced some form of unwanted sex—43 percent with steady dating partners. "Parents need to reiterate the fact that there are guys out there who don't have a full set of values and who will take advantage of them," says Dr. Olkowski. Caution them to be careful of date-rape drugs, such as flunitrazepam (Rohypnol), an illegal drug that can be slipped unknowingly into someone's drink and leave the victim disoriented and with a decreased ability to resist or even remember an attack.

Teach respect. Today, sexual pressure comes from a number of forces at work in your teen's world, says Carol Watkins, M.D., a psychiatrist in Baltimore. Some popular music, for example, promotes female sexual submission. Don't let your son fall prey to those beliefs. Teach him from

(continued on page 70)

Teen Pregnancy

Terrified and trembling, your teen speaks one word that sends your entire world crashing in: pregnant. A serious consequence of dating, teen pregnancy is, unfortunately, a fact of life for many American families. Nevertheless, when it happens to you, you're likely to feel alone, angry, and as confused as your teen.

To help sort out your feelings, you and your teen should get crisis pregnancy counseling, says Geeta Swamidass, executive director of Living Well Medical Clinic in Orange, California. "It's not the end of life, but it is traumatic. Call a place that will allow you to talk."

A hospital or community-based organization can help you locate local programs that offer crisis pregnancy counseling for teens. Such counseling centers can also provide information on abortion, adoption, and keeping the baby.

Whether the pregnancy involves your daughter or your son's girlfriend, you'll probably need to guide them in choosing the proper course of action. Below is an outline of the options they'll be faced with and some things to consider before making a choice.

Abortion

Your daughter should know that: Abortion laws can be fairly complicated and will vary depending on the state your child lives in. Matters such as parental consent, required waiting periods, and the times during which an abortion can be performed are regulated by the political system in your state. The procedure is safe and is simplest during the first 12 weeks. The longer a woman waits, the more emotionally difficult it will be to handle, says Nedda de Castro, a licensed social worker in New York City who specializes in teen pregnancy and parenting.

Your son should know that: He shouldn't try to pressure his girlfriend to abort the baby. From a legal standpoint, the decision rests entirely with the mother. Furthermore, women who are co-erced into having an abortion tend to face emotional fallout later, says Maura Quinlan, M.D., associate professor in the department of obstetrics and gynecology at Emory University School of Med-icine and medical director at Grady Teen Clinic, both in Atlanta.

Adoption

Both parties should know that: Although adoption is the least common choice, especially among urban teens, it nevertheless should be considered carefully as an alternative. "There's an old-fashioned assumption that you give away the baby and that's the end of it," says de Castro. Today, adoption agencies allow teens to select the parents. What's more, birth parents can opt for an open adop-tion, which enables them to have contact with the adoptive family.

Keeping the Baby

Your daughter should know that: No matter how young she is, by law she will be considered the baby's guardian. That means she, not you, is responsible for the care and medical needs of the child. To ensure a healthy baby, she'll need good prenatal care—preferably through a clinic specializing in teens. She must eat a balanced diet and abstain from cigarettes, alcohol, and, of course, drugs. While many girls who keep their babies don't finish high school, a girl who makes it a priority to finish her education can often find a way to do so, says de Castro.

Your son should know that: Even if he doesn't want the baby, or he breaks up with his girlfriend, in many states he is legally bound to support the child financially. He may also have the right to share custody. How much your son will be required to pay will be determined by state guidelines. Those guidelines vary but are generally based on the needs of the child and the ability of the parent to pay. A child support order is usually established in court or through an administrative hearing.

a young age that girls should be respected for who they are. And teach your daughters to respect the integrity of their bodies so they do not feel compelled to submit to sexual pressure. Surround both genders with positive role models, like youth group leaders, who can reinforce your messages about respect.

Discourage perilous partners. If your child wants to date someone who is on drugs or someone who is much older, you may need to inform the police, says David York, cofounder of Toughlove International in Doylestown, Pennsylvania. But remember, if your teen's boyfriend is on drugs, she is likely to be using drugs also. Assume that she is and contact a local drug counseling center for help.

When an older man shows interest in your daughter, statutory rape may be a risk. Call your local district attorney's office to find out what legal recourse you have in your state, recommends York. Keep in mind that police won't make an arrest until a crime has been committed, says Trudy Delgado, victims assistance officer with the 35th District of the Philadelphia Police Department. But, police can send out a community relations officer to speak to the man and spell out plainly the consequences of having sex with a juvenile.

Beware of cyberdating. While the movie *You've Got Mail* may have romanticized the concept of cyberdating, the truth is that it can be risky business. Your teen could put herself in jeopardy by arranging to secretly meet a computer pal or by giving up too much information about her whereabouts. The FBI recommends the following to reduce your children's risk of being victimized.

- Talk to them about sexual predators and online dangers.

- Keep the computer in a common room where the screen is visible to all family members.

- Use parent controls that limit your child's access to Internet sites, and monitor her use of chat rooms.

- Maintain access to your children's online accounts and randomly check e-mails.

- Caution your children never to arrange a meeting with people they've met online, post pictures of themselves, or give out identifying information to people they don't know.

Beware of stalkers. A 1998 survey of 8,000 men and 8,000 women in the United States found that 1 out of every 12 women and 1 out of every 45 men had been stalked during their lifetime. If a former boyfriend follows your teen, makes harassing phone calls, vandalizes your property, or engages in other threatening behaviors, you'll need to protect her. Caution your child that the first step to take anytime someone is following her is to pick up the phone and call the police, says Delgado. "Make a police report, and the police will take it from there," she says. Police will probably recommend that you document all incidents in a journal that can serve as future evidence, and that you seek a restraining order against the stalker. How that order is enforced depends on your state laws, but it could forbid the stalker to make any contact with the victim. Until the stalking stops, your child will have to take safety precautions such as always carrying a cellular phone, changing her routine daily, and never going out alone.

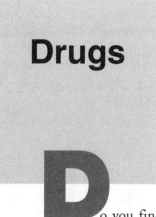

Drugs

Do you find yourself wondering whether your children have been tempted by drugs and alcohol? Yours seem like good kids, but you can't watch them all the time. If you are worried about your children and drugs, you should be. Substance abuse is a major adolescent health problem.

Substance abuse—whether alcohol, drugs, or cigarettes—is dangerous because of its direct health consequences, but it is also entwined with other behaviors that contribute to the leading causes of death among young people: car crashes, accidents, homicide, and suicide.

The risk for drug abuse increases as teens get older. Although about

3 percent of 12- to 13-year-olds use drugs, the rate for 16- to 17-year-olds is almost 20 percent. Understanding the risk factors for substance abuse, knowing how to identify the warning signs that your teen might be using drugs, and having a plan in place for helping your teen resist substance abuse will help protect your teen.

"The best way to educate your children about drugs and alcohol is to educate yourself," says Luisa del C. Pollard, chairperson of the Substance Abuse and Mental Health Services Administration (SAMHSA) Hispanic/Latino Initiative in Rockville, Maryland. "The more you know, the more comfortable you will be and the better you will be able to communicate to your teen how to resist drugs and alcohol."

To further educate yourself, read on to learn about the major types of drugs that threaten your children. You'll also find some basic guidelines for keeping your kids off drugs and expert advice on what to do if your child is abusing drugs.

The Threats

Tobacco. Teens who use this addictive substance are at risk for a number of other dangerous risk behaviors. A government study found that teens who smoked cigarettes were more than 10 times as likely to use illegal drugs and more than 15 times more likely to abuse alcohol than those teens who didn't smoke.

Alcohol. This is the substance most commonly abused by teens—and they are starting as early as age 12.

Marijuana. While it relieves tension and produces a dreamy state in the user, it can also set the stage for future nightmares for both you and your child. Why? First of all, marijuana is known as a "gateway drug"—that is, it is often the first step toward the use of harder drugs, such as cocaine and heroin, which are physically addictive and can kill your child. Also, studies have shown that teens who start using marijuana when they are young often develop problem behaviors as they grow older: They are more likely to drop out of school, abuse alcohol, and have multiple sex partners without condoms, which puts them at risk for AIDS and other sexually transmitted diseases. Teens who use marijuana are also at an increased risk for becoming depressed and thinking about suicide. As if that weren't enough, long-term abuse of marijuana may cause lung disease or cancer.

Cocaine. This nasty white powder stimulates the brain to produce pleasurable sensations that make a user feel more confident and energetic. There are many ways in which this drug can be abused: intravenously (by vein), snorted through the nose, or smoked. Crack is the street name for smokeable (or freebased) cocaine, which is inexpensive but delivers an immediate and powerful "hit." Almost as immediate as the hit is the user's addiction. The short-term effects of cocaine use include dilated pupils, increased alertness, and decreased appetite. Long-term use can lead to addiction, paranoia, hallucinations, stroke, and heart attack. Users who take cocaine intravenously are also at risk for acquiring AIDS from sharing contaminated needles.

Inhalants. These are found in common household products like cleaning fluids, typewriter correction fluid, felt-tip markers, aerosol sprays, paints, and lacquers. To use an inhalant, teens spray the substance (usually from an aerosol can) into a plastic or paper bag or onto a rag. Then they immediately start sucking in air from the bag or rag. Inhalants deliver a high by depriving the body of oxygen (suffocation) or causing the heart to beat rapidly and erratically. Abusing inhalants can cause nervous system damage, memory loss, liver and kidney damage, impaired perception and muscle coordination, and often death. A user who inhales a substance out of a paper or plastic bag to increase the concentration of fumes also greatly increases the chances of suffocating.

Club drugs. These substances are commonly found at dance clubs, all-night parties, and "raves." There is a wide variety of these drugs, and using them can have serious health consequences, even death.

Here are a few of the popular ones that you should be aware of.

- Ecstasy, which chemically is known as methylenedioxymethamphetamine or MDMA, has properties similar to the stimulant amphetamine and the hallucinogen mescaline. It's usually taken orally in a tablet or capsule and is extremely dangerous in high doses. It can lead to heart attack, stroke, and seizures.

- Grievous Bodily Harm, also known as GHB and Liquid Ecstasy, is produced as a clear liquid, a white powder, a tablet, or a capsule. It has a relaxing effect at lower doses, but higher doses can result in coma or death.

- Ketamine, known as Special K or Vitamin K, is an injectable anesthetic used for humans and animals. It's produced as a liquid or as a white powder that's smoked with marijuana or tobacco products. In some cities, it's injected intramuscularly. At higher doses, it can cause potentially fatal breathing problems.

- Roofies, Rophies, and Roche are all street names for flunitrazepam (Rohypnol), a sedative that is not approved for use in the United States but is used in Europe. It's tasteless and odorless, and it dissolves easily into carbonated drinks. One of its effects is anterograde amnesia, which means the user may not remember what happened while she was taking the drug. Because of this, this drug is used to spike the drinks of unsuspecting women so they can be raped while under its effects.

Okay, So What Can I Do?

You may be asking yourself this by now, and the answer is, fortunately, a lot. Studies show that children consider their parents—not their friends, teachers, or messages in the media—the biggest influence in their choosing not to use drugs. Although a discussion with both parents is the most effective method, single mothers should not despair; many teens find it easier to talk to their mothers than their fathers about drugs and are more likely to go to their mothers when they need advice. And there are a lot of parenting strategies you can employ to keep your kids drug-free. Here's what the experts recommend.

Educate them. Use the scary information about the drugs mentioned in this chapter to stress to your kids what a danger these drugs really are. This often isn't enough, however, says Carmen Colón, a counselor for the Hispanic Urban Minority Alcoholism and Drug Abuse Outreach in Cleveland. Most teenagers have the mixed blessing of a strong sense of invincibility that can make even frightening statistics go in one ear and out the other. In many cases, though, teens *do* have a tremendous fear of losing face or becoming unpopular with their peers. You can appeal to that side of your kids by pointing out some of the less attractive facts of drug use: for example, that smoking gives you wrinkles and yellow teeth, that people who use inhalants can suffer permanent brain damage, and that

Signs That Your Child May Be Using Drugs

T rying to figure out if your child is using drugs or just going through a difficult phase of adolescence is a big challenge sometimes. According to the National Center on Addiction and Substance Abuse at Columbia University in New York City (CASA), there are some signs you can watch for that might indicate your child is involved in drugs. The more of these signs you see, says Alyse Booth at CASA, the more concerned you should be that your child may have a problem.

- Low grades or poor school performance

- Withdrawal, isolation, depression, or fatigue

- Aggressive, rebellious behavior

- Truancy

- Excessive influence by peers or a new group of friends

- Hostility and lack of cooperativeness

- Deteriorating relationships with family

- Loss of interest in appearance and personal hygiene

- Loss of interest in hobbies and sports

- Changes in sleeping and eating habits

- Evidence of drugs or drug paraphernalia

- Physical changes such as red eyes, runny nose, frequent sore throats, rapid weight loss, or bruises from falls

drinking binges often end with the indulger in the graceless position of throwing up.

Know the age of introduction. While every child's experience is different, some huge changes take place in our kids' social worlds between the ages of 12 and 13. At this point, most kids are moving from elementary to middle school—and the exposures to drugs that they invariably find there. Statistics show that the proportion of teens who say that they could buy marijuana if they wanted more than triples from age 12 to 13. A 13-year-old is almost three times as likely to know a teen who uses acid, cocaine, or heroin as a 12-year-old is.

Believe that your child is going to be exposed. Never assume that your child's school is drug-free. The fact is that most schools are not. According to the National Center on Addiction and Substance Abuse at Columbia University (CASA) in New York City, 11 percent of school principals say that their schools are not drug-free. However, 66 percent of the students say the same. In light of the odds that there are going to be drugs in the school, it's better that you take for granted the fact that your kids *are* going to be exposed to them and start working with them on making smart choices.

Make the rules crystal clear. "The old adage that kids are looking for boundaries is very, very true," says Susie Carleton, R.N., a coordinator for the Addiction Technology Transfer Center in the department of psychiatry at the University of California, San Diego. "If your children find that the boundaries set for them are ambivalent, they'll bang up against them until they either find a firm limit or discover that there really isn't a rule for that particular situation after all." Lay down very specific rules and the consequences for your child if he breaks them, she recommends. Once you've done so, be sure to follow through each time.

One frequently sore subject with kids who have been caught using drugs is the privacy of their rooms and belongings. "I don't recommend invading your child's privacy lightly," says Carleton, "but you can make it clear that though the child has his room where he is entitled to privacy, that room is a part of your house and available to you if you feel it is important."

Spend time with your child one-on-one. Studies have found that the best way to reach an adolescent who is involved with drugs is usually to work with him face-to-face, one-on-one. Schedule time to do something with your at-risk child, just the two of you, and take advantage of opportunities to spend time with him on the spur of the moment, too. Don't spend it all lecturing or talking about drugs, Carleton recommends, but instead focus on strengthening your relationship with activities or time spent that you can both relax and enjoy. Above all, don't underestimate your own importance in your child's decision making. "Even though peer groups are extremely powerful in the short-term decisions your kid is going to make, all the research indicates that parents are the first and foremost influence on the decisions their children make," she says. "So even if it seems as though your child is not listening to your input and advice, keep talking, spending time with him, and offering it anyway."

Start a family meal tradition. It seems too simple, but the fact is that kids who eat dinner with their parents 6 or 7 nights a week are less likely to get involved with drugs than their peers who don't. A study conducted by CASA found that 93 percent of teens who eat dinner with their families that often say they haven't smoked a cigarette in the last month. That number drops among teens who eat with their families less often. The same is true for drinking: More than half of students who eat dinner with their parents 6 or 7 nights a week haven't been to drinking parties in the past 6 months.

Worship together. Another surprising statistic about teens who get involved with drugs is that 56 percent of those who attend worship services with their parents four or more times a month say that they will never use an illegal drug. Just 15 percent of teens who attend services less than once a month say the same.

Push activities that respect the body. "When we survey kids who are athletic and involved in activities that challenge them physically, many would never consider smoking a cigarette or using illegal drugs," says Alyse Booth, vice president and director of marketing for CASA. "They've developed too much of a regard for their bodies to be willing to damage them with drugs."

Don't leave the after-school hours unsupervised. Kids who say that they "just hang out with friends" in the after-school hours are at higher risk for getting involved with drugs than kids who have activities and supervision during that time. "This is a time when it's daylight, and a lot of parents aren't thinking about the potential for their kids getting into trouble," says Booth. "But kids who are not engaged during those hours are at high risk for getting into trouble not only with substance abuse but also with violence and sexual activity."

Teach your kids not to be manipulated. According to CASA, one of the most effective ad campaigns against drug use in recent history is a series that points out how teens are being manipulated by big tobacco companies for profits. Teenagers and even younger kids know what it's like to feel manipulated, and most hate to think of themselves as being used by anyone, says Booth. She recommends talking with your kids about the calculated campaigns of tobacco companies, about liquor distributors that indirectly market to children, and about the biggest manipulators of all—drug dealers. If your teenager starts to feel like a consumer who's being taken advantage of, he may see drug use in a whole new light.

Create a parenting co-op. Getting together with the parents of the kids your teen spends time with can be one of the best resources that parents have, says Carleton. "By bringing together the parents of kids in a group that spends time together, parents can pool their resources both for keeping track of where the teenagers are and what they're doing and to come up with appealing supervised activities and events that the kids can participate in," she explains. The younger your kids are when you start this practice, the better.

Reinforce good behavior. In struggles with kids who are using drugs or are at risk to do so, it's easy to become solely focused on bad behavior and on punishments and restrictions, says Booth. But the fact is that most kids respond better if those rules and consequences are balanced with rewards and reinforcement when they do the right thing.

Carleton recommends using personal rewards rather than monetary ones as often as you can. "Compliment your children, tell them you are proud of them, fix their favorite meal—whatever you can do to make them feel good about following your rules, making smart decisions, and being a participating member of your family," she says.

What to Do If Your Child Does Use Drugs

This may be one of the toughest situations a parent can face. Whole books have been written on this subject, so obviously this chapter won't be able to address everything you need to know. But following are some good starting points in winning the war on drugs in your family.

Recognize the problem early. This may sound obvious, but the first step in helping a child with a drug problem is admitting that there is one, says Pollard. "Often parents don't want to talk about their children's drug abuse because they are embarrassed, they think they will grow out of it, or they don't know who to ask for help," she says.

Once you admit it, you need to get involved—the sooner the better, says Florence Morehead, manager of the Monterey Bay Teen Challenge drug and alcohol rehabilitation program in Watsonville, California. "Your child needs to know that you are aware of what is going on in his life and at what level you are unwilling to tolerate it."

Get help sooner rather than later. When your child has a drug problem that is affecting your family's well-being, it's better to seek help early on than to wait until the problem escalates, says Carleton.

"When you have a child who refuses to accept a family's rules or who shows signs of drug abuse, you can't get help too soon," says Morehead. Ask your child's school counselor, pediatrician, or the family's clergyperson for advice on finding a qualified professional.

Don't withdraw your support. Emphasize to your child who is using drugs that it is his behavior and not him personally that you are not going to tolerate. "Let him know that you are there and you love him," says Morehead. "But also tell him that you aren't about to sit back and watch as he throws away his potential, and so you will take whatever steps are necessary to help him stop using drugs."

Limit their access. "The fact is that kids who are taking drugs, especially if they are taking them repeatedly, have abused a trust you put in them," says Morehead. "Do not give them windows of opportunity where they are unsupervised or left in situations where they are likely to make foolish choices." Enlist the help of friends and family if necessary to help you keep on top of your child's schedule.

Eating Disorders

What mother doesn't worry whether her baby is getting enough to eat? Eventually, most children learn to eat their vegetables, and mothers turn their focus to other parenting concerns, like homework, sibling squabbles, and after-school schedules. But in some families, a serious and frightening struggle begins to emerge in late childhood or adolescence when a child develops an eating disorder.

Experts believe that eating disorders afflict approximately 5 million Americans each year, especially adolescent girls and young women. Boys can have eating disorders, but this is rare. Puzzling, frustrating, and potentially life-threatening, eating disorders include a number of separate kinds of problems.

- Bingeing. In this case, the adolescent eats much more food in a limited period of time (say, within 2 hours) than most people would eat—that is, a whole box of cookies or a gallon of ice cream, perhaps after a day of eating hardly anything. In addition, she experiences a lack of control over the eating. She can't stop, even if she wants to.

- Purging. After bingeing, or even after a normal meal, the child induces vomiting or takes laxatives, diuretics, or enemas to get rid of calories from the food she has eaten.

- Fasting. The adolescent goes for long periods of time without eating or eating very little food.

- Excessive exercise. She may run for hours every day or do hundreds of repetitions of calisthenics in an attempt to burn calories from food she has eaten.

- Unusual eating patterns. The child eats in a certain, overly restrictive way. For instance, she might eat one piece of dry toast every day for breakfast and one piece of lettuce with no dressing for lunch. She might count out 19 pieces of dry cereal to eat or cut pieces of rice in half.

- Distorted body image. Bruce Arnow, Ph.D., associate professor of psychiatry at Stanford University School of Medicine, describes it this way: "A child or teenager who is getting very, very thin might complain about her stomach pouching out or her thighs being too big. Even though the parents and the doctor disagree, she really sees herself this way, as if she were looking at herself in one of those mirrors at amusement parks that make you look beanpole thin or round like a cannonball."

Dr. Arnow adds an important point, however: A child does not have to be thin to have an eating disorder. In fact, about half of people with bulimia are within 10 percent of their ideal body weight, just a bit on the thin side, or slightly heavy.

Defining the Problem

Eating disorders are illnesses that doctors diagnose because of specific symptoms. Your adolescent might have an eating disorder if she:

- Is thin, 15 percent below her ideal body weight for her age and height

- Refuses to gain enough weight to be in the normal range

- Is very afraid of gaining weight or being fat

- Perceives herself to be fat, even though she is not

- Evaluates herself mostly in terms of her body shape and weight

- Doesn't acknowledge the seriousness of being so thin

- Has missed menstrual periods (as a result of hormone deficiencies caused by not eating enough nutritious food)

- Forces herself to vomit or uses laxatives or diuretics to lose weight

She also may have physical symptoms such as fatigue, constipation, dental cavities, dry skin and hair, hair loss, fragile bones, soft furlike hair on her back, or sores on the back of her hand (from forcing herself to vomit).

Which Eating Disorder?

If a person displays symptoms such as being excessively thin (15 percent or more below ideal body weight), missing three menstrual periods, being intensely afraid of becoming fat, and experiencing body image distortion even if she is extremely thin, she may meet the criteria for diagnosis of a rare and extremely dangerous eating disorder, anorexia nervosa.

If she regularly eats huge quantities of food, punctuated by periods of fasting, throwing up, using laxatives, or exercising furiously to work off the excess calories, the diagnosis is bulimia.

A third eating disorder, binge-eating disorder, includes regular bouts of eating large quantities of food, but no purging. Still, the child will have negative feelings and unusual eating behaviors. She might eat very quickly, eat until stuffed, eat even if she isn't hungry, eat alone, or feel disgusted or guilty after eating too much.

Why Does This Happen?

Eating disorders arise from a complex mixture of contributing factors, explains Sara Forman, M.D., instructor of pediatrics at Harvard Medical School. Among the causes are the following:

- Biology. These problems can run in families. Studies of twins show that heredity may play a role. Also, certain brain chemicals may be at different levels in people who develop eating disorders.

- Psychology. An eating disorder is a form of psychiatric or psychological illness. People simply cannot will themselves to think about food in a normal way and recover from an eating disorder without help. Other mental disorders in people with an eating disorder may be present as well: depression, anxiety, and obsessive-compulsive disorder. Eating disorders also may occur in people with certain personality traits. They may be sensitive, or perfectionists, for example.

- Social environment. Adolescents who live in societies that place a great deal of emphasis on body image, especially thinness, are more likely to develop eating disorders. Their families may highly value physical appearance or perfection or struggle with issues like divorce or family strife.

- Developmental insecurity. Adolescent eating disorders most often develop at two critical times: at ages 13 to 14, during puberty; and at ages 17 to 18, when young people are facing important decisions about leaving home, getting jobs, and perhaps going away to school.

Parents Can Help

Families can play a role in averting eating disorders, helping uncover the problem once it exists, finding help, and supporting the adolescent through what can be a long recovery. Here are some practical things you can do for your child.

Get help right away. An eating disorder is a serious illness—and may be fatal. If you think there is a problem, particularly with anorexia, schedule an appointment with a physician immediately. But your child and your entire family will also need help from a mental health professional: a psychologist or psychiatrist. Social workers and nutritionists may also be needed.

Confronting an eating disorder in your child takes a great deal of courage. Many families feel embarrassed about or ashamed of the destructive behavior. They often try to deal with it for months before seeking professional help, says social worker Gina Andrews-Duarte of Galveston, Texas, who counsels people with eating disorders and their families.

She recalls the parents of a bulimic girl who were so desperate to control her obsessive eating that they finally put a padlock on the refrigerator. But the girl's problems were not confined to her eating, as is typical, since eating disorders can often be symptoms of more complex emotional issues. It wasn't until the girl literally pushed over the refrigerator in her rage that they sought outside help.

Dr. Forman stresses that the consequences of not getting help early are dire. Anorexia nervosa can be fatal in as many as 1 in 20 cases.

Even with recovery, it can cause permanent bone loss, leading eventually to osteoporosis, a disease of fragile bones. Long-term anorexia nervosa can also damage the heart, brain, and other organs. Bulimia can lead to tooth loss, heart rhythm abnormalities, and lasting intestinal problems.

Join in the therapy. "The best chance we have in treatment today of overcoming anorexia among adolescents is catching it early and involving the whole family in the treatment," says Dr. Arnow.

Be willing to change. Dr. Forman is especially hopeful of a patient's recovery from an eating disorder when each family member is willing to examine how his or her own attitudes or behavior might have unintentionally contributed to the problem. In these families, the desire to help the teenager who is suffering overwhelms any feelings of defensiveness or anger.

Foster your child's self-esteem. Make it a practice to highlight wonderful things about your adolescent that have nothing to do with her body. Praise such things as schoolwork and accomplishments in art, sports, or music.

Don't tease. Adolescents often feel self-conscious about their bodies. Don't let anyone in the family make fun of a child who is struggling with weight or the changes of puberty. Reassure girls especially that physical changes, such as a filling-out of the hips, are normal as a girl becomes a woman.

Debunk media images. Many girls want to look like rail-thin models, television stars, and popular musicians they see in magazines, on billboards, and on TV. Point out to your children that starvation isn't beautiful. Make note of famous people who are beautiful and normal in weight.

Discourage dieting. "Innocent dieting is the precursor to a lot of this," says Dr. Forman. If you, your child, or another family member struggles with a weight problem, encourage healthy, consistent eating and exercise—not fad dieting or extreme restrictions of food.

Maintain good communication. Talking frequently with your preteen or teenager about school, friendships, dreams, and disappointments sends the message that you care. Eating disorders sometimes emerge in troubled or chaotic households, says Andrews-Duarte. A child with an eating disorder may be trying to control some aspect of her life or may need acknowledgment as a full human being.

Don't demand perfection. People with eating disorders may be remarkably critical of themselves as they constantly strive for goals that are unattainable. Mothers can help by admitting that they remember making mistakes during the upheaval of adolescence, explains Andrews-Duarte, and by reminding their daughters that they aren't perfect now. Forgive your children their mistakes. Seek professional help so everyone can find peace and understanding through this vulnerable process. Tell your children that you love them no matter what.

Above all, do not give up hope. More than half of cases of bulimia and anorexia can be completely cured, and another 30 percent of people have a partial recovery, according to a report published in the *New England Journal of Medicine.* (For tips on healthy weight loss, see the Overweight chapters on pages 118 and 445.)

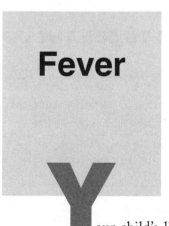

Fever

Your child's little pajamas are all wrinkled, his face is reddened, and the hair over his forehead is soaked in sweat.

When your child appears feverish, the first instinctive reaction from you is probably to try to cool him down. But a child who is hot may not have a high temperature and, even if he does, bringing down the fever is not always the best solution, says A. Gayden Robert, M.D., a pediatrician and chief of general pediatrics at the Ochsner Clinic in New Orleans.

Any worried mother will call the doctor as soon as a fever starts climbing, and with reason. It is important to discover what is causing the fever. This does not mean, however, that you have to make the fever go down immediately.

"Fever is a symptom, not a disease," explains Dr. Robert. The pediatrician points out that fever is generally caused by a viral or bacterial infection, such as measles or flu. "It is a defense mechanism that helps the child fight the infection."

Many doctors agree, however, that you may need to treat the fever so that the child can rest more easily. If he is crying or is very irritable because of the fever, you definitely want to bring it down so that he is more comfortable, says Carol Kilmon, R.N., Ph.D., professor of nursing at the University of Texas Medical Branch at Galveston. Therefore, here is how to deal with high temperatures so that you can make your child more comfortable.

WHEN TO SEE THE DOCTOR

Generally, fever does not require medical attention, but there are some warning signs that indicate a need to see a doctor, according to A. Gayden Robert, M.D., a pediatrician and chief of general pediatrics at the Ochsner Clinic in New Orleans.

If you are worried about your child's fever, consult your physician. You should *always* call him, however, when your child is feverish and:

- Cries inconsolably

- Is confused or delirious

- Is having a convulsion or just had one

- Has a stiff neck

- Is having difficulty breathing, even though his nose is clear

- Has persistent vomiting or diarrhea

- Has had the fever for more than 72 hours

How to Take Your Child's Temperature

Time your reading. Body temperature fluctuates during the day, points out Sanford Kimmel, M.D., a pediatrician and professor of family medicine at the Medical College of Ohio in Toledo. Generally, it is higher at the end of the afternoon or beginning of the evening and lower in the morning. It can also vary because of exercise or very hot foods. To get an accurate reading, you should take your child's temperature 30 minutes after he has quieted down or 30 minutes after he has had a hot meal or drink, advises Dr. Kimmel.

Take the temperature correctly. The temperature of a baby is measured more accurately with a rectal thermometer, which is shorter and has a thicker bulb than an oral thermometer, says Dr. Kimmel. Cover it with petroleum jelly, then insert the thermometer slowly, no more than 1½ inches, and keep it carefully in that position for at least 3 minutes. To do this, place the baby on top of the dresser table or on your lap in the diaper-changing position, and lift the baby's legs to facilitate access. You may want to lay your child on his stomach, across your lap; separate his buttocks and insert the thermometer.

Use an oral thermometer when your child is ready. When a child is 4 or 5 years old, he can generally cooperate in holding an oral thermometer under his tongue for at least 4 minutes, says Dr. Kimmel. Digital thermometers are fast, accurate, and a little safer than the traditional ones of glass and mercury. They are also very expensive. Just be sure that your child sits calmly, because any activity will increase the temperature.

Evaluate the result. Although 98.6°F has long been considered the classic "normal" oral temperature, some people routinely have a higher temperature. So your child could have a slightly higher reading and still be perfectly healthy. Your child has a fever if his temperature is above 100.4°F measured rectally, 99°F measured under the arm, or 100°F measured orally, says Dr. Robert.

How to Bring Fever Down

Give your child acetaminophen. Pediatric acetaminophen (such as Children's Tylenol) will help to reduce the fever, says Beth W. Hapke, M.D., a pediatrician in Fairfield, Connecticut. This product comes in liquid form for babies and preschool-age children. It is sold as chewable

A Different Type of Fever

Your child's fever has remained high for 3 days, but your pediatrician has told you not to worry. All of a sudden, on the fourth day, the fever comes down and a rash appears on your child's torso, neck, arms, and legs.

Call the doctor, but don't get distressed. It is not the appearance of a new disease but a sign that the cause of your child's fever was a harmless condition called roseola, says Daniel Bronfin, M.D., professor of pediatrics at Tulane University in New Orleans.

"Roseola is not always possible to diagnose before the rash appears, but when we see a playful child 1 or 2 days into a fever of 103°F to 104°F without other symptoms, we suspect it is roseola," says Dr. Bronfin.

Roseola is caused by a virus, and it appears with greater frequency among children 6 months to 2 years of age. No medicines are required, and you should try to lower the temperature only if your child is uncomfortable, says Dr. Bronfin. You should be aware, however, that you can lower the fever only a few degrees.

Even if it appears that your child is more irritable, the rash does not cause itching or discomfort, and he does not require treatment. It will disappear in a few hours or, at the latest, in a few days. Once the rash appears, this illness is no longer contagious.

tablets for older children. Check the instructions on the package to determine the correct dosage for your child's age and weight. If your child is younger than age 2, consult your physician.

Physicians warn that you should never give aspirin to a feverish child because it has been linked with a serious disease called Reye's syndrome.

Try giving your child a sponge bath. Give your child a lukewarm sponge bath for 15 to 20 minutes, says Lynn Sugarman, M.D., a pediatrician with Tenafly Pediatrics in Tenafly, New Jersey.

Place your child in a bathtub with lukewarm water, and sponge the water over his arms, legs, and body. "As the water evaporates, the body cools off, which helps reduce the fever," explains Dr. Sugarman. Do not use water so cold that the child shivers. Shivering, in fact, will make the body temperature increase, which defeats the purpose of the sponge bath.

If you do not want to take the child out of bed to bathe him, you can loosen his clothing and sponge him with the help of a basin.

Leave the alcohol in the medicine cabinet. In the past, mothers would rub feverish children with alcohol, but doctors today discourage this practice. "Besides causing chills, alcohol can be absorbed by the skin and cause a toxic reaction in your child," says Dr. Robert. Also, breathing the vapors can irritate your child.

Offer your child many liquids. A child with fever breathes more rapidly than normal, so he loses a lot of fluids. If he has diarrhea, the loss is even greater. "Be sure that your child sips some liquid—whatever his stomach will tolerate," advises Dr. Kimmel. "Prepare cold drinks, not hot, and give him small amounts frequently instead of having him drink a lot at one time."

Any beverage for children is all right as long as you avoid giving your child cola, tea, or coffee, because these are diuretics, which promote the loss of fluids. You can add some variety if you give him soup, a frozen ice pop, or gelatin. As for nursing infants, their regular feeding provides them with sufficient liquid. If your baby has had diarrhea for more than 24 hours, ask your doctor about giving him Pedialyte, an oral electrolyte solution available at drugstores, suggests Dr. Kimmel.

Keep your child's clothing light. A child wearing flannel pajamas or wrapped up in a blanket will overheat, making the fever worse. "Keep your child in light clothing and make sure that he sleeps covered by a thin blanket or sheet," advises Dr. Sugarman.

Make meals optional. If your child has a fever and does not want to eat, do not force him, says Dr. Kimmel. On the other hand, if he asks for pizza, no problem. "If the child has a craving for some food, it is likely that the appropriate thing to do is to give it to him," he says.

A child with an upset stomach or a stomach virus, however, will

A Feverish Attack:
A Frightening Experience

I f your child has ever had a feverish convulsion, you will not soon forget it. It starts with a rapid increase in temperature, generally from an infectious disease such as tonsillitis, which apparently causes a change in the electrical patterns of the brain.

Feverish convulsions appear in 1 of every 25 children, and in some cases the feverish child falls unconscious. Other attacks may emulate an epileptic attack where arms and legs contort without control. Some other attacks are noticed because of the lack of attention on the part of child. You should always get in contact with your physician when your child suffers any type of convulsion.

When the convulsion starts, follow these recommendations, advises John Freeman, M.D., professor of neurology and pediatrics at the Johns Hopkins Hospital in Baltimore.

- "Just turn your child on his side and be sure that he can breathe freely," says Dr. Freeman. This way, saliva or vomit will not block the windpipe.

- Move all dangerous objects out of the way.

- Do not try to keep your child's mouth open; he will not swallow his tongue.

- If the episode lasts for only 5 to 10 minutes, call your doctor as soon as it is over.

- If the episode lasts for more than 10 minutes, or if your child has trouble breathing, take him to a hospital where he can receive anticonvulsant medicines.

probably prefer something simple, like cookies or toast with a little bit of jam. Other "comfort foods" like oats and applesauce, bananas, and pudding are also good options, says Dr. Kimmel. Avoid fruit juices, however, as they can contribute to the diarrhea.

Don't expect a normal temperature. Neither acetaminophen nor the sponge bath will bring back the child to normal, says Daniel Bronfin, M.D., professor of pediatrics at Tulane University in New Orleans. "If the fever was 104°F," he says, "you may be able to bring it down to 101°F."

Keep your child at home. It is best to keep your child at home while he has a fever. "The rule of thumb here is that the child may return to school once the temperature has remained normal for 24 hours," says Dr. Robert. "Even if we don't know for certain, we believe that if the fever is gone, then the infectious agent is gone as well."

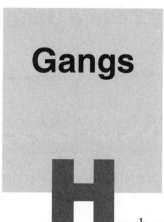

Gangs

How do your children view gang members who strut down the street in low-hanging khaki pants, pausing to flash a gang sign to another member? Are they seen as menacing or protective? Cool or ridiculous? Flush with drug money or heading for lives burdened with arrest records or gunshot wounds? Or even death?

These are issues to discuss with your children, since the self-image that gang members try to convey is often at odds with the reality of the lives they lead.

"The breeding ground of all gangs is exclusion," says Sergeant Richard Valdemar of the Los Angeles Sheriff's Department. "An individual feels threatened by poverty, ignorance, or some form of victimization, real or imagined. He finds other individuals who feel the same way, and their feelings are fed by an anti-establishment culture, drugs, crime, and racial separatism." Motivated by a desire for power and vengeance, the gang lashes out at outsiders at first, but eventually turns on itself as competing factions break away.

A 1998 U.S. Department of Justice survey of 2,668 law enforcement agencies concluded that 28,700 gangs and 780,000 gang members were active in the United States that year.

Gangs are as diverse as the neighborhoods in which they flourish. At one end of the spectrum are those involved with highly organized criminal businesses. At the other end are smaller, neighborhood-based gangs

Signs That Your Child May Be in a Gang

There is no simple list of telltale signs that a child is in a gang. Many identifying signs come and go, even within a particular gang. Gangs in your city may wear a glove on the left hand or don black trench coats. They may have spider tattoos on one leg, or they may wear the gear of a certain sports team.

But lots of kids today have tattoos and admire the Oakland Raiders, and they are certainly not all in gangs. So keep in mind that these are merely guidelines. You can find out from your local police department or nonprofit antigang organizations which symbols pertain to the gangs in your city.

Be alert if you notice any of the following:

- Symbols drawn on your child's notebook covers, backpack, or body. Gang "tags" may look like letters or shapes, but the pattern will be copied repeatedly and may represent a code for your child's gang name.

that may sell and use drugs but are bound by a sense of power, unity, and fierce loyalty. The price, however, is unspeakably high. What seem at first to be bonds of friendship or support become handcuffs on a youth's future. Independence and achievement fall to empty vows of loyalty. In the extreme, the brutality of gang life leads to prison, disability, or death.

Listen, for example, to Alva Luz García, a 24-year-old from Dallas who has spent the last 8 years in a wheelchair. At age 16, while 5 months pregnant, she was shot three times, including once in the throat, leaving her paralyzed from the waist down.

She had joined the Mystic Knights, a small Dallas gang, at 13,

- A change in behavior. Is your child evasive about how he spends his time? Is he increasingly contemptuous of your rules and more attached to outside friends than family?

- Signs of drug use. Does your child come home "high"? Have you found drugs or alcohol in his room?

- Declining school performance. A drop in grades or a sudden disinterest in outside activities such as sports may indicate a problem.

- Clothing associated with gangs. Some gangs wear bandannas, beads, baggy pants, sports jerseys or hats, certain athletic shoes, certain colors, or distinguishing jewelry. If known gang members in your area wear something distinctive, don't assume that your child is now wearing it simply because it is in style.

- Injuries from a beating. Initiation into most gangs means being beaten up, or "jumped in." Your child could also be beaten because he is not in a gang. You need to find out what happened.

"jumped in," or initiated with a beating, by her older brother's girlfriend. "My parents didn't have a high school education. All they knew how to do was work and work and work. My mother worked nights, and she was so sleepy that all I ever saw her do was cook and clean and work."

In a family with nine children, money and tempers were short. "They would slap us, but they didn't know how to speak with us. They didn't help us with homework or talk to us about our friends or about puberty or anything. They put clothes on our backs and food on the table," she says.

"I was interested in sports. I had dreams of being a model or a Dallas police officer. But I didn't have anybody to communicate with me, so I turned to my brothers (who were in gangs) and my friends," says García. "I didn't know I was going to be sitting in a chair the rest of my life."

Prevent Trouble Before It Starts

Former gang members and gang counselors say that the main key to keeping your child out of a gang is to provide an alternative life from the very beginning. Here are their suggestions.

Talk and talk and talk. Former gang members say that their parents did not know their friends, did not ask much about school or their activities, and did not notice early signs of drug use or gang involvement until it was too late. "Pay attention to your kids and spend time with them. Don't let your kids go to waste," says Javier Solis, a former gang member, now disabled from a gunshot wound, whose gang involvement ended his dreams of enlisting in the military.

Make time for family. Children don't reveal their troubles and triumphs on command, at a certain moment set aside for quality time. So enlist your son's or daughter's help when you're folding laundry, chopping vegetables, washing dishes. When hands are busy, talk flows. (Make sure the TV is off.)

Fill up your child's schedule. "Get up to the school and find out every after-school activity there is," recommends Robert J. DeSena, founder of the Council for Unity, a gang violence prevention movement based in Brooklyn. "Sign up your child for tutoring, recreation, arts and crafts, basketball, whatever." What DeSena calls "the time factor" is a huge contributor to gang involvement. He believes that every child and teenager should be busy with a structured, supervised activity between 2:00 P.M. and 8:00 P.M.—peak hours for crime.

Establish safe havens. Make sure that your child has a secure place to go when school is not in session. Besides activities, YMCAs and other community organizations offer consistent, safe supervision by adults who understand kids and who have a stake in seeing kids succeed. At the YMCA, 8.5 million kids under age 18 receive computer training and participate in job skill sessions, camps, and activities from dance to martial arts. Many programs offer free transportation, and no child is turned away because his family can't pay.

Support your child. Often what draws kids to gangs is approval, says DeSena: "You were in trouble, and they bailed you out." Once that happens, "the pull of the street is like a vortex, and it will be very hard to get them out." When your child does something good, be generous with praise. Let your child know that you are there in times of trouble, too, providing both discipline and love.

Don't abandon them when they make mistakes. Growing up is hard to do, and adolescents will surely stumble along the way, says Carmelita Gallo, director of programs and product development for the YMCA of the USA. "Kids value the fact that an adult doesn't give up on them. They think, 'I messed up, and I don't know why I did it. Are you still there for me?'"

Establish rules and consequences. Even very young children should know your rules and what happens if they are broken. Very small children may need a time-out from activities, while older children may need to be restricted from television or may need favorite toys or privileges taken away. Serious misbehavior calls for serious consequences, insists Del Hendrixson, director of the Bajito Onda Foundation, a Dallas-based organization that offers shelter from gangs in the form of job skills and support. She describes one family who removed every piece of furniture from a teenager's room and made him earn it back, starting with the privilege of sleeping in a bed. Was that extreme? "I don't think so," she says. "You are the parent. You make the rules."

Form a network of moms. In today's chaotic world, no mother can know everything going on in a child's world, much less supervise her child every minute of every day. Exchange phone numbers with mothers of your children's friends. Work as a team to explore activities for your children and teens. Trade advice and make rules together.

Be vigilant. Know what is in your child's room, on the covers of his notebooks, and in his backpack. It doesn't mean that you have to snoop; just be alert. Especially know what gangs are in your neighborhood. Be familiar with their members and their signs, which might be as simple as a black T-shirt with a certain logo, or a hand gesture. "You have to be incredibly vigilant," says DeSena. "There are vultures out there. If you let your child get too close, you will be fighting for the kid's soul."

Nurture your child's strengths. Every child has a talent. Find your child's special gift and do everything in your power to help it develop. García loved gymnastics. Her parents couldn't afford a special school, but perhaps they could have found a YMCA program that would have been free. Solis loved soccer, but his parents never came to the sign-up day for after-school sports. A budding artist can be painting at the Boys and Girls Club or tattooing a gang symbol into a friend's wrist. As a parent, you need to guide that choice.

Envision a better future for your child. Every child has dreams. What first-grader doesn't want to be a firefighter or a singer or a professional soccer player when he grows up? But too often, parents get wrapped up in the difficult job of making ends meet, and they forget to share in their children's dreams. Don't dismiss as nonsense a little boy's dream of becoming an astronaut; tell him to do well in math and make a project for the school science fair. Read your little girl's mock newspaper and tell her she can be a real reporter if she becomes a good reader and writer. Point out role models who grew up in your neighborhood: doctors, business owners, law enforcement officers, and members of the military who stayed in school and realized their ambitions.

Don't be in denial. If your child is wearing ganglike clothing, displays gang signs, and is increasingly secretive, and you suspect that he may be involved in drug use or criminal activity, pay attention to your gut feelings. Your child is probably in a gang. "It's a problem that isn't going to go away by itself. You have to face it and get help," says Deputy Sylvia Ramos of the Los Angeles County Sheriff's Department STAR program (Success Through Awareness and Resistance).

Don't buy the "protection" explanation. Some mothers believe that their children have no alternative but to join a gang, since they think that local schools are completely dominated by warring factions. "It's a question I get all the time, and it's a myth," says Sergeant Valdemar. "Even in the worst schools and the worst neighborhoods, like the one where I grew up, fewer than 10 percent of kids get involved in gangs." Gangs only force newcomers to join when they have been hanging out with them, dating girls in the gang, or seeking out the gang for protection. Kids who steer clear of relationships with gang members will never be forced to join, he says. The two former gang members interviewed for this book both admitted that joining a gang was a choice. Peers around them made the opposite choice and avoided the violence and angst that they encountered as a part of gang life.

Finding a Way Out

Just as not every child must join a gang, not every gang member must remain in a gang. Although gangs can threaten dire consequences to those who leave, some gangs generally do not hunt down members who have left their fold, in contrast to gangs such as the Crips and Bloods, which may kill expatriates, says Hendrixson.

If your son or daughter is in a gang, do not lose hope.

Get help. Helping your child escape gang life is not easy. You must find ways to motivate your child to want to leave. Then you must understand the dynamics of the gang to figure out how a break can be made without endangering your child, your other children, or you. Whom can you turn to?

- Community antigang programs. Bajito Onda Foundation, based in Dallas, and the Council for Unity, based in Brooklyn, are only two of the many nonprofit organizations that exist to help gang members pull away and find another life through peace, job training, and the love and support of friends. Through these organizations, you can meet former gang members who can explain how they cut their ties to gangs. To find the names of organizations like this in your community, call the United Way or your local Boys and Girls Club, both listed in the telephone book under Community Service Organizations, Human Service Organizations, or Youth Organizations.

- Churches. The Roman Catholic Church and other churches and religious organizations have been very involved in gang prevention and helping gang members to get a fresh start. Each archdiocese has its own separate program. Ask for more information at your local parish, or call your local Catholic Charities' office of family life.

- Schools. The guidance counselors at your child's school are excellent resources. They can help you work with your child and can tell you how to reach local agencies that offer support and shelter to people trying to escape the grip of gangs.

- The police. Many times people are reluctant to contact the police because they think that they will be exposing themselves or their children to arrest. But many police departments now have prevention officers whose job it is to keep kids out of trouble, not put them in jail. These officers may work in the schools, talking to children about ways to stay off drugs and stay out of gangs. They may be able to give you advice over the phone without even knowing your name.

Consider a move. A move will only be successful if it is your child who desperately wants to leave gang life. The impetus has to come from him. If you move because you want to force your child to leave a gang, he will just join up with another gang or start a new one, warns Enid Margolies, Ph.D., director of education, safety, development, and support for the New York City schools.

But if the desire is there to start a new life, relocating to a new setting may help a child re-establish himself. You may have a relative in another city or outside the United States whom he could stay with, or the whole family may want to consider a move.

Hay Fever and Allergies

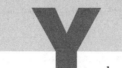**Y**our daughter's nose does not stop running, and it itches like there's no tomorrow. She has no fever, but she's sneezing continuously, and her eyes are teary, red, and swollen. Of course, she feels miserable.

"Hay fever," you think, and you may be right (although, generally, children under 5 are not allergic to pollen). So, what does she have if it is the end of winter, when there are no blossoms?

Instead of having hay fever, your daughter may be allergic to something besides the pollen that floats in the atmosphere during the year, such as dust mites, mold, or animal dander. When a child is allergic to something she inhales, her body perceives the inhaled substances as viral or bacterial invaders. As a defense, her body sends assassins called histamines. Normally, this reaction helps quite a lot because histamines generally finish off the invaders that could make her sick. But, when there really isn't a virus or bacteria to eliminate, and instead there's only mold or pet dander, the histamines trigger disagreeable side effects, among them congestion, itching, runny nose, and sneezing.

So, what can you do? Many allergy specialists agree that allergy prevention starts at home. "We place a great emphasis in avoiding contact with the allergen, which is an effective and inexpensive way to treat allergies," says Peter LoGalbo, M.D., professor of pediatrics at the Albert Einstein College of Medicine of Yeshiva University in the Bronx.

The first step is to go to the allergist's office, where your child can be tested to find out what allergens are causing the problem. Once your child's allergies have been diagnosed, here is what you can do to solve the problem.

WHEN TO SEE THE DOCTOR

If keeping your child away from what causes her allergy is not adequate to relieve the symptoms, your physician will recommend other measures. "The second line of defense is medicine, which can be effective but may have side effects. Finally, we turn to allergy shots if the first two fail," says Peter LoGalbo, M.D., professor of pediatrics at the Albert Einstein College of Medicine of Yeshiva University in the Bronx.

You can also treat your child with over-the-counter products, but you should first ask your physician about the quantity and type of medicine to use.

"Antihistamines work better when your child has symptoms such as sneezing, itching, and watery eyes," says David Tinkelman, M.D., professor of pediatrics at the Medical College of Georgia in Augusta. But antihistamines may make your child drowsy, reduce her ability to concentrate, or cause dry mouth.

"On the other hand, decongestants will help open a stuffy nose but will not help with a runny nose or with sneezing. They can suppress the appetite or cause insomnia, nervousness, or irritability," says Dr. Tinkelman.

Many over-the-counter preparations are combinations of antihistamines and decongestants. These can provide relief but can also cause more side effects. Your physician will tell you what you can try or order another treatment if those over-the-counter products don't work out.

But never allow your child to use over-the-counter nose drops, warns Gail G. Shapiro, M.D., clinical professor of pediatrics at the University of Washington in Seattle. These drops cause the lining of the nose to shrink. They may provide temporary relief, but the inflammation will appear again, and it will often be worse than when it started. There are prescription drops that work well, points out Dr. Shapiro, so consult your doctor if your child requires additional relief from hay fever.

Help with Dust Mite Allergies

Prepare to implement changes. "Many children are allergic to the droppings of the house dust mite, a microscopic insect that lives where dust collects, such as on upholstery, pillows, stuffed animals, and carpets," says David Tinkelman, M.D., professor of pediatrics at the Medical College of Georgia in Augusta. To reduce contact with the mites, you should make some modifications to your furniture and, possibly, change how you clean the house.

Cover the mattress with plastic. Wrap your child's mattress, box spring, and pillow with vinyl-backed covers, available at department and discount stores. "Companies that sell items for allergies have some very elegant ones, but the inexpensive vinyl covers are quite appropriate for children," says Gail G. Shapiro, M.D., clinical professor of pediatrics at the University of Washington in Seattle.

Stick adhesive tape over the zippers. Dr. Tinkelman recommends finishing the treatment by putting adhesive tape over the zippers of all the covers. That way the mites that are inside the bed and the pillow won't be able to come out. Both duct tape and wide, heavy duty plastic sealing tape will work well.

Get rid of feathers and down-filled quilts. "Pillows and comforters filled with feathers and down are a paradise for mites," says Rebecca Gruchalla, M.D., professor of internal medicine at the University of Texas in Dallas. "Instead, change to cotton blankets and foam or polyester pillows, which are washable."

Use hot water. Wash all of your child's bed linen frequently in very hot water, says Dr. Shapiro. Hot water kills mites and eliminates droppings. Use the hot-water wash-and-rinse cycle. Be sure to wash all of the bedding, including the mattress cover and the blankets as well as the sheets. The best bet is to wash the bedclothes every 1 to 2 weeks.

Careful with the floor covers. Carpets and rugs are a mite's favorite hideaway. "Remove the carpet from your child's room," says Dr. Gruchalla. "Instead, use a cotton scatter rug that can be washed regularly in hot water."

Treat the remaining carpets. Perhaps it is not practical to remove all the carpets from the rest of your house, but you can keep them free of allergens. Treat them with Allersearch ADS, a 3 percent tannic acid solution, recommends Dr. Shapiro. Often, it is used with Acarosan, a product that reduces the mite population in the carpets, according to Dr. Shapiro. Both products should be applied every 3 months to be effective, in keeping with the instructions on the package. Both of these products are available by mail order from Allergy Control Products, 96 Danbury Road, Ridgefield, CT 06877.

Change vacuum cleaner bags. While it's important to vacuum frequently, you first need to make one important change. "Substitute regular vacuum cleaner bags for bags made of a special paper that traps mite particles," says Paul Williams, M.D., professor of pediatrics and allergy at the University of Washington in Seattle. "When you use a conventional bag to vacuum, you are actually collecting allergenic particles and tossing them back into the air, which worsens the situation." The special bags for catching allergens (one of the brands is Hysurf) can be purchased at a few stores where vacuum cleaners are sold or at National Allergy Supply, 1620 Satellite Boulevard, Suite D, Duluth, GA 30097.

Eliminate curtains. "Curtains and blinds are great trappers of dust," says Dr. LoGalbo. It's a good idea to replace them with washable curtains, but it is even better to install pull-down shades that can be wiped off easily, says Dr. Gruchalla.

Eliminate mites from stuffed toys. Since there may be an abundance of dust mites in a flock of stuffed toys, the best thing is to remove them from the child's bedroom. But if your child is very attached to some special stuffed toy, you can remove the mites from it with a heat or cold treatment, according to Dr. Tinkelman. "Dust mites cannot survive in extreme temperatures," he says. "Soak the stuffed toy in the hot-water cycle of your washing machine, or put it inside a plastic bag and leave it overnight inside the freezer."

You may want to allow your child to choose another stuffed toy occasionally to interchange favorites. If you buy any more, make your life easy and choose those that can withstand machine washing and drying.

Consider changing where your child sleeps. Your child should not sleep in the lower bunk or in a canopy bed, says Dr. Tinkelman. "Children love bunk beds and canopies, but so do dust mites," he points out. Mites live both in the upper mattress of the bunk and in the dust that collects on the canopy.

Pay attention to closets. "Closets are rarely cleaned or aired, and as a result they tend to be dust mines," points out Dr. LoGalbo. Any closet that is used by your child must be vacuumed every time you vacuum the rest of the room. If you have rarely used closets filled with papers or old toys, keep the closet door closed all the time.

Solve it the dry way. "Mites love humidity," says Dr. Williams. "If you can maintain the level of humidity below 50 percent, you have solved a great part of your problems with mites. Get a dehumidifier for your child's bedroom."

Minimize Mold

Buy a humidity meter. Mold thrives where there is a high level of humidity, according to Dr. Williams. To stop mold allergens, measure the humidity in your house and use a dehumidifier, says Dr. LoGalbo.

Air out. "Let fresh air circulate through the house, especially in bathrooms and kitchen where mold tends to develop," says Dr. LoGalbo. Window or ceiling fans help air circulate.

Remove the books from the bedroom. "Mold spores are known to live in books," says Gilbert Friday, M.D., professor of pediatrics at the Center of Asthmatic and Allergic Diseases in the Children's Hospital of Pittsburgh. "For those children allergic to mold, it is best to keep books in a bookcase with glass doors or all together outside. At the very least, dust books frequently."

Use cleaners that kill mold. "Choose cleaners such as Lysol that inhibit the development of mold," suggests Dr. LoGalbo. You can also make a mold-fighting mixture by adding a few tablespoonfuls of commercial chlorine to a bucket of water. Use a brush soaked in this solution and scrub damp areas and other surfaces to discourage mold. (Use rubber gloves to protect your hands from the chlorine mixture.)

Keep your children away from leaves. There is a lot of mold in piles of fallen leaves. Discourage your allergic child from playing in or rolling around near the piled leaves, advises Dr. Shapiro.

Control Pet Allergies

Out with the pets. Children may be allergic to dander, the dead skin from your pets. Cats, in particular, are responsible for the worst problems because they lick themselves so often that when the saliva dries, its allergens go into the air, says Dr. Friday.

"Ideally, family pets, such as dogs or cats, should live outside," says

Dr. Williams. If your pet cannot live outside, you should look for another home for that animal.

Ban pets from the bedroom. If moving a pet outside is not practical, and your family cannot bear to give away the animal, set some limits over its territory. It's most important to keep the pet out of your child's bedroom, says Jonathan Becker, M.D., a pediatrician at the University of Washington in Seattle.

"Pets such as hamsters and gerbils should also be removed from the bedroom because their droppings may promote the development of fungi or mold to which some children are allergic," says Dr. Friday. "Even birds may present a problem because the flapping of their wings releases a fine powder of bird allergen into the air."

Keep the cat out of the basement. Do not relocate your cat to the basement if you have forced-air heat, says Dr. Friday. "In a house with forced-air heat, the cat allergen—which is very light—would go right up through the heating system and spread all over the house."

Bathe the cat. "Preliminary research suggests that if you bathe your cat every week for at least 8 weeks, just with plain water or shampoo and water, you will remove the surface allergens produced by the cat's saliva. Unfortunately, you should continue bathing the cat every week from then on, to get continued benefit from the treatment," says Dr. Shapiro.

The problem is that it's difficult to get most adult cats to endure one bath, let alone a bath once a week. You will have more success bathing your cat if you start when your pet is just a kitten.

Prevent Problems with Pollen

Take advantage of the air-conditioning. Your child will not be able to avoid all contact with pollen, which prevails during spring and late summer. But her nights can be more restful if you have air-conditioning in her bedroom, according to Dr. LoGalbo. "It is not easy to resist the temptation to keep windows open when the night air outside is cool," he admits, "but this would allow pollen to come into the bedroom, and your child will wake up feeling awful."

Schedule time for games outdoors. Noon is the best time for children prone to hay fever to play outside. "In the morning, there is a very high concentration of pollen," says Dr. Friday. "As air warms up, it raises and takes pollen away. In the afternoon, when air cools, pollen comes back down. So, the best moment to let children play outdoors is precisely between the morning and the afternoon."

Close the car windows. "You will get a greater concentration of pollen if you drive with the windows down," says Dr. Friday. "If your allergic child is in the car, the best thing is to use the car's air-conditioning during the pollen season."

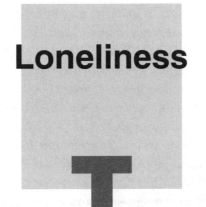

Loneliness

Twelve-year-old Amy comes home every day after school and sits in her room watching TV or playing video games. She doesn't ever call anyone on the phone and has friends over only occasionally. She's shy and doesn't like sports. When her mother asks who she hangs around with at school, she shrugs her shoulders and mentions one or two names. And now her mother's worried. She wonders if her daughter is lonely or just prefers to be alone.

If your child is like Amy, you may be ruminating over the same question. The truth is, some children just don't feel a sharp need for lots of social interaction. So, if your son or daughter acts like Amy and doesn't seem at all unhappy about being that way, she's probably not lonely, says Dorothy Lowery, a school psychologist in Radnor, Pennsylvania. "The child or adolescent who is lonely wants to be with others and feels hurt because they are unable to make that connection," she explains.

To help come to a determination, look at past behaviors, says Muriel Savikas, Ph.D., a child psychologist in Manhattan Beach, California, and author of *Guilt Is Good!*. A child who has always been content to come home and play quietly may simply prefer being by himself to being with friends.

Take steps to remedy the situation when your child makes a sudden shift toward solitude, or if he seems withdrawn or complains regularly about minor infirmities. "Big indicators of problems for kids is if they are physically ill with headaches or stomachaches, or if they are going to the nurse a lot," says Dr. Savikas. "That's because it's safer for kids to have physical ailments than emotional problems."

In some cases, loneliness will be easy to recognize. For example, if you move into a new neighborhood, or if your child changes schools or even has a falling out with friends, he may be clearly forlorn. There are also times when loneliness might be masked. Adolescents often put on a good face, says Cathleen A. Rea, Ph.D., a clinical child psychologist in Newport News, Virginia. It's important, therefore, to look for signals that indicate feelings of loneliness. If your child becomes moody or exhibits some symptoms of depression (see "Get Help for Depression"), he may need help making friends.

For advice on helping your child overcome loneliness, read the following tips. Since children of different ages often have different needs, the tips are divided into three categories: those appropriate for all children, those specific to younger kids, and those geared to helping adolescents and teens.

For All Children

Children of all ages may have a tough time making and keeping friends. Some have poor social skills, like being overly aggressive or too shy. Others may need more avenues for meeting other children. Whatever the case, you can take measures to bolster your child's social skills and get him better integrated. Here's how.

Get him to the doctor. Before you make any assumptions about the emotional well-being of your withdrawn child, schedule an appointment for a checkup, suggests Dr. Savikas. "Whenever you see mood swings or a change in behavior, the first thing you want to do is rule out anything physical."

Watch your child play. "Parents, if they are trying to understand why their child is lonely, need to be able to face the fact that there's often a reason why their child isn't liked or accepted by others," says Lowery. The starting point, then, is to observe how your child or adolescent interacts with other kids.

Get Help for Depression

A child or teen who is lonely and becoming isolated may be suffering from depression. Many teens experience brief bouts of depression, then bounce out of depression without treatment. But you should seek professional help when depression interferes with your child's ability to function. Here are a few telltale signs.

- Complains often of vague physical ailments such as stomachaches, headaches, or fatigue

- Performs poorly in school or is frequently absent

- No longer enjoys things once considered fun and shows no interest in being with friends

- Has outbursts of shouting and unexplained irritability or crying

- Shows extreme sensitivity to rejection or failure

- Exhibits heightened irritability, anger, or hostility

- Has persistent boredom or low energy levels

- Threatens to run away from home

- Makes a major change in eating or sleeping habits

- Speaks of suicide or behaves self-destructively

If you suspect that your child may be experiencing depression, ask your pediatrician for a referral to a child or adolescent psychiatrist who can make a diagnosis. Treatment usually includes individual or family therapy, or antidepressant medications.

If you have a preschooler or an elementary-age child, you can invite another child over to play, then supervise them. Does your child refuse to share, act bossy, or get angry or teary when he doesn't get his way? If so, pull him aside and give him some feedback, suggests Lowery. If you have an adolescent, take him and a group to a football game or the mall, and keep your ears tuned to the conversation. Is your son teasing others or being insensitive when others talk? Is your daughter too catty? If you observe troublesome behavior, bring it up afterward. Say, "I notice that you were doing this and maybe Joe doesn't like it," suggests Lowery.

Help your child develop realistic expectations of others. Does your child argue a lot with other kids or complain about being disappointed by friends? He may be expecting too much from his peers, Lowery says. Try to get him to approach friendships more realistically. Ask him to name specific ways he can trust his friends. Maybe one boy is good at being on time but not at keeping secrets. Let your son know that he can't expect his friends to be good at everything. If you see your child routinely demanding too much of his peers, he may be transferring unmet needs onto his friends. Therefore, it's especially important that you, as a parent, take time to be more nurturing and make an effort to meet your child's needs.

Enlist your child in extracurricular activities. Team sports, the marching band, scout troops, and youth groups can all provide children with an opportunity to interact with others in a supervised setting. Try to help your child find something he enjoys, but don't be surprised if you meet with some resistance at first. Kids who are feeling lonely often don't have a lot of energy to seek out their own activities. So, lay out a lot of options, focusing on those you know will be most appealing, and allow your child to choose one.

Know your child's style. Kids relate to groups in two ways. Some prefer one-on-one relationships that build into groups. Others feel most comfortable joining a group and from there developing individual friendships, says Dr. Savikas. Get to know your child's style and work within it. Don't, for example, sign your daughter up for softball when she knows no one else on the team and doesn't relate well to groups. Instead, encourage her to join with a friend. By the same token, get your child involved in group activities if he is awkward at meeting new friends on his own and feels more secure in a group setting.

Limit isolating activities. Kids who spend hours after school playing computer games or watching TV can become socially isolated. "TV is fine if it's a family event, and video games if they're interactive," says Dr. Savikas. But you should restrict the amount of time your kids spend doing those things alone, she advises. Keep TV viewing and computer game playing down to about an hour per day, and then encourage your child to participate in more social pastimes.

Consider peer counseling. When your child has lots of trouble fitting in, you should ask the school to include him in a peer-counseling class. Offered by many school districts nationwide, peer-counseling programs enable students—under the guidance and supervision of a teacher—to counsel each other. "These classes help students explore why problems are happening, with the people they are having problems with," says Dr. Savikas.

Be there. "There are many reasons why kids are lonely these days, but a major reason is that their parents aren't available," says Byron Egeland, Ph.D., professor of child development at the Institute of Child Development at the University of Minnesota in Minneapolis. Working parents and single parents often have no energy left at the end of the day to devote to their children. If you feel that this is a problem in your family, what should you do? "Make your kids your top priority, no matter what," suggests Dr. Egeland. "Kids need attention and nurturance from their parents, and there is no substitute." In fact, he says, young children need close contact with their parents for a variety of reasons, including the development of self-control—an essential trait, since kids who lack it often behave in a way that alienates others.

For Young Children

In the preschool and elementary years, your children are developing rudimentary social skills. If they are friendless, it may be because they are shy, or bossy, or alienate their peers for other reasons. Your guidance can go a long way toward helping them. Here's how.

Be a role model. A young child who lacks the social skills to make friends can benefit from your example. So, extend yourself, advises Dr. Savikas. Get to know the parents of other children his age and invite them over. Not only will that allow your child to witness firsthand how you make friends, it will also provide him with a playmate.

Role-play. If your youngster routinely turns friends off because he doesn't share well or play nicely, you can better his social skills through role-play. Practice sharing, taking turns, and compromising. Elementary-age children who are shy may need assistance initiating a conversation. Give them some tips and let them practice asking you questions about yourself, as if they were getting to know you.

Treat attention deficit disorder (ADD). Kids with ADD are prone to impulsive behavior and often have difficulty taking turns. This can alienate other children, says Lowery. (See the symptoms for ADD in "Attention Deficit/Hyperactivity Disorder: What to Look For" on page 36.) If you believe that your child may have ADD, ask the guidance counselor for a referral to a mental health professional who can diagnose this condition and recommend treatment, either through behavioral strategies or medication.

For Adolescents and Teens

Even a child who was well-integrated in elementary school may begin to feel lonely in the middle school and high school years. Reasons vary. Kids who can't keep up with the academic demands of these grades may believe that they are different from their peers, and that leads to feelings of loneliness, says Dr. Rea. In fact, teens tend to feel lonely or rejected anytime they are different. As a parent, you can play a vital role in keeping your kids connected, and it's crucial that you do so, because teens who become alienated or depressed are at risk for suicide. (For more information, see "Suicide Watch.") Lonely teens may also turn to drugs and alcohol as a quick ticket to fit into a group, explains Lowery. Here are some ways you can keep your teens from turning loneliness into tragedy.

Seek support groups. If your child is gay, he is likely to feel very alienated. You can help him by being available for him, seeking counseling if you need it, and finding him support groups. Similarly, gifted children can be as mentally distant from their peers as mentally retarded children are. Having your gifted child placed in a gifted program can diminish his sense of isolation, says Lowery.

Find a place where they can fit in. "Some kids feel set apart because

Suicide Watch

Suicide is the third leading cause of death among U.S. teens. If your child is lonely and depressed, he could be at risk. According to the National Institute of Mental Health and the American Academy of Child and Adolescent Psychiatry, a child who has suicidal feelings will exhibit many of the same symptoms associated with depression. He may also become violent and rebellious, exhibit a marked personality change, begin using drugs or alcohol, and grow intolerant of praise.

Your teen could be planning to commit suicide if he:

- Complains of being a bad person

- Says things like "Nothing matters" or "I won't be around much longer"

- Becomes suddenly cheerful after a period of depression

- Has bizarre thoughts or hallucinations, indicating psychosis

Most communities have 24-hour crisis counseling networks for people in danger of suicide. Check your yellow pages for local suicide hotlines, or ask your school guidance counselor or physician for a referral.

---

they are different," says Dr. Rea. "Find things that interest them." If your daughter likes to write, see the guidance counselor about having her work on the school newspaper. There, she'll meet peers with a similar interest, and she won't feel so isolated.

Some kids can also benefit from the camaraderie they encounter from a part-time job, Lowery says. She counseled one gifted student who had difficulty making friends after he transferred to a new high school. He enjoyed biking, so he got a job at a bike shop and discovered a whole new avenue for making friends.

Go one-on-one. Once a week, do something alone with your teen, recommends Dr. Rea. Take him to breakfast, or play a game of miniature golf together. "When they act as if they don't want you around, be there anyway," she says. If you remain well-connected with your teen, you'll be better able to read the signals when he's lonely and to keep him from becoming alienated.

Chauffeur him to karate classes. A teen who is lonely, different, and lacks confidence may benefit from a self-defense class, such as karate or tae kwon do. There, he'll gain the skills he needs to help build confidence, says Dr. Rea.

Mother your child's friends. Your son is rejected by many of his peers at school, so he starts hanging around with a crowd you don't like. What can you do? If you try to cut him off from his friends, he'll find sneaky ways to be with them. Instead, Dr. Rea suggests that you invite those kids over so often that they start seeing you as their second mom. That way, you're not only supervising their activity, you're developing a relationship with them that can, ideally, be beneficial. "These are all kids who are looking for a home and a family. Start parenting them in a way they are not getting at home," says Dr. Rea.

Let others know. The two boys responsible for the tragedy at Columbine High School in Littleton, Colorado, were angry, alienated youths. Kids who become alienated and isolated can lose their abilities to stay grounded in reality, explains Dr. Rea. What's more, alienation is usually accompanied by deep-seated anger, creating a potential for violence. If you are worried that your child is becoming alienated, seek help. Ask your guidance counselor or physician for a local mental health agency where your teen can get counseling. But don't stop there. "Let a lot of people know you've got a kid in trouble so people can reach out and shelter this child and protect him from himself," says Dr. Rea. Family members, close friends, clergy, and teachers can all act as resources to help your child.

Night Terrors
and Nightmares

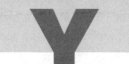

ou're awakened by a blood-curdling scream. You race to your child's room to find her sitting bolt upright in bed, howling, her eyes wide open and filled with terror. You call her name, but she stares right through you, as if you weren't there. She may begin thrashing and striking out. She may even try to get out of bed. Then as suddenly as it began, the "spell" is over, and she's sound asleep.

"Most parents who witness this say that the child looks like she's possessed," says Barbara Howard, M.D., assistant clinical professor of pediatrics at Duke University Medical Center in Durham, North Carolina. "But there's a perfectly rational explanation. The child is experiencing a night terror."

Though night terrors may sound like something that requires professional help, they are actually normal and fairly common in children. Experts say that they occur during the deepest part of the sleep cycle, about an hour or two after the child falls asleep.

"Normally, this is the point where the child cycles into a lighter sleep where dreams occur," says Ronald Dahl, M.D., associate professor of psychiatry and pediatrics at the University of Pittsburgh Medical Center and director of the Children's Sleep Evaluation Center at Western Psychiatric Institute and Clinic, both in Pittsburgh. "But particularly if the child is very tired, a split may occur. Part of the system says that it's time to go into light sleep, but another part says, 'No, I'm still tired.' So part of the brain stays deeply asleep while another part goes into a high-arousal state."

The child who is having a night terror is not awake, yet not quite asleep, notes Dr. Dahl. And the "terror" aspect of this phenomenon really only registers on the parents. The child herself is not conscious, nor does she remember playing out this scene from *The Exorcist* the next day, says Dr. Dahl.

Nightmares, on the other hand, are very frightening for children. "A nightmare is essentially a dream that is sufficiently scary to wake a child up," says Dr. Dahl. "In fact, the child may wake up quickly, become fully awake, and have trouble getting back to sleep. She may be a little confused, but she'll probably be coherent. A nightmare is likely to occur late in the night or early in the morning, in the second half of the sleep period."

Both night terrors and nightmares tend to run their course and disappear over time. But there are a few techniques that you can use to make things easier for your child.

Coping with Night Terrors

Stay calm. "Remind yourself that although a night terror looks scary, it's not a seizure. It's not a terrible thing," says Dr. Dahl. "Night terrors are very common and normal, especially in kids between the ages of 3 and 5."

Stand by until it's over. Though it may be difficult to watch your child screaming, there's really nothing you can do to stop a night terror, says Dr. Howard. "But you can make sure that the child is safe when it's happening by restraining her if necessary. Children do sometimes hurt themselves thrashing or running around. And it's almost impossible to wake them."

Don't mention it. "Don't talk to your child about the episode the next morning," says Dr. Howard. "And don't let siblings talk to her about it either. Kids don't remember night terrors. But if they find out later what they did, they may get upset about being out of control."

Try a preventive wake-up call. "If your child is experiencing terrors, you could try waking her up about 30 minutes after she goes to bed and then letting her go back to sleep," says Dr. Howard. "That breaks up the sleep cycle and tends to interrupt the pattern of the night terrors."

Make sure your child is getting enough sleep. "Increase the total amount of sleep your child is getting," suggests Dr. Dahl. "If she's fairly young, it might mean letting her go back to taking daily naps. For an older kid, try letting her sleep longer in the morning or put her to bed a little earlier."

How to Stop a Sleepwalker

Sleepwalking, like night terrors, usually happens when a child is in transition from very deep sleep to light, dreaming sleep, says Ronald Dahl, M.D., associate professor of psychiatry and pediatrics at the University of Pittsburgh Medical Center and director of the Children's Sleep Evaluation Center at Western Psychiatric Institute and Clinic, both in Pittsburgh.

"This is a very difficult transition for young children to make, and they often do strange things, like sleepwalking or talking in their sleep," says Dr. Dahl. If you have a sleepwalker, safety is the primary concern. Here's what the experts recommend that you do.

Wake the child up. "You can often wake a child up from sleepwalking and guide her back to bed," says Barbara Howard, M.D., assistant clinical professor of pediatrics at Duke University Medical Center in Durham, North Carolina.

Increase sleep time. "Being overtired is a major factor in sleepwalking," notes Dr. Dahl. "Ninety-nine percent of children experiencing these partial arousals do better after increasing the total amount of sleep."

Install a gate. "Install a portable folding gate or a screen door to block the doorway so she can't get out," suggests Dr. Howard. "These are better than locking the door, and you can hear her if she gets up." You should also place a gate across any stairway.

Change bed arrangements. "If your child is sleeping in a bunk bed, make sure you take her off the top bunk," says Dr. Dahl.

The reason for this, Dr. Dahl explains, is that the more tired a child is, the more difficult it will be for her to switch from deep sleep to light sleep. "The classic time for night terrors to occur is when young children first give up their daily naps," he says. "The first time a kid stays up for 12 hours or more, there's more pressure on her sleep system than she's ever had, and it drives her deeply into sleep, deeper than she's ever been. At the end of that first deep sleep cycle is when she's most likely to have a night terror."

Think happy thoughts. "If kids are worried, anxious, or a little bit more fearful than usual as they fall asleep, they're more likely to have these events," says Dr. Dahl. "Ask your child if anything's worrying her just before she falls asleep. Often a child who is well-behaved but shy and inhibited by temperament will get into the habit of lying in bed and worrying.

"Helping the child establish a positive routine at bedtime can reverse that," he says. "Have her focus on positive thoughts about the good things that have happened to her that day. Help her feel safe and secure. That seems to cut down on night terrors."

Talk over fears during the day. "Help your child express her worries and fears during the day rather than letting them surface at night," says Dr. Dahl. "Often a child who gets night terrors has a small, specific, but irrational fear that's worrying him. As soon as she expresses her fear and understands that it's not worth worrying over, the night terrors go away."

Don't make it a habit. "Be careful to avoid what's called secondary gain, which means the child gets some benefit from having had a night terror," says Dr. Howard. "Even though the night terror was unintentional, if the child wakes up and finds the parent there, concerned about her and giving her a lot of attention, it can seem like a reward. That can reinforce and perpetuate the problem. So it's important not to coddle the child too much by waking her and giving her something to eat or drink, for instance."

Dealing with Nightmares

Turn on the light. If a child wakes up with a nightmare and comes running to your room, be prepared to listen and find out why the child is afraid.

"Most kids want their parents around," says Dr. Dahl. "Some don't need much more than your reassurance that everything is all right." But sometimes, you may have to go back to the child's room, turn on the light, and show her there's nothing there. "The child really needs to spend more time with you until she winds down," he says.

Break the rules now and then. Your child may want to spend the rest of the night in your bed, even if it's not usually allowed. "It's okay to occasionally break the rules if the child is badly frightened," says Dr. Dahl, "though you may have to nip that behavior in the bud before it becomes a bad habit. Most kids will go back to their beds without protest the next night if you remind them of the rule."

Give the child a nightmare protector. A flashlight or a "protective" stuffed animal can be very soothing to a child plagued by nightmares, says Sheila Ribordy, Ph.D., professor of psychology and director of clinical training in the department of psychology at DePaul University in Chicago and a clinical psychologist specializing in treating children and families.

"For a child, it's important to feel she has some control over her nightmares," she says. "Children need to have a sense that they are powerful people so things aren't so scary for them."

Have a bedside chat. "If a child is having a lot of nightmares, you may need to help her relieve some of the stress that comes up during the day," says Dr. Howard. "Children these days are under enormous stress. Often they're watching violent movies or TV programs. Sometimes they're subjected to a bully at school or at day care. Or they're being asked to toilet train or deal with a new sibling or give up their room." Since these stresses can lead to nightmares, it helps if you can talk to your child about what's happened during the day, according to Dr. Howard.

Follow a calming bedtime routine. "Your child's experience at bedtime should be a calming one," says Dr. Howard. She suggests including a story, a song, or cuddly animals in the routine.

Children who are having nightmares may develop a fear of falling asleep, and a bedtime routine that includes books or music can help. "Playing music or story tapes gives them something to focus on other than the fear of nightmares that might be coming," says Dr. Ribordy. "Often these activities are distracting enough to help them fall asleep easily."

Overweight

What if you knew your child had a disease that would cut short his life or make him suffer from heart and breathing problems, diabetes, and back pain? Of course, you would do anything you could to prevent this disease.

What people are slow in realizing is that America's youth is in the midst of an unrecognized epidemic of such a disease: the "disease" of obesity. A nationwide study shows that one in every five children between the ages of 6 and 17 is already overweight or at risk of becoming obese. Obesity is a stepping-stone to diabetes, high blood pressure, heart disease, sleep difficulties, and bone and joint problems.

Besides the serious physical consequences of being too heavy, being overweight can be emotionally painful, stresses Hilda M. Ramos, a social worker who works with overweight kids at Mount Sinai Hospital in Chicago. "The younger kids are preoccupied with other things, but as they get older, it becomes very sad. These kids become very, very depressed."

But What Is "Normal" and What Is "Overweight"?

This is a very tough question, and the experts don't all agree. Here are some of the most common ways of determining whether a child is overweight.

Height and weight charts. Most pediatricians will track your child's growth on a chart that accounts for natural development in a growing child and compares that pattern to other children of the same age. If your child is in the 20th percentile for height but the 95th percentile for weight, it means that among 100 children, only 19 would be shorter than he is but 94 would be thinner. Such a disparity over time would indicate that the child is overweight.

Body mass index (BMI). This measurement has been used more and more in recent years to determine whether someone is overweight. It's based on a formula that compares your child's height and weight to the national norms. For every height there is a corresponding weight and BMI. Different people that are the same height will weigh more or less and thus have a higher or lower BMI. Generally, the higher your BMI, the more likely you are to be overweight.

To calculate your child's BMI, you'll need to do a little bit of math. First, multiply your child's weight in pounds by 705. Assuming your child weighs 100 pounds, 705 multiplied by 100 is 70,500. Then measure your child's height in inches. Let's assume that your child is 52 inches tall. Multiply that number by itself (52×52). You get 2,704. Then divide the weight sum (70,500) by the height sum (2,704). The result, 26, is your child's BMI. If it's slightly between 25 and 30, then some doctors would consider your child to be overweight.

If you're not too mathematically inclined, certain Web sites will automatically figure out your child's BMI for you. To find one, go to an Internet search engine and type "calculate" and "BMI" in the Search box.

Skinfold measurements. Mostly used in research studies, this method involves using a tool to see how much skin can be pinched from key areas of the body, such as the upper arm.

Visual signs of obesity. Sometimes your kid's physical appearance is enough to make the diagnosis. Gwendolyn Wright, M.D., a pediatrician at Mount Sinai Hospital in Chicago, tells parents to look at their children's bellies. Does the area around the navel look fat? "If so, the child is fat," she says.

Medical warning signs. Children and teens who are overweight may already have high blood cholesterol levels and blood pressure—meaning, they are at risk for heart disease. They may already have the form of diabetes that used to be seen only in obese adults. Other weight-related health problems that kids may have include bowing of their legs, or other orthopedic problems, and sleep apnea.

The bottom line is that there is no one absolute way to tell whether your child is overweight. The best advice is to listen to your doctor, who is trained to evaluate all of the evidence and advise you whether your child needs to stop gaining weight so quickly or even lose some pounds.

Food for Thought

As soon as you realize that your child is overweight, you can begin to help. The first step is to rethink menu choices, not only for your child but also for your whole family.

Don't rush it. Weight control is a lifetime effort built on small changes in the diet that can be adopted over time. "Fad diets don't work," insists Dr. Wright. She encourages healthy eating instead of dieting, aiming at a weight loss of no more than ½ to 1 pound a week.

Start the day right. Don't serve meat at breakfast. Instead, make oatmeal, whole wheat toast, and nonsweetened cereals the cornerstones of the morning meal. Include juicy, vitamin-rich fruits as well.

Make dinner a family affair. A recent study from Harvard Medical School found that adolescents who regularly eat dinner with their families have healthier eating habits. They are more likely to eat more servings of fruits and vegetables each day, get important nutrients, and eat less sugar and fat.

Pack the lunch. Even though it's nice when preteens and teens take over the lunch-making chore, they aren't necessarily mature enough to make sensible decisions about what to put in the bag. Reclaim the job yourself, tucking in a healthy sandwich on whole grain bread, several pieces of fruit, vegetable sticks (celery, carrots, bell peppers), and water or 100 percent juice.

Stick to the menu. "Parents should be in charge of what food is offered. If your kids don't eat it, that's okay. But they should not be given something else instead," advises William H. Dietz, M.D., Ph.D., a pediatrician and director of the division of nutrition and physical therapy at the Centers for Disease Control and Prevention in Atlanta. Too often, parents worry that their kids haven't eaten enough at a meal, so they allow them to eat chips or other high-fat, low-nutrition foods instead.

Be master of the fridge. "Let's face it, teenagers want it easy," says Ramos. "When they come home from school, they're hungry. Whatever they see first in the fridge is what they're going to eat." Your job is to be the controller of the refrigerator, stocking it with what you'd like them to eat (fresh fruits and vegetables, diet sodas, and so forth), so they don't duck out the door for the nearest convenience store and its enticing pastries and candy bars.

Give them water. It's too bad water doesn't have the same cool advertising campaigns as soda and juice, which are filled with calories and not much nutrition. Remember, clear sodas are just as sugary as dark colas, unless they're diet sodas. So serve eight glasses of water a day instead. You'll save money while you save calories.

Celebrate salsa. Rich in antioxidants, brimming in flavor, salsas of all kinds are natural health foods. Spoon salsas over potatoes instead of butter and sour cream. Use them to smother lean cuts of grilled meat. Dip into them with homemade, low-fat chips made from tortillas sparingly brushed with oil and baked.

Lighten up your dairy ingredients. Serve your teens skim or 1% milk, not whole milk. In recipes, substitute fat-free half-and-half for heavy cream. Use fat-free sour cream for the fat-laden regular version. (No one will be able to tell the difference!) And switch to fat-free sweetened condensed milk instead of the regular kind for making rich-tasting flan and other desserts without the heavy calorie load.

Gobble up turkey. Substitute poultry for high-fat cuts of meat: turkey sausage for pork sausage, ground chicken or turkey for ground beef. But be a careful label reader: Some ground turkey breast is even higher in fat than beef. Go for the package with the lowest total fat.

Trim your chicken. Dark meat and chicken skin are where the fat lurks, so make your chicken dishes from skinless breasts. As with beef, you should cut off all visible fat before preparing your dish.

How to Get Them Moving

Exercise, like healthy eating, needs to be a family affair. Think about ways to enhance your daily life by doing something physical rather than sitting around. Here are some ideas to get you started.

Leave the car at home. Walking your children to school or doing nearby errands as part of a family walk can make exercise a part of your everyday life, providing benefits for you as well as your overweight child. For teenagers, don't be a full-time chauffeur. Encourage them to walk to friends' houses, the mall, or school. Or help them save up money to buy a bicycle.

Teach by example. If you spend 1 to 2 hours a day engaged in some kind of physical activity (walking, bicycling, gardening, playing outdoor games with your kids), your child will follow your lead.

Get to know the "off" button on your TV. Dr. Wright says that studies prove a direct correlation between weight in kids and how much TV they watch. Limit television watching gradually at first, perhaps to 1 to 2 hours a day. You may want to make a deal with your kids: an hour of TV in exchange for an hour of activity, whether that means walking, playing basketball with friends, or inline skating.

Make summers count. Steer your teen toward an active summer job as a camp counselor or a worker for the local parks and recreation department. He'll get valuable experience and references. It'll be more fun than working behind the counter of an ice cream store—and less tempting, too.

Tap into community fitness programs. In the wintertime, check out local YMCA or Boys and Girls Club activities. These centers often offer swimming, martial arts classes, volleyball, basketball, and other activities in a safe, supervised environment. No one is turned away because they can't pay.

Consider sports. Some kids enjoy participating in after-school sports programs or organized athletics, such as soccer. If your child enjoys being part of a team, by all means register him. But Dr. Dietz cautions against forcing unenthusiastic children to be involved in organized sports, where gifted athletes soon dominate the playing field while other children sit on the bench.

Suggest salsa . . . or swing. Swing, salsa, and merengue dancing are enormously popular among teenagers and provide social interaction as well as healthy fun. Check out local classes through the YMCA, the parks and recreation department, and your local school. Many schools have dance clubs that meet after school.

Support Strategies

Overweight children often suffer from low self-esteem. They may be subjected to teasing by their classmates. Worst of all, they may begin to think of themselves only in terms of their weight, forgetting their positive qualities. Ramos offers these tips on how to be supportive of an overweight adolescent.

Take it seriously. Don't dismiss your child when he expresses concern about weight. "Listen. Try to understand," advises Ramos. But if a physician agrees that the child is overweight, be supportive and try to help the adolescent eat healthy, nutritious meals and get more exercise.

Don't reward with food. If your adolescent makes you proud, say so. Set a time to spend special time with him, shopping or going for a walk. Or reward him with extra privileges.

Be adaptable. When your son or daughter pushes aside your lasagna in favor of a slice of whole grain bread and a salad, remember that it's the food that's being rejected, not you. Remind yourself that keeping your child healthy is the most important thing you can do as a mother.

Ask for help. As you gradually shift the family toward healthier eating patterns, include your teenager in meal planning, grocery shopping, and preparation. Your efforts will convey your commitment to helping your child lose weight, and the time spent together will enrich your relationship. "Bring the family together in the kitchen," urges Ramos. "When everybody's busy doing something, kids will open up and talk."

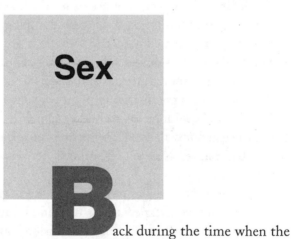

Sex

Back during the time when the Monica Lewinsky scandal erupted, parents all over the country found themselves scrambling for answers to their kids' questions about the affair. Psychologist Ana Nogales, Ph.D., didn't want to keep her daughters, Gabriela, 13, and Natalie, 10, in the dark. So she sat them down for a frank discussion.

"I told them there are many levels of sex and that it's a way adults communicate with their bodies in a very intimate relationship," recalls Dr. Nogales, founder of Nogales Psychological Group in Los Angeles and author of *Dr. Ana Nogales' Book of Love, Sex, and Relationships*. She gradually led into the fact that sex is pleasurable, and there are various ways of experiencing that pleasure. And when she got to the nitty-gritty, her kids laughed and said, "Eeew!" She laughed with them.

Talking to kids about sex may be the most dreaded task in all of parenthood, but experts agree that it has to be done. How else will they learn about the birds and the bees? School sex education classes are generally sparse on details, says Dr. Nogales. And information gathered from friends or popular media is likely to be dubious at best. So, if you want to make sure that your kids have access to the right information about sex, the job of telling them falls on you.

Tips for "The Talk"

This is, of course, easier said than done, and it's difficult to know where to begin. Some experts suggest educating kids about sex from a very early age, but what do you do if you haven't discussed this topic and are broaching it with your adolescents for the first time? "Start with your own feelings and limitations," suggests Dr. Nogales. "Tell them, 'I always felt so embarrassed to talk to you about sex, but now I want to do it, and I'm willing to do it.' When we talk about our own limitations, our children will appreciate that and understand."

Principles are a good starting point for your talk, says Dr. Nogales. When she spoke with her own children about the Monica Lewinsky affair, she began not with details, but with principles. Let them know right off the bat that sex is an act of intimacy between two people who love each other.

Other important topics to discuss in the beginning of the talk are your values and your expectations of your children. What values you choose to relate will be a personal decision, but don't limit yourself to blanket statements that promote virginity and oppose premarital sex, says Dr. Nogales. "Teach them about respecting themselves and their bodies," she recommends. Responsibility is another value you should address. Advise your children that sharing their bodies must be a responsible decision that can only be made after they've shared all other aspects of a relationship, such as ideals, philosophies, and thoughts.

After this, the next step would logically be the anatomical basics. Since you obviously have kids, you shouldn't have a lot of trouble with this part. But there are other, more complicated issues you need to dis-

Some Common Myths

I n the absence of adequate information about contraception, teens may fall prey to "You can't get pregnant if . . ." folklore. Here are a few myths you should warn your teen about.

You can't get pregnant if . . .

- *. . . you have intercourse during your period.* It is rare for women to conceive while they're menstruating, but not impossible, according to psychiatrist E. James Lieberman, M.D., clinical professor at the George Washington University School of Medicine in Washington, D.C.

- *. . . you have sex for the first time.* That's simply not true. Women who use no contraception can and do become pregnant the first time they have intercourse.

- *. . . you haven't had your first period.* Since you are fertile 2 weeks before your first period, you could become pregnant if you have unprotected intercourse.

- *. . . you jump up and down after sex.* This offers no protection.

- *. . . neither of you has an orgasm.* Even if a small amount of semen leaks out of the penis, the sperm, once in the vagina, can enter the uterus and fertilize an egg.

- *. . . you douche with soda immediately after intercourse.* Douching with soda involves shaking up a bottle of carbonated cola and allowing it to shoot up into the vagina. While this may not be harmful, it, like other douches, does not protect against pregnancy.

cuss, like contraception and disease, and for this you may need some extra information. To help you, this chapter covers each of these topics, first explaining why it is so critical to talk with your children about sex, then giving you the basics so you can give them accurate, practical information from the pros.

Pregnancy and Contraception

The first thing to recognize is the obvious: Sex can lead to teen pregnancy, and many teens are sexually active. By the time they are 17, more than half of all American teenagers have had sex, with 16 being the average age of first intercourse for girls, and 17 for boys. Given this, it's not surprising that the United States has the highest teenage pregnancy rate of all the developed countries.

The best way to stop pregnancy, besides abstinence, of course, is contraception. You may feel, however, that talking to your kids about contraception will encourage them to have sex, and so you may feel inclined to avoid that topic. But that's a mistake, say experts like Debra W. Haffner, president and chief executive officer of the Sexuality Information and Education Council of the United States in New York City and author of *From Diapers to Dating: A Parent's Guide to Raising Sexually Healthy Children*. "It's important that your children know your values about premarital sex," she acknowledges. "But if they're not going to listen to you, they need to know how to protect themselves from pregnancy and how to protect their lives."

Contraception Basics

So let's assume that you're taking the plunge with this theme. One of the first things that you should keep in mind is that while there are many contraceptives on the market, not all are recommended for teens. Teenagers generally fare better with methods that require the least personal compliance, says Maura Quinlan, M.D., associate professor in the department of obstetrics and gynecology at Emory University School of Medicine and medical director at Grady Teen Clinic, both in Atlanta. For space reasons, this chapter does not give all of the varied methods for contraception. Instead, it focuses on the birth control methods commonly used by teens so that you can discuss them with your children.

Some family planning clinics and county health departments provide these at low cost, or they may even be free to qualifying low-income families.

Male Condoms

- Description: A thin sheath, usually of latex, placed over the penis during intercourse to prevent the sperm from entering the vagina. Condoms are readily available in supermarkets and drugstores. Latex condoms, when used correctly, provide protection against sexually transmitted diseases and therefore should be used even when other methods are in place.

- Estimated effectiveness: 86 percent. They are more effective when used in conjunction with spermicides.

Oral Contraceptives

- Description: Pills containing a combination of estrogen and progesterone to suppress ovulation. Skipping pills sharply decreases their effectiveness. Nevertheless, they are the most popular method among teens, and they offer other benefits, such as regulating periods. Side effects could include nausea, changes in menstruation, weight gain, and, very rarely, high blood pressure, blood clots, and stroke. Available by prescription only. A pelvic exam is needed to get a prescription, but many clinics don't require them immediately for young teens.

- Estimated effectiveness: over 95 percent

Depo-Provera

- Description: One of the most ideal methods for teens, because it requires no daily compliance. It consists of an injection of progesterone that must be given by a health professional every 3 months. Users may experience irregular bleeding at first. After several months, periods will stop completely.

- Estimated effectiveness: over 99 percent

Emergency Contraception

- Description: High-dose birth control pills. It is appropriate to take only in cases of an emergency, such as when a condom breaks or when, for some reason, no contraception was used, explains Dr. Quinlan. It won't affect an established pregnancy and must be given within 72 hours of unprotected sex in order to prevent a pregnancy. It is taken in two doses and is available by prescription only. May cause nausea and vomiting. Teens can call the toll-free emergency hotline number (888) NOT2LAT to find a doctor or clinic that will provide it.

- Effectiveness: 75 percent

Sexually Transmitted Diseases and Your Kids

Besides pregnancy, the other big concern with regard to discussing sex with kids is disease. Approximately 3 million teens contract sexually transmitted diseases (STDs) in this country every year. Those diseases include, among other things, HIV, which has become the sixth leading cause of death among young people ages 15 to 24.

Sexually transmitted diseases can lead to cervical cancer, infertility, and even death. Inform your teens about the dangers of three STDs most common among young people: chlamydia, human papillomavirus (HPV), and human immunodeficiency virus (HIV), recommends David Celentano, M.D., professor of epidemiology at Johns Hopkins University School of Public Health in Baltimore.

Chlamydia. An estimated 4 million people are infected with chlamydia each year, primarily adolescents and young adults. About 75 percent have few or no symptoms. Untreated, chlamydia can lead to pelvic inflammatory disease in women, potentially causing chronic pain or permanent damage to the reproductive organs. It can be effectively treated with prescription drugs.

HPV. This disease may cause genital warts but often has no noticeable symptoms. In women, it can lead to the development of cervical cancer, which is responsible for 4,500 deaths each year. HPV often resolves itself, but if it progresses, surgical treatments can be used to eradicate affected cells.

HIV. Most people with HIV, which causes AIDS, are between the ages of 25 and 40. Nevertheless, it's still a concern for teens. "We don't generally know when people become infected," notes Dr. Celentano. "Presumably most 25-year-olds with HIV were infected as teens."

How to Protect Your Children

Keep pushing the condom message. What's the most important thing to tell your child about prevention of STDs? "Condoms, condoms, condoms," says Dr. Celentano. "Parents need to teach kids that sex is having intercourse with a condom every time." This lesson you teach your kids can make a big difference. One study of 372 sexually active adolescents ages 14 to 17 found that teens who had discussed condom use with their mothers before their first sexual encounters were three times more likely to use condoms than those who hadn't.

To protect against STDs, only latex condoms are effective. And while little research has been done on female condoms, they are generally considered safe as well.

Tell them to beware of so-called safe sex acts. Many people believe that they can't become infected with HIV through oral sex. Now, research suggests that's not true, says Dr. Celentano. While oral sex may be safer than vaginal or anal sex, it still presents a risk, and teens should be wary of engaging in oral sex with anyone whose sexual history is unknown.

Explain about avoiding multiple partners. Teens often place themselves at greater risk for STDs because they tend to switch sexual partners. Let your teens know that the more partners they have, the greater their chances of contracting a disease.

Parenting Strategies

Okay, let's say the big talk (or talks) is over. As we're sure you well know, just talking is not going to do the trick. Here are some strategies that you should keep in mind to help your kids forestall early sexual involvement.

Don't leave 'em alone. "I think most teenagers get pregnant between the hours of 3:00 and 5:00 in the afternoon," says Dr. Nogales. She encourages working moms to find ways to ensure that their adolescents are

properly supervised. Involve your teen in district-run after-school programs. If none are available, band together with other parents to create
your own programs. Parents who work part-time or varying shifts can
take turns hosting after-school homework sessions or cooking classes.

Maintain curfews. Curfews have a dual purpose, says psychiatrist E.
James Lieberman, M.D., clinical professor at the George Washington
University School of Medicine in Washington, D.C., and coauthor of
Like It Is: A Teen Sex Guide. They teach children responsibility, and they
limit the amount of time kids spend at night with friends—or with a
girlfriend or boyfriend. A good rule of thumb is to start with a relatively
early curfew, say 9:30 or 10:00 P.M. "The way they earn a later curfew is
to keep an earlier curfew," Dr. Lieberman suggests. "A later curfew is
kind of a reward for responsible behavior." Make the curfew earlier
whenever your adolescent comes home late or behaves irresponsibly.

Set out the welcome mat. Get to know your child's friends. Invite
them over, even put yourself out a bit, recommends Dr. Lieberman.
That way, you can keep a good handle on who your child's influences
are. But beware: If you openly disapprove of your teen's friends, you'll
invite rebellion. If you fear a friend could be a bad influence, talk to your
teen about peer pressure and specific safety issues, like wearing seat belts
and not drinking and driving—as well as alcohol, drugs, and sex.

Set some house rules. "Don't bring your boyfriend/girlfriend into
the bedroom" is a wise rule to institute, recommends Dr. Nogales. You
can give teens space to be alone together, she says, but make it clear that
a bedroom is a private place and that the family room or backyard is
more appropriate. Another good rule: Don't permit your children to en-
tertain friends when you or your spouse isn't home.

Be firm but not strict. Parents who institute a number of strict rules
send their children a message they'll read as "You don't know how to
make your own decisions. You're dumb. You will just go out and make
the wrong decisions," says Dr. Nogales. All too often, children take that
message to heart and do make unwise decisions. For example, if parents forbid a young teen to date until he is 16, the child is likely to do
it behind the parents' back and possibly make some poor decisions
about sex. "We need to teach our children to think for themselves," Dr.
Nogales says.

Sibling Rivalry

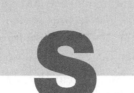

So, your kids don't exactly get along like the Waltons. Okay, so they get along more like the World Wrestling Federation. This is normal, right?

Wrong. Although parents can't necessarily recreate the warm, fuzzy feelings the siblings on Walton's Mountain had for each other, there are certainly many ways to avoid full-scale warfare among brothers and sisters. "You can easily make their interaction a better experience by what you do," says child and family psychologist Barry Ginsberg, Ph.D., executive director of the Center of Relationship Enhancement in Doylestown, Pennsylvania.

"There are no easy answers, but it's important to remember that some conflict can be constructive—provided it doesn't get out of hand," says Dr. Ginsberg. "Stresses and fights occur because that's how we negotiate a new, more stable level of relationship. But kids tend to be clumsy at this, and so they need their parents' help."

Here are a few ways to maintain the peace in your household.

Set clear limits. You may not be able to stop your children from arguing, but you can keep disagreements from escalating into brawls, says James Bozigar, a licensed social worker and coordinator of community relations for the Family Intervention Center at Children's Hospital of Pittsburgh. "Make it clear that hitting and the behaviors that often provoke it—name calling, taunting, attacking personal weaknesses—are off limits," he says. "You can say, 'You don't have to love your baby sister, you don't even have to like her, but you must stop hitting her.'"

Call a family powwow. If you're trying to establish new guidelines for behavior, it's better if the siblings themselves play a role in figuring out what those guidelines would be, says Adele Faber, coauthor of *Siblings without Rivalry*. Faber, who conducts nationwide workshops on sibling relationships, recommends calling a family meeting to do just that.

"Open the floor to discussion," she says. "When it's a rule the child has helped fashion, he'll want to try to make it work. But if it's a rule imposed from on high, he'll be more likely to test or challenge it."

Reinforce the family's new guidelines. If the rule is "no hitting," the disciplinary action for infractions should be a time-out, says Mark Roberts, Ph.D., professor of psychology at Idaho State University in Pocatello. Dr. Roberts and his colleagues have studied which techniques are most effective in stopping sibling aggression. "Calling a time-out wins hands down," he says. "When the kids begin to fight, parents should say, 'No hitting in this house. *You* sit on this chair, and *you* sit on that chair.' The chairs should be up against walls and around the corner from each other so the kids can't see each other. Wait 2 to 5 minutes, then talk with the kids about their argument. They will probably have cooled off, so this is a good time to discuss alternatives to fighting."

Substitute words for fists. Brothers and sisters who fight often don't know how to share, take turns, consider others' feelings, or negotiate— all skills they're going to need to form relationships outside the home, says Faber. "So one of the rules that is especially helpful is, 'Say it with words, not with fists,'" she says. By using language to express their anger, siblings take the first step on the road to mutually respectful relationships.

Says Faber: "The sweetest thing I heard was from a mother who had tried this method. She called me and said, 'I passed by the kids' room today and saw my older child with his fists raised about to clobber his younger sister. She looked up at him and said, "Michael, use your words." He stopped, with his fists in midair, and said, "Get out of my room!" She said, "I'm going." I was so pleased.' I told that mother, 'Now, *that's* civilized behavior.'"

Don't ask who started it. The usual response to the question, "Who started it?" is a two-parter: "He did." "No, she did." But you don't want to play judge or jury, says Faber. "You won't get to the bottom of it. The bottom is bound to be murky. Often you'll hear, 'I had to hit him because I could tell he was about to hit me.' It's better to say, 'Boy, you two sound angry at each other.'" That statement diminishes rage and provides an opening for a discussion of the children's real grievances. "So, Adam, you're upset because you want to watch TV. And, Jim, you're upset because you need quiet to study. What can be done in a case like this?"

Reflect feelings back to the child. Very few kids are really happy about sharing their parents' love and attention with someone else, even if that someone else is related to them. Negative feelings toward siblings are normal, says Faber. "It's important to allow those negative emotions to surface. Feelings that are banished don't vanish. They either go underground and get expressed in dreams, nightmares, headaches, and stomachaches, or they're acted out in punches or pinches," she says.

Faber suggests listening to your child's feelings and then reflecting them back in a way that acknowledges the child's mixed emotions about a sibling—who is, after all, both an interloper and a playmate. "A father in one of my workshops listened to his son's long list of objections to his new baby sister. Then he reflected back to the boy, 'Sounds to me as if part of you wants her out of here forever. And part of you is sometimes glad she's here.' Periodically over the next few weeks, the little boy said, 'Daddy, tell me again about my two feelings.' I think that child is well on his way to emotional health," says Faber.

Create a special time for one-to-one parenting. "When a new sibling arrives, reserve special times when you can fully commit yourself to being with the older child," says Dr. Ginsberg. "Don't allow any external events to change this. The older child needs to be confident that he will have his special time alone with the parent."

Ask the older child to give you a hand. An older sibling will feel more involved in things if you give her a simple job to do, like bringing you diapers. "This will increase the child's sense of importance and responsibility," says Dr. Ginsberg. "You can say, 'Now that we're busier with the new baby and you're older, you can have this job that will help out around the house.'" Just be sure the task is meaningful—not some busywork invented simply to make the child feel better. "That's phony, and kids can see right through it," Dr. Ginsberg says.

Look for patterns. Sometimes, sibling fights exhibit a pattern, says Dr. Ginsberg. "Once you see the pattern, you can head off clashes by structuring—that is, shaping the situation in advance for the best kind of interaction possible," he observes.

"For example, if your children always fight when they get home from school, it may very well be to get your attention," Dr. Ginsberg says. "They've been away from you all day. If you're busy in the kitchen when they get home, they may feel this is the only way to get to you." So what can you do? "You can structure things differently by preparing dinner before your kids come in, and giving *them* your time and attention," he says. "Or include them in the meal preparation process so they're there with you."

Figure out a way to say "You're special." "Children need to be seen and enjoyed as separate individuals," says Faber. "If you were to say to your husband, 'Who do you love more, your mother or me?' and he replied, 'Honey, I love you both equally,' he would be in big trouble. But if he said, 'Honey, there's no comparison. My mother is my mother and you're my beloved wife,' he'd be on safe ground."

The same policy works for kids. For example, when little Amy asks, "Who do you love best?" you can answer, "Each of my children is special. You are my only Amy. No one has your thoughts, your feelings, your smile, your way of doing things. Boy, am I lucky you are my child."

Respect sibling differences. While it may seem "fair" to give each child the same number of pancakes in the morning, this "fair" treatment doesn't recognize that each child's appetite may be different, says Faber. "If you hear, 'Hey, you gave him three pancakes and you only gave me two,' respond with, 'Oh, are you still hungry? Do you want a whole pancake or just a half? A whole? Well, one whole pancake coming up.' What you've done is shift the message from 'You are getting as much as your big brother' to 'I am meeting your individual needs.'"

Stomachache

It is six o'clock in the morning, and the faint voice heard from the bunk is apologetic: "Mommy, my tummy hurts." And maybe you think: Is it really hurting, or is it just an excuse for not going to school?

If your child is younger than 12 years old, it is almost a certainty that his stomach does hurt, says Catherine Dundon, M.D., a pediatrician in Goodlettsville, Tennessee, and mother of two children. "Children younger than 12 don't have the ability to pretend that they are sick," she says. If your child tells you that it hurts, you can assume that it does.

Many times, stomachache in children is the result of indigestion, constipation, or nervous agitation, says Dr. Dundon. If symptoms are severe, you should call the doctor promptly. If not, there are many things that you can do to take care of that tummy. Here is what physicians recommend.

Apply heat. Many children feel that heat gives them great relief when their tummy hurts, says Bruce Taubman, M.D., professor of pediatrics at the University of Pennsylvania in Philadelphia. A baby may feel comfortable if you place a hot-water bottle on your legs and then place him tummy-down on the bottle. Older children can use a heating pad, but it has to be set to a low temperature and be used only when an adult is

WHEN TO SEE THE DOCTOR

"Many parents fear that it is appendicitis every time their child complains about a stomachache," says Bruce Taubman, M.D., professor of pediatrics at the University of Pennsylvania in Philadelphia. "But a child with appendicitis would not be walking around and saying, 'My tummy hurts.' Your child would have a very severe pain."

"You have to take a child who cannot get up or who writhes with pain immediately to the doctor," says Don Shifrin, M.D., a pediatrician in Bellevue, Washington. "The same has to be done for a child who—in addition to the pain—has fever with nausea or vomiting not associated with meals. A child who develops pain, significant discomfort, or vomiting after falling or being hit in the abdominal area should also be examined." If your child shows these symptoms, you should call your physician immediately to get an appointment. Or if the pediatrician is unavailable, take your child to the emergency room as soon as possible.

present. (A child should lie not on the heating pad but on his back, with the pad on his abdomen, explains Dr. Taubman.)

Let your child rest. "It is also a good idea to rest the intestines," remarks Dr. Taubman. Put off solid food for 24 hours. "Give your child many liquids, such as mineral water, water, the sports drink Gatorade, and chicken broth," says Dr. Taubman. But keep all the rest in the pantry.

Manual Therapy for a Tummy That Aches

When a child has a moderate stomachache rather than a severe one, massage is a good way to relieve him, says Ann Linguiti Pron, a certified registered nurse practitioner in Willow Grove, Pennsylvania, especially if the cause of the pain is gas, constipation, or colic.

Even when the child is a baby, suggests Pron, you should tell him that you are going to massage his tummy to help him feel better. Then, start massaging slowly and carefully in a clockwise circular movement, which imitates the movement of food and gas through the digestive system, says Pron. If you do it correctly, she adds, you may not only relieve your child's pain but also help whatever is *causing* the pain to move toward the exit.

Here are some ways to help relieve pain.

- Have your child lie on his back. Rub a quarter-size dab of vegetable or massage oil between the palms of your hands to warm it up. With your oiled hand, massage the abdomen in a clockwise circular movement, starting just below the rib cage, going around to the groin, and back up across the abdomen, says Pron. Continue with the

Give your child a painkiller. "Infant acetaminophen (Children's Tylenol) will reduce the pain," says Dr. Taubman. Look in the package for instructions on the correct dosage for your child's weight and age. If your child is younger than 2, consult your physician.

Be careful with codeine. One thing that you *should not* do in case of abdominal pain is give your child medicines with a codeine base that were left over from a former sickness, warns Don Shifrin, M.D., a pe-

circular movement for several minutes and then change hands.

- With the child still on his back, place a hand horizontally just under the rib cage and slide it downward toward the groin, as if you were sweeping grains of sand from the abdomen. Alternate your hands rhythmically to massage the abdomen with steady sweeping strokes. Repeat several times, then go back to massaging the abdomen with a gentle circular movement.

- If your child has not eaten during the last hour, you can also try raising his legs while you do the sweeping movement described above, says Pron. Hold his feet with one hand and lift them almost to a 90-degree angle while you continue sweeping with the other hand. It is easy to lift the feet of a baby or small child. If your child is older, you can ask him to lie down and bend his legs with his feet on the floor.

- To give an infant additional relief from gas or colic, help him bend his knees instead of lifting his legs, suggests Pron. Lift one leg and gently bend his knee toward the abdomen, then quickly release it. Do the same with the other leg. Then, bend and release both legs together. Repeat the exercise and then massage your child's tummy again.

diatrician in Bellevue, Washington. It is possible to alleviate the pain temporarily, but you can also conceal the progress of a serious disease such as appendicitis, an obstruction, or an infection.

Give your children time. "As our lives speed up, one thing we do not give our children is the necessary time to go to the bathroom," says Dr. Dundon. In fact, the way we hurry our children, both at home and at school, is producing more cases of constipation, she says.

"I see at least a child per week in the office that has withheld his bowel movement for so long and so often that his intestine has expanded, and he has lost already his ability to move waste through it," says Dr. Dundon. As a result, waste impacts itself in the intestine and the fluid of the upper part of the intestine filters through what is impacted and leaks onto the child's clothing. "A child that has impacted feces will frequently suffer from abdominal pain after eating," she says.

The way to prevent both the problem and the pain is to give your child 5 to 10 minutes of *uninterrupted* time in the bathroom during the morning, suggests Dr. Dundon. "Do it as part of the routine, like brushing teeth," she says. Make your child sit on the toilet and read a book or listen to a story. Don't allow anyone to enter and pressure your child. Just allow him the opportunity and let nature take its course.

Give your child much love. "If your child is not constipated or vomiting, the abdominal pain could be caused by stress," says Dr. Dundon. "Pain from stress is something that we adults generally feel in our heads, and the children feel it in their stomachs." Some causes for stress can be a change in the family or a death.

How can you help? "What a child with a stress-related stomachache needs is love," says Ann Linguiti Pron, a certified registered nurse practitioner in Willow Grove, Pennsylvania. The frequent cuddling, hugs, and kisses are sufficient to alleviate a tight abdomen and take away the pain, she says.

Ask about school. "If a child continues complaining from abdominal pain during the week, however, there could be a problem at school that your child has not been able to express in words," says Pron. "Your child needs to talk with you and perhaps with his teacher or a guidance counselor."

So, drop everything you are doing and, if necessary, get to work a little bit late, but sit down and talk with your child. The problem may be as simple as a bully at the bus stop, a teacher who scolded him, or a seat assignment that forces your child to sit at a desk near somebody of the (gross!) opposite sex.

Any one of these situations can make your child want to avoid school, says Dr. Dundon. "But even if 'school phobia' is the culprit, when your child says that his tummy aches, it is true. And he does not need you to tell him that it is not so. That will only hurt him again."

Instead, advises Dr. Dundon, if your child complains of abdominal pains before going to school, offer him hugs and praises when he finally manages to get himself moving. Then, once he's off to school, call his teacher. If she knows that the child is having stomachaches before going to school, she may be able to reduce the stress load at school by not calling on him in class, by moving Johnny the bully to the other side of the classroom, or by offering your child more support and recognition than she might normally give in a busy classroom.

Herbal Options

In the other parts of this book, which offer tips for dealing with the adults in the house, you'll notice that the general health recommendations include some herbal recipes. In this part we haven't done that because we want to give you some overall guidelines about giving herbal remedies to kids before getting into specific herbal tips for your little ones.

First of all, although some herbalists believe that kids can be given medicinal herbs, we advise you to *never* give them to your children unless you consult their pediatrician first and get his approval. The tips we offer in this section are designed for kids who are at least 8 years old. If your son or daughter isn't a baby but has not yet reached that age, you should consult your pediatrician before giving them any of the following remedies. The fact is, there has been very little research done on the effect of medicinal herbs on kids. Therefore, you need to be very cautious when using these remedies. Always clear up any questions you may have with your pediatrician beforehand, and stop using any herbal remedy if you notice that your little one has a negative reaction.

That said, here are some herbal healing options.

Give ginger tea as needed. Ginger is a powerful stomach soother, says Robert Jay Rowen, M.D., a holistic physician at the Complementary Medicine Center in Anchorage, Alaska. Pick up the tea at any health food store or well-stocked supermarket and let it steep for about 10 minutes, then let him sip it slowly.

You can also make tea from fresh ginger. Finely chop or grate 1 teaspoon of the root, put it in a mug, and fill the mug with freshly boiled water. Cover it with a saucer and steep for 10 minutes. Let the tea cool slightly and let him sip it slowly.

Baby a belly with some peppermint. This herb is great for soothing the stomach, says James S. Sensenig, N.D., a naturopathic physician and professor at the University of Bridgeport College of Naturopathic Medicine in Connecticut. "Mint has a very relaxing effect on the gut because it stops muscle spasms in the digestive tract," he says.

Pick up some real peppermint tea at a health food store or grocery store. Check the label to be sure it contains real peppermint, not just peppermint flavoring. Add 1 cup of boiling water to 1 teaspoon dried leaves and steep for about 5 minutes. Strain out the herbs and serve at least ½ cup, suggests Kathi Keville, an herbalist in Nevada City, California, and director of the American Herb Association. Commercial peppermint tea bags or even peppermint candy may help, too, she says.

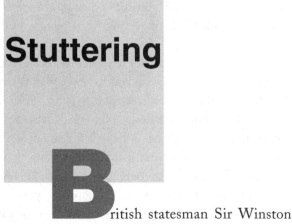

Stuttering

British statesman Sir Winston Churchill was a stutterer, as were scientist Sir Isaac Newton and writer W. Somerset Maugham. So are singer Carly Simon and actors Bruce Willis and James Earl Jones. That your child is in such distinguished company may be small consolation, though. Stuttering is a problem that can affect your child's social life, her school performance, and her self-esteem.

There are many theories on why people stutter, but none is conclusive. One thing that is clear is that stuttering—or disfluency, as the experts call it—is a problem of childhood. "Ninety percent of the people who are going to stutter start to do so by the time they're 7," says Edward Conture, Ph.D., professor of speech-language pathology and chairperson of the department of communication sciences and disorders at Syracuse University in New York and one of the nation's leading experts on childhood stuttering.

There is good news: Most children who begin to stutter gradually stop. Therapy with a trained speech and language pathologist tends to be quite successful, says Barry Guitar, Ph.D., professor of communication sciences and disorders at the Eleanor M. Luse Center for Communication Disorders at the University of Vermont College of Arts and Sciences in Burlington.

Intervention, however, needs to be undertaken early, says Dr. Guitar, himself a stutterer. "With the majority of kids under age 5, treatment helps so much that they will either overcome their problem or have only a minor disfluency. If the stuttering is severe, treatment is usually successful in helping the child learn to deal with it so it doesn't interfere with communication."

What You Can Do

Though stuttering generally requires professional help, there are many supplemental things that parents can do at home to help their child overcome this relatively common problem. Here are some simple techniques suggested by the experts.

Talk like Mister Rogers. That means slow down and speak clearly. Although many parents find this television personality's delivery annoying, his rate of speech does closely match kids' speech-processing abilities, according to Dr. Guitar. "On the other hand, if a child is listening to an adult speaking at a very rapid rate, the child will also try to speak rapidly and may become discoordinated," he says.

By slowing down, you're modeling a way of speaking that your child is realistically able to achieve, adds Dr. Conture. "It also provides the child with sufficient time to smoothly and easily generate her own speech. Initially, in a conversation with your child, you may only need to do this for about 5 minutes. Then you can probably go back to a more typical speaking rate, provided you don't talk too rapidly."

Take the pause that encourages. Don't be too hasty in responding to a child's comment or question, says Dr. Conture. "Pause for 1 to 2 seconds before you respond," he says. This will underscore the calm, slow pace of conversation and make it easier for the stuttering child to keep up her end of the conversation.

Set aside a special time to chat. Life is busy for everyone these days, and parents can't always drop everything and engage in slow, measured conversation. "But it helps if a child knows that she has a certain time each day when the parent is going to listen to her. Even if you can only set aside 5 to 10 minutes, that can compensate for the fact that life is too busy and rushed," says Dr. Guitar.

Let the child talk about her feelings. When you set aside some time to be with your child, let the child direct the conversation, says Dr. Guitar. Children who are going through a tough period may have a lot of feelings and thoughts that have gone unexpressed, he notes. These quiet times with you, when the child is in charge, may give her the sense of security she needs to express herself. "It can really be magical if you create an environment where the child feels free to talk about feelings and where all feelings are considered okay and normal."

Use the salt shaker trick. A child who stutters may get shut out of fast-paced dinner conversations. One way to make things easier is to give dinner-table talk a special structure, says Dr. Guitar. "One family used a salt shaker that was passed around the table. If you had the salt shaker, it was your turn to talk, and no one could interrupt you. This kind of structure is good for the stutterer because she doesn't feel she always has to struggle to get a word in."

Avoid "simultalk." "Try not to talk over the end of your child's utterance," says Dr. Conture. Though you sometimes may be tempted to finish your child's long, labored sentences; complete her thoughts; or interrupt her in a rush to get the conversation moving, let her finish. Otherwise you could possibly make her stuttering worse.

Don't be so picky. Kids who stutter need to know that they don't have to be perfect, that they can make mistakes and still be okay. Many of these children worry more about how they talk than what they say. "They worry about being perfect in talking, rather than just talking," says Dr. Conture. "Parents can help, though, by not being so picky about everything—the child's room, her fingernails, her homework, her

False Starts Can Be Normal

Your 3-year-old can't seem to get out a thought without countless false starts. Each sentence she utters seems to double back on itself as she edits and re-edits every phrase. Occasionally, she trips over a word. Is your child a stutterer?

There's a good chance she's just experiencing the normal period of disfluency many children go through sometime between the ages of 18 months and 6 years, says Barry Guitar, Ph.D., professor of communication sciences and disorders at the Eleanor M. Luse Center for Communication Disorders at the University of Vermont College of Arts and Sciences in Burlington. "Children with normal disfluency problems will repeat words or syllables once or twice, li-li-like this," he says.

When is there cause for worry? "We get concerned when kids repeat parts of words more than once or twice," says Dr. Guitar. "There's also some cause for concern if a child gets stuck on a word and it just won't come out, or if the child appears to be struggling, showing physical tension as she speaks."

If you suspect that your child could be a stutterer, contact a trained speech and language pathologist who specializes in stuttering. Both the American Speech-Language-Hearing Association, 10801 Rockville Pike, Rockville, MD 20852, and the Stuttering Foundation of America, PO Box 11749, Memphis, TN 38111-0749, can make referrals.

chores. Give the kid some slack," he says, "so she can learn that she can screw up and make mistakes and the world doesn't end."

Let speaking skills come naturally. Parents who are constantly correcting speech mistakes or stressing verbal skills can worsen their child's stuttering problems. "Take away any pressures," says Dr. Guitar. "Kids will develop language and speech skills on their own just by hearing conversation. They don't need to grow up in households where there's a lot of time spent learning vocabulary and the names of all the dinosaurs."

Make the teacher your ally. It's important that your child's teacher understand how to handle speech problems. "Giving oral reports, volunteering answers in class, and reading aloud are all difficult things for the stuttering child. Don't ask the teacher to excuse your child from these activities," says Dr. Guitar, "but open up communication so the child feels comfortable talking to the teacher about it. Kids who stutter will have good days and bad days. Your child may want to strike a deal with the teacher that she's only called on when her hand is up, so her good days can be taken advantage of and her bad days forgiven."

Teen Rebellion

Slamming doors. Missed curfews and plummeting grades. Emotions that are so turbulent and hostile you can't help wondering what this angry teenager standing in front of you did with the sweet, loving child you thought you'd raised.

Welcome to the "trying teens." As generations of parents can attest, adolescence and teenage rebellion are among the most difficult challenges that families face. While some teens make a relatively smooth transition into adulthood, others seem to go out of their way to make life—yours no less than theirs—as difficult as they possibly can.

Teenage rebellion is so common that psychologists often sum it up with this phrase: "All families some of the time, some families all of the time," says Michelle Wierson, Ph.D., associate professor of psychology at Pomona College in Claremont, California.

Rebellion and Risks

Children come into adolescence with a strong belief in the family's attitudes and values. Within a few years, they're challenging just about everything and everyone. You can think of it as the teenage equivalent of the "terrible twos": They go through a phase in which they reject their parents' rules and expectations in order to forge their own identities. For girls, the rebellious years start around ages 12 to 13. Boys start a little later, usually around 14 to 15.

"People have to expect rebellion from every teenager," says Dr. Wierson. "Having a good relationship prior to the teenage years is not a buffer from conflict in adolescence. Likewise, having conflicts does not mean there is something wrong with your relationship."

Most teenagers manage to get through this rebellious phase without serious (or at least permanent) repercussions, if you don't count a few fender benders and perhaps a minor brush with the law. But rebellion can potentially lead teens in dangerous directions. According to government surveys, about 50 percent of young people have experimented with alcohol. About 11 percent have used illicit drugs in a given month. And among the 15.3 million new cases of sexually transmitted diseases that occur each year, at least 25 percent are reported among teenagers.

Preparing for the Worst

The best way to deal with teenage rebellion is to anticipate the problems long before they start and to share your concerns with your children, says Dr. Wierson. At the beginning of adolescence, for example, sit down with your child and take a look into the future. Admit your concerns by saying, "I'm not looking forward to all the fights we will have, but I'm sure we're going to have them." Putting the cards on the table will help your children understand that you're aware of them as individuals, and that you're expecting to work through the problems together.

Having regular conversations about potential problems helps in another way, too. Teenagers crave autonomy and independence. Making them a part of the decision-making process gives them a sense of responsibility for the outcome. After all, it's harder for teenagers to rebel against rules and expectations that they played a part in creating.

Finally, parents need to remind themselves that no matter how wild their teenagers seem, with their crazy hairstyles, unusual clothing, and emotional ups and downs, the changes they're witnessing are almost always temporary. Research has shown that once the rebellious phase winds down, most young people reverse course and begin adopting many of the attitudes their parents wanted them to have all along.

Getting to that point, of course, can be incredibly frustrating. The challenge for parents is to prevent temporary conflicts in the family from escalating to the point that they become lifelong problems—either because family relationships are damaged to the breaking point or because the children took ever-increasing risks and finally got hurt.

Hot Tempers, Cool Planning

Here are a few ways to help your children—and yourself—get through this difficult time.

Don't sweat the small stuff. Even for parents who came of age in the permissive 1960s, it can be difficult to just stand by as children dye their hair green or wear clothes that look like army tents. But unless children are doing something flagrantly inappropriate—like going to church while wearing a skintight micro-miniskirt—you don't want to insist they dress a certain way, says Dr. Wierson.

Part of being a teenager is the desire to do what all the other kids are doing, says Dr. Wierson. Another part is the desire to do things they know their parents will dislike. Letting them rebel in small ways will help reduce the urge to rebel in other, more harmful ways.

"Teenagers need to feel as though they have the choice to be different from their parents," Dr. Wierson says. "This gives them the sense that they're making their own decisions."

Make your presence felt. One reason teenage rebellion sometimes spins out of control is that many parents simply don't interact with their children as much as they could. According to the U.S. Census Bureau, more than a quarter of the children in the United States live with one parent. Single parents can still be accessible for their children when they're washing the dishes or reading the paper, says Dr. Wierson.

But even in two-parent families, teenagers are often left alone a lot of the time. "Kids need a lot of supervision," says Dr. Wierson. "When they're alone with friends, a lot of things just seem to happen." Ways to supervise your children include spending time watching TV together rather than letting them hole up in their rooms. Or inviting their friends over to hang out rather than shoving them all out the door. Or even sim-

When Rebellion Goes Too Far

It's never easy to tell when a child's normal rebellious behavior is starting to cross the line into something more serious that requires a professional's help. According to Phyllis York, cofounder of Toughlove International, a program for troubled teens, the warning signs include:

- Staying out all night

- A sudden drop in grades

- An entirely new circle of friends

- Verbal or physical abuse

- Frequent lying

- Lack of motivation and laziness

- Signs of alcohol or drug use

Any one of these signs means that your child may be getting into more trouble than you can handle alone. You may want to consult a family therapist. Or call Toughlove at (800) 333-1069 to locate a chapter in your area.

pler, periodically poking your head in their rooms to talk or just stopping them in the hall to ask how their day went.

Discuss punishments before the crimes. Regardless of the infraction—missing curfew, skipping class, or having friends over when they shouldn't—teenagers often respond to criticism with a couple of universal themes: "It's not fair" or "You never told me."

So tell them. Sit around the table and ask them to discuss the types of trouble teenagers get into. Then assign certain punishments. Thirty minutes past curfew? A day without television. Didn't turn in homework? Grounded for the weekend.

"You're giving the kid a heads-up about what to expect," says Dr. Wierson. Discussing the issues together helps neutralize the "it's not fair" refrain. "Your child will know that if he gets caught, this is what's going to happen. The responsibility is on him," Dr. Wierson explains.

Get together with other parents. For parents dealing with their first teenager, it's not always obvious what constitutes fair expectations and appropriate punishments. "It's useful to get together with your friends and compare notes," says Dr. Wierson.

Keep the rules flexible. Making rules isn't a one-shot thing. A curfew that's right for a 13-year-old might be too restrictive when your child turns 14 or 15. Parents need to be constantly looking at family rules, making them more lenient as their children mature—or more restrictive when the kids aren't coming through.

Similarly, there will always be times when rules need to be bent a bit—giving a later curfew when a special event is taking place, for example. You can get additional mileage by linking the extra privilege to extra responsibility: "Yes, you can stay out until midnight on Saturday, but only if the kitchen is clean before you leave."

"Kids who think the rules will never change, or who have no sense of control over earning a change, are more likely to sneak around or violate limits," Dr. Wierson explains.

Be careful about giving ultimatums. Parents say all sorts of things when they get angry. Ultimatums given in anger, however, have a way of backfiring. When your teenager has missed curfew for the third night in a row, for example, you might hear yourself saying, "One more time, and you'll be grounded until August." Now, you have two choices: Enforce the punishment, which essentially means that *you're* grounded until August, or back down, in which case your child has learned not to take you seriously.

It's always better to try to anticipate problems and plan the corresponding punishments when you're not angry, says Dr. Wierson. Or at least think long and hard before giving an ultimatum. You don't want to threaten a punishment if you're not willing to carry through.

Back off when you need to. It's normal to say things that you don't really mean. If you feel you've made a mistake and were too harsh, it's fine to revisit the issue. This doesn't mean backing down when your child is being obnoxious, Dr. Wierson adds. Even if you feel that you made a mistake, you don't want to be coerced with threats, tantrums, or other typical teenage behavior. "What I recommend is setting up a way in which they can earn a lighter punishment," Dr. Wierson suggests.

Suppose, for example, you grounded your child for a month for some infraction. Tell him that you've thought it over and have decided to reduce the "sentence" by a week *if* he does something for you, like picking up the living room for a week or keeping his room clean.

Give yourself room to think. Teenagers have a gift for pushing their parents' buttons. Rather than reacting on the spot (and saying something you'll later regret), tell your child, "This is a problem, and we'll need to think about the punishment for a while," says Dr. Wierson. This gives you time to plan your response. At the same time, the delay will make your child sweat a little, which isn't a bad thing under the circumstances.

Walk away from conflicts. Teenagers who are in bad moods may not listen to logic. "Within reason, it's fine to stand back and let them blow off steam. Confronting them will probably make the situation worse," says Dr. Wierson.

Just don't stick around and watch while your child is sulking, yelling, or generally acting up. If you do, your child will get the idea that his behavior is influencing your decisions. Instead, leave the room. Better yet, suggest that he go for a walk or watch TV for a while. "Teenagers often know what they need to do in order to calm down and feel a little better," says Dr. Wierson. Once tempers have cooled, you can revisit the issue and find a resolution, she says.

TV Addiction

Alex's family was planning a very special trip by station wagon all over the country. When Alex, who was only 6 years old, found out there would be no TV for 3 weeks, he could not believe it. "So, what am I going to do?" he protested.

Whenever Tracy, 10, comes into her bedroom, she turns the TV set on. It is as automatic for her as turning on the light. Whether she is doing her homework, playing with her friends, or talking on the phone, her TV is always on.

Both Alex and Tracy are TV addicts. In a certain way, they are as dependent on the images appearing on the screen as many adults are on cigarettes or alcohol. And the consequences could be serious.

Many studies have demonstrated that children who watch TV a lot are fatter and less fit and have higher cholesterol levels than children who watch less TV. Some experts consider that watching TV in excess can encourage a more tolerant attitude toward violence as well as promote aggressive behavior.

If it concerns you that your child is watching too much TV, here are some tips to get rid of the television habit.

Record the number of hours. "Write down how much TV your child is watching daily," suggests Nicholas A. Roes, chairperson of the American Educational Association and author of *Helping Children Watch TV*. It may surprise you to see the number of hours he is watching TV in a week. Once you are aware of the magnitude of the problem, you will be more able to make changes, Roes says.

Short-circuit the electronic babysitter. "Don't get into the habit of using the TV set as a babysitter, no matter how busy you may be," says Marie Winn, who has written a book on this problem. Instead, introduce some active pastimes that your child can carry out when you are not able to supervise him.

How to Convert an Enemy into an Ally

I f used intelligently, television can be turned into a positive and educational force in the life of your child, says Nicholas A. Roes, chairperson of the American Educational Association and author of *Helping Children Watch TV*. These are some of his suggestions.

- If your child enjoys watching game shows, make them a family activity. Choose some subjects that appear frequently in these programs and spend time together looking them up in an almanac or the encyclopedia to prepare for next week's program. Then tune in to the program and allow your child to answer each question and keep his own score.

- To encourage critical judgment, ask him for a report on the TV programs, in the same way he prepares reports on books at school. Depending on your child's age, each report may contain comments on facts related to the plot, the sequence of events, the development of characters, the scenery, the music, and the special effects.

- If you see violence in a program you and your child are watching, discuss alternatives; that is, what nonviolent means the characters could have used to solve their problems.

- Suggest that your child write letters to the producers, sponsors, and TV networks to express his feelings about various programs.

You can provide him with a wide variety of drawing materials, for instance, or buy some easy musical instruments that he can play on his own. If you read to your child—and do a lot of reading yourself—you would be encouraging him to be entertained by books as much as by television.

Schedule something for your child that is worth watching. "Check the channel listings with your child every weekend and choose programs for the coming week that you would feel comfortable having him watch," says Carole Lieberman, M.D., professor of psychiatry at the University of California, Los Angeles. "Choose those programs that are educational and nonviolent, that support the type of values you want your child to have."

If the program is part of a series, watch at least one episode with your child to make sure it's really suitable. *Important:* As soon as the selected program is over and before your child gets hooked on the next one, turn the TV off, says Dr. Lieberman.

Take a day's rest. "Designate 1 day a week only as a Day without TV," suggests Winn. "Some families do that on a Saturday or Sunday, as part of their Sabbath observance." Make it clear that everyone, including mom and dad, will have to find more creative ways to occupy their time during that day.

Make time for homework. To ensure that your children do their homework, try to establish the rule that there will be no TV in the evenings on weekdays, which, according to Winn, is the most difficult rule to enforce. Discuss this rule first during a family meeting to make your child understand why you give it so much importance.

"Children do not necessarily watch TV over the whole weekend to catch up on what they missed on weekdays," says Winn. In fact, if they are unaccustomed to watching during the week, they will most likely look for other activities in their free time once Saturday arrives.

Try a "TV Turn-Off Week." Occasionally, you can present your children with the challenge of keeping the TV off during a whole week, suggests Winn, who has organized TV Turn-Offs in the United States. "That's when you'll see how dependent your family is on TV." The insight may be sobering, but it could help you set limits in the future, she points out.

Most likely, your kids will suffer to a certain extent from withdrawal.

They will probably beg you for permission to watch "just one" favorite program. But remain firm.

"Just be sure you present this as an experiment or an adventure, never as a punishment," says Winn. "As an additional incentive, think of some reward for the weekend. Perhaps you decide to take a special family trip, buy a new game or some other toy."

Take advantage of the videocassette recorder. "When you increase the use of videotapes, you will gain greater control over what your children watch and when they watch it," says Dr. Lieberman. Besides, if a problematic or confusing issue arises in the program they are watching, you can press the pause button and talk with your children about it.

"You can also fast-forward the tape if there are offensive commercials," she adds. Or you can choose to watch one of those commercials with your child, and then stop the tape to teach him to be more skeptical concerning advertising. "You may want to discuss how the ad is suggesting that if the child gets this toy, he will be the most popular kid on the block," suggests Dr. Lieberman. You may point out how unrealistic that subtle message is.

Do not allow the TV to take away your child's sleep. Establish a regular bedtime schedule for your child that does not change from night to night depending on when certain programs end, advises Bobbi Vogel, M.D., a psychotherapist and family counselor in Woodland Hills, California. And do not place a personal TV set in your child's bedroom, unless you want to completely lose control over what and when he watches.

It is not good as background. Do not allow your child to leave the TV on as background noise, advises Dr. Vogel. "It is too visually stimulating," she explains. When you go check on him, he is going to be watching it instead of just listening to it. If he likes to hear something while drawing or doing other activities, have him listen to a record or the radio.

Vomiting

Was it too much cake and ice cream at your first-grader's birthday party? Something in the sausage pizza? Or that third ride on the merry-go-round? What prompted that colorful return of lunch may keep you guessing. But one thing you know for sure: You hope it doesn't happen again.

And in most cases, it won't. "Most vomiting is caused by gastroenteritis," says Marjorie Hogan, M.D., an instructor of pediatrics at the University of Minnesota and a pediatrician at the Hennepin County Medical Center, both in Minneapolis. "That's a viral infection of the gastrointestinal tract, which is simple and self-limiting." In other words, it probably won't last long.

On the other hand, if vomiting does continue, it could lead to dehydration. "Vomiting a few times is usually no big deal," says Dr. Hogan. "Kids usually have enough fluid on board. It's when vomiting persists, when it's accompanied by diarrhea, or when the child is a baby or toddler that you need to be careful."

Older children are more able to tell you when they're parched and thirsty. "With infants," says Dr. Hogan, "it's hard to know when they've crossed that line. That's why you need to contact a doctor immediately."

Most children need some parental comfort, since vomiting can be pretty scary. And while you're nursing your child back to a state of settled stomach, try these tactics.

Give that tummy a rest. "The first thing to do is to stop putting things in the child's stomach. Give it a rest," says Loraine Stern, M.D., associate clinical professor of pediatrics at the University of California, Los Angeles, and author of *When Do I Call the Doctor?* That also goes for babies who are still breastfeeding or bottlefeeding, says Dr. Stern.

Why Babies Spit Up

If you're the first-time parent of a newborn, there's one very important thing to remember: Spit happens.

Many babies have a condition known as gastroesophageal reflux, says Marjorie Hogan, M.D., instructor of pediatrics at the University of Minnesota and a pediatrician at the Hennepin County Medical Center, both in Minneapolis. That means the sphincter muscle at the bottom of the esophagus isn't working well yet, so breast milk or formula sloshes back up, creating that foolproof identifying mark of a new parent, the shoulder splotch.

There are a few ways to minimize spitting up until the baby's esophageal sphincter tightens up.

Handle gently. Don't jostle the baby during or after a feeding. Don't automatically fling him to your shoulder and start to burp him, says Loraine Stern, M.D., associate clinical professor of pediatrics at the University of California, Los Angeles, and author of *When Do I Call the Doctor?*

Follow baby's cues. "Pay close attention to the baby's feeding cues," says Dr. Hogan. "Feed at his tempo, stop when he seems to want to stop, and when he wants to take a rest, take a rest. Don't try to feed past fullness."

When in doubt, call the doctor. "Babies who spit up a lot can sometimes absorb fluid in their lungs, which can lead to lung disease," says Dr. Hogan. "Your doctor can also tell you if your baby is growing well and if the spitting up is caused by an obstruction. If a baby is vomiting a lot, don't deal with it at home. See a doctor right away."

WHEN TO SEE THE DOCTOR

If your child has been vomiting, you need to be alert to signals that he is becoming dehydrated. If the child refuses fluids, stops urinating, cries without tears, has dry mucous membranes, or appears lethargic, listless, drowsy, or confused, he may need to be taken to the hospital and given fluids intravenously or put on a special oral rehydration program. In any case, call the doctor if the vomiting persists for more than 2 to 3 days, which increases the likelihood of dehydration.

You should also be on the lookout for symptoms of more serious illnesses or injuries. These include:

- Projectile vomiting in a baby, especially under 4 months of age. This forceful vomiting may be a symptom of pyloric stenosis, an obstruction at the end of the stomach that prevents food from passing through.

- Vomiting accompanied by fever. This can be a symptom of meningitis, bowel infection, or some other serious condition.

"Just skip a regular feeding until the stomach seems to settle." Offer oral rehydration fluids such as Pedialyte, instead, in small, frequent sips. You can ask your pharmacist for these drinks, which basically contain sugar, salt, and a few other nutrients and are available at most drugstores.

Offer reassurance. "Vomiting can be very scary to a child," says Dr. Hogan. "Assure him that he's going to be all right." A young child may want you to hold him and stay with him for a while. For older children, it's comforting to be tucked into bed until they feel better.

Start foods slowly. Wait for your child to express an interest in eating, then start with clear liquids, says Dr. Stern. Your main objective

- A hard and bloated stomach in between episodes of vomiting. This could indicate an intestinal or stomach obstruction that could lead to life-threatening problems—so immediate attention is a must.

- Vomiting after recovering from a viral infection. This could be a symptom of Reye's syndrome, an inflammation of the brain and liver that can be fatal.

- Vomiting after a head injury. This may signal a concussion or bleeding in the brain.

- Vomiting yellow or green liquid (bile) repeatedly. This sometimes means that there's an obstruction in the stomach.

- Vomit that resembles coffee grounds. This usually means there is blood in the stomach, a sign of internal bleeding.

- Vomiting after an accident involving the stomach, especially a bicycle handlebar injury. Even if the vomiting occurs a week or two later, you should call the doctor. This kind of vomiting may mean that there's a bruise in the intestines.

is to avoid dehydration. Many children can't tolerate water after vomiting but will suck on ice chips or even a cold, wet washcloth. Offer juices (unless there's also diarrhea), ice pops, oral rehydration liquids, and gelatin, suggests Dr. Hogan. If the clear liquids stay down, you can offer dry toast or crackers. "Avoid milk and milk products, though, which aren't well-tolerated."

Pour a cola. Things do go better with Coke. This is an old home remedy that has stood the test of time. "There's something about lukewarm Coca-Cola Classic that makes it stay down better than most things," says Dr. Stern. "Serve it lukewarm and a little bit flat. Stir it a little to make the bubbles disappear."

Ask about this OTC remedy. "If, after waiting a few hours, you've given the child sips of liquids and those don't stay down, an over-the-counter antinausea medicine called Emetrol may help," says Dr. Stern. Consult your doctor first, however—and ask for the proper dose for your child's weight and age.

Trust your child. Whether he says he wants tea and toast or a pepperoni pizza, serve it up. When children are ready to eat again, it's best to go with what they feel they can eat, says Dr. Hogan. With younger, less verbal children, however, stick to bland foods such as toast, crackers, rice, or potatoes at first. If the child's stomach tolerates those foods, you can gradually introduce others.

PART THREE

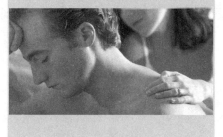

Mom's Medicine
for Men

Abdominal Fat

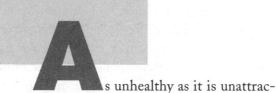

As unhealthy as it is unattractive, the potbelly has long been the bane of men who love to eat and don't get enough exercise. They *know* they should lose it. They *want* to lose it, but it's not easy. In a typical survey, abs were the overwhelming choice of respondents asked to name the area of the body they most wanted to tone.

It's a simple equation: A guy (or woman, for that matter) who takes in more calories than he burns will put on weight. And for a guy, one of the first places you see the added pounds is on the stomach. A big part of this story is genetics. Just as women are predisposed to packing extra weight on their hips and waists, men tend to store it in their gut . . . prominently, for all the world to see.

Despite all the jokes about big bellies, they are a serious problem. Study after study tells us that fat between the shoulders and hips (read: abdominal fat) is bad news for the heart. It helps raise cholesterol levels, which blocks arteries and leads to coronary heart disease. Fat around the midriff has been linked to insulin resistance, which can raise blood pressure. There's also evidence to suggest that it puts people at increased risk for diabetes. Felicia Busch, R.D., a dietitian in St. Paul, Minnesota, calls it the most critical weight to lose. "You can be only 10 to 15 pounds overweight, but if it's all in the abdomen, it's much more serious than if you were 30 to 40 pounds overweight with the pounds spread out," she says.

Goodbye, Gut

Well, you obviously can't "cure" your husband's big belly as you could a bee sting. You also can't make him lose it if he doesn't want to. However, if he really wants to lose it, with Mom's Medicine you can give him support and some simple, practical ways to lose that belly.

Have him start with the basics. Any exercise that moves the body through space will help lose that gut, says Peter D. Vash, M.D., executive medical director of Lindora Medical Clinics in Costa Mesa, California. "Isometrics with weights is great for building muscle mass and certainly shouldn't be ignored, but if you want a toned stomach, you have to lose fat mass. And you do that by regular and frequent aerobic exercise—anything from treadmill walking or running to swimming or cycling," Dr. Vash says. Advise your man to aim for a minimum of 30 minutes, 4 days a week, he adds.

Don't let him crash-diet. It may seem that cutting back on how much you eat is the quickest way to get rid of a potbelly. But it's not. Dieters who severely restrict their caloric intake may lose fat, but they can actually lose *muscle* as well.

In a study done at Tufts University in Boston, 11 men and women age 60 and older were divided into an exercise group and a diet group. Members of the exercise group rode stationary bikes for two 45-minute sessions to burn 360 calories a day, and closely monitored their diets to be sure that they ate exactly the same amount of calories as they did before the program began. To make the match even, the dieters ate 360 fewer calories a day than before.

After 12 weeks, the dieters had lost an average of about 11 pounds, but more than 6 of those pounds were muscle. The exercisers dropped an average of 16 pounds, all of it fat. The moral of the story: If your guy's cutting calories, he should cut only between 200 and 400 calories a day, says William J. Evans, Ph.D., director of the nutrition, metabolism, and exercise laboratory at the University of Arkansas for Medical Sciences in Little Rock. Any more than that and he risks losing muscle, warns Dr. Evans, who conducted this study.

And if someone is trying to lose weight, muscle can be his best friend. That's because even when he's not using his muscles, they burn more calories than fat does. So the more muscle he has, the easier it is to lose weight.

Help him do crunches correctly. Abdominal crunches won't melt belly fat; only sufficient aerobic exercise and proper nutrition will. But they are a great exercise for strengthening the muscles below the belly fat. And that can certainly aid his appearance and help keep his back healthy. But he has to do crunches properly. He shouldn't get locked into "the 'more is better' way of thinking," says Ann Marie Miller, a certified personal trainer and fitness training manager at New York Sports Clubs in New York City. "Doing 500 crunches quickly and in haphazard fashion won't do as much good as 20 done with perfect form. There are no ab muscles in the neck or legs, but I still see guys jerking their heads and swinging their torsos. The goal is to stimulate as many muscle fibers as possible, and this is done by executing crunches slowly."

Here's how your husband can get the most out of his crunches, Miller says. He should lie flat on his back, arms folded across his chest or hands behind his head, elbows out. Then he should bend his knees at a 45-degree angle, feet flat on the floor. Slowly, he should curl his torso upward. He needs to lift his shoulders off the floor while his lower back remains flat on the floor. His rib cage will move toward his pelvis.

Suggest that he break up his aerobic workouts. Two or three short bouts of exercise throughout the day can help melt that belly fat away. "Breaking up workouts helps to increase fitness while expending more calories at the same time," Dr. Evans says. Because the man is not doing the activity for as long, he can "keep up the intensity throughout the workout without getting as tired," Dr. Evans explains.

Dr. Evans recommends that your husband try working two or three 20-minute sessions into his daily routine 5 days a week. A morning jog and a brisk walk at lunch will suffice. He should just make sure that he's doing aerobic exercise—the kind that gets the heart pumping and the lungs huffing and puffing. "Aerobic exercise is probably the very best way to target abdominal fat," says Dr. Evans. "It is the only kind of exercise shown to pull fat stores more directly from the abdominal region."

Have him try squats. The exercise known as squats engages lots of muscles—the gluteus maximus (the largest buttocks muscle), quadriceps, hamstrings, inner thighs, outer hips, abdominals, lower back, and shoulder girdle—all the while elevating the heart rate. "There's no such thing as spot reduction; you have to work your entire body to lose the belly," says Annette Lang, a certified personal trainer at Equinox, a fitness club in New York City.

Lang offers the basic free-standing squat as an excellent starter exercise. Show him these instructions on how to do it: Stand with your legs at least shoulder-width apart and your feet slightly pointed out to keep your hips, knees, and ankles in alignment. Cross your arms in front of your chest. As you slowly lower your body, keep your abs and lower back stable. Make sure that your rear end goes back, rather than your knees going forward or extending out over the tips of your toes. It should feel as if you're sitting in an imaginary chair. Lower your butt until your thighs are parallel to the floor, then slowly rise back up. Start out doing 8 to 12 repetitions every day, work up to two or three sets, and add dumbbells or a barbell later. Keep in mind that you should always check with your doctor before starting a new exercise program.

Suggest eating lean. Fatty foods equal a fat stomach. It's a no-brainer, but it's so important. And it's easier for men to make the small dietary changes that add up over the long haul than it is for women, Busch says. "Ironically, the fact that men, in general, have worse eating habits gives them lots of room to improve. Switching to low-fat milk and salad dressings, eating pretzels instead of potato chips, and skipping the cheese on sandwiches all are very small changes that can make a big difference over time," she says.

Tell him to tighten up. Lang likens this to the way you would instinctively tighten up if someone tried to punch you in the stomach.

A tip that Busch gives her patients is to get in the habit of consciously holding in their stomachs as they walk. "Or when he's driving, he can suck in his gut at every stoplight. These are just a couple small things he can do to engage his abdominals as much as possible in order to tone the underlying muscle," Busch says.

Limit his drinks. Not only is alcohol calorically dense, it also targets the abdomen—hence the term *beer belly*. If he really wants to keep his waistline under control, he has to cut back on the booze. Busch recommends that when you go out, his first two drinks should be club sodas or something else nonalcoholic. "Not only does this help fill him up before he's touched any alcohol but it also prevents him from lowering his inhibition, which always makes it easier to overdo it on the food and drink," she says. (For more information on weight loss, see the Overweight chapter on page 445. Although the tips in this chapter are in the section for women, men can also use them effectively.)

Back Pain

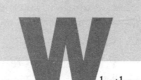

hether he is a warehouse worker hefting boxes onto a truck or a telemarketer rooted to a chair, headset, and computer, your husband will probably have a case of serious back pain sometime in his life. About 80 percent of people do.

The back isn't a single anatomic entity like an arm or a foot but rather a complex column of bones, disks, and muscles designed to hold the torso erect. Consequently, the causes of back pain are numerous: pinched nerves, weak abdominal muscles, loss of flexibility, tight leg muscles, a big gut, trauma, sitting too long, poor overall fitness, and herniated disks.

Your husband's first bout of back pain will likely clear up within a month or so, no matter what he does, says Philip Greenman, D.O., professor of osteopathic manipulation and physical medicine at Michigan State University in East Lansing. But if he's had back pain once, he has a 50 percent chance of having it again.

"Back pain is notoriously recurrent, and the second and third incidents tend to be more severe than the first," says Dr. Greenman. "It's hard to treat, and that's why a better focus is on prevention."

Some Common—And Uncommon— Solutions to a Common Problem

Here's a mixed-medicine approach of conventional and alternative cures you can try to help your husband with back pain.

Lay him down. Tell him to lie on the floor on his back, bending his knees at a 90-degree angle and resting his legs on a chair, suggests Dr. Greenman. "This position takes all pressure off the back, disks, and nerves," he says. "It usually gives the relief you're looking for." He should do this for 20 minutes every couple of hours.

Have him check his legs. He may think that the problem is in his back, where the pain is, but it could be in his legs. After sitting or bending all day, his leg muscles may be extremely tight or unbalanced (meaning that some muscles may be loose and relaxed while others are contracted or in spasm). Tight leg muscles pull oddly on the torso and put pressure on the back and abdominal muscles, says Jerome F. McAndrews, D.C., spokesman for the American Chiropractic Association. To rebalance his calf muscles, he should stand flat-footed on a stair step in flat, comfortable shoes with the balls of his feet on the very edge and his heels in the air, advises Dr. McAndrews. Holding on to a railing for support, he should slowly lower his heels until he feels a tightness up the back of his legs. Advise him to hold for a few seconds, repeat 5 to 10 times, and do as needed during the day, says Dr. McAndrews.

Advise him to stretch his legs. The previous tip also applies to those muscles running down the backs of his thighs. Sitting for long periods—the bane of office workers—shortens the hamstring muscles in the backs of the legs, which then yank on the pelvis and make other muscles compensate. He can work his hamstrings by standing up and placing one heel on a steady chair or end table. (He should hold on to a nearby table or chair for balance.) Then he can keep this leg straight and lean forward until he feels a pulling sensation in the back of his thigh. He should hold this position for about 30 seconds and then switch to the other leg, suggests Dr. McAndrews. He can do this a few times a day, especially after

WHEN TO SEE THE DOCTOR

Have your husband see the doctor immediately if he experiences any of the following: fever; severe, debilitating pain; numbness; pain that is considerably worse when he's lying down; pain radiating down a leg; loss of function in his leg (such as not being able to rise up on his toes); loss of bladder or bowel control; or recent unexplained weight loss or pain that persists for more than a week.

he's been sitting for a long time. He shouldn't try to "lock" the extended leg when first attempting this stretch. As the muscles stretch out, "locking" the leg will come naturally, advises Dr. McAndrews.

Herbalize him. Although the herb valerian is best known as a mild sedative to treat insomnia, its soothing qualities can provide pain relief for a backache triggered by overworked, spastic muscles, says Jacqueline Jacques, N.D., a naturopathic physician in Portland, Oregon. Give him two 250-milligram capsules four times a day or 20 drops of tincture every 2 hours. Muscles in pain tend to tense up. An animal study showed that compounds in valerian relaxed smooth muscle cells, and relaxed muscles tend to heal faster, says Gayle Eversole, Ph.D., a certified nurse practitioner and herbalist from Everett, Washington. "It also quiets the part of the nervous system that causes the sensation of pain," says Dr. Jacques. The sedative effects of valerian also come in handy, since back pain tends to keep people tossing and turning at night. Unlike over-the-counter sleep aids, it won't leave him with a hangover effect the next morning.

One big problem with valerian, though, is that it reeks. The yellowish green oil from this relaxing root contains the same aromatic properties as human sweat. Unless he can endure its nasty smell and taste, it would be better for him to take a capsule of valerian rather than a tincture, says Jacob Schor, N.D., a naturopathic physician in Denver. "If my patients opt for the tincture, I just tell them to pinch their noses and swallow," he says. It's okay for him to take valerian for back pain until his symptoms subside.

Note: A tincture is a highly concentrated herbal liquid. It's made by soaking leaves in alcohol or glycerin—which extracts the herb's medicinal properties—for at least 6 weeks. Tinctures are sold in health food stores in small bottles with eyedroppers to give doses. Be sure to store them out of the reach of children.

Cure it with a cayenne cream. Creams and ointments containing cayenne stimulate the release of the body's own painkillers, says Dr. Jacques. Scientists believe that the active substance in cayenne, capsaicin, also interferes with the action of the body's pain messenger, called substance P. Rub the sore area with red-pepper ointment three or four times a day. Use a standardized ointment containing 0.075 or 0.025 percent capsaicin. He won't get relief with the first application, says Dr. Jacques. It takes a few applications to wear out those pain messengers.

A SOOTHING SOLUTION

To ease your husband's back pain quickly, apply a compress soaked in a blend of pain-relieving essential oils and water, says Jacqueline Jacques, N.D., a naturopathic physician in Portland, Oregon. This recipe combines the healing powers of peppermint, bergamot, and lavender to stop muscle spasms and quiet pain and inflammation. Adding Epsom salts to the water helps promote absorption of the essential oils through the skin. The magnesium in Epsom salts also acts as a muscle relaxant.

To make the compress, dip a small kitchen towel or a washcloth into the solution and wring it out. Apply it directly to the painful area for 15 to 20 minutes two or three times a day.

Use cold water for treatments for the first 24 hours after the onset of pain. Later, you can use warm water to make the solution or reheat leftover solution before using it. For added relief, have him lie on his back with his feet elevated while the compress is in place to help relieve the pressure on his lower back, says Dr. Jacques. Here's the recipe:

1	tablespoon Epsom salts
1	gallon cold water
3	drops peppermint essential oil
3	drops bergamot essential oil
4	drops lavender essential oil

Mix the Epsom salts into the water, then add the peppermint, bergamot, and lavender oils and stir gently. Store extra solution in a dark glass container away from heat and light.

After you use the cream, be sure to wash your hands with soap to avoid a very uncomfortable burning sensation if you happen to touch other parts of your body. Also, never put the cream on a rash or open wound. It's safe to use this remedy for long periods of time, but if pain persists for more than 3 to 4 weeks, have him see a doctor.

Warm him up. A heating pad, a hot compress, or a warm bath or shower relaxes muscles and brings fresh, healing blood to the injury, says Dr. Greenman. He can take a 10-minute warm shower, or you can apply heat with a heating pad or hot compress for 15 to 30 minutes or until the area has a pink blush, and then remove. Don't do it any longer than that or you'll make matters worse, Dr. Greenman warns. "People will lie on a heating pad for hours and then won't be able to move. That's because the area is just congested with blood," he says. "You should apply heat just a few times a day for short periods."

Increase his circulation. Another way of getting fresh blood to an injury is taking the herb ginkgo, says Alison Lee, M.D., a pain management specialist and acupuncturist with Barefoot Doctors, an acupuncture and natural-medicine resource center in Ann Arbor, Michigan. This herb has been shown to dilate blood vessels and may theoretically increase bloodflow to his aching back, says Dr. Lee. You can buy the herb in capsule form in health food stores and over the counter in many drugstores. Dr. Lee recommends a product with standardized extract. Follow the package directions for dosage information.

Also, in some cases, a combination approach may be useful. Whereas ginkgo biloba increases bloodflow, curcumin can add an anti-inflammatory effect, suggests Dr. Lee. Curcumin, a highly concentrated form of turmeric sold in health food stores, is a potent anti-inflammatory medicine that is very effective for a soft-tissue injury such as a sore back, says Dr. Lee. Look for a product (capsule form) with standardized extract of 95 percent, and follow the dosage recommended on the label.

Tell him to get a move on. The old prescription for backache was several days of bed rest, recalls Dr. Greenman. But since most back pain is from muscle strain, tightness, and spasms, being immobile just makes people weaker and more prone to further injury. And bed rest also can help convince him that he really is sick and unable to help himself, says Dr. Greenman. The sooner he gets moving, the sooner he'll feel better. So have him get up and do some walking and a little stretching. Just make sure he doesn't overdo it.

Baldness

Man's battle with baldness began long before "rugs," plugs, and Rogaine. Through the ages, men have rubbed their scalps with a variety of stuff—including chicken droppings—in an attempt to keep their hairlines from retreating. But there's still no magic potion. Two out of three American men develop some form of baldness, and half of them are markedly bald by age 50.

Androgenetic alopecia, the medical term for male-pattern baldness, is the condition responsible for 95 percent of hair loss in men. It can begin as early as puberty, starting with loss of hair from the top of the head or a receding hairline. Eventually, all that may be left is a monklike fringe around the sides and back of the head. Male-pattern baldness is thought to be caused by a combination of two factors: heredity plus a sensitivity to dihydrotestosterone (DHT), which is derived from androgen, a male hormone. It's thought that DHT shuts down the hair follicles on the scalp in men who are genetically predisposed to going bald, says Richard S. Greene, M.D., a dermatologist in Hallandale, Florida, who has performed more than 9,000 hair transplants. Less common causes of hair loss include high fever, some medications, chronic illness, and major surgery.

How serious this problem is depends on his attitude. Some guys have an easy-come-easy-go attitude about their hair, while others equate a balding pate with the passing of their youth and vigor. The seriousness of the problem also depends on how far he's willing to go to get his hair back, since some treatments involve considerable expense and risk.

How He Can Stop the Loss

Advise him to try Propecia. This is the brand name of finasteride, a compound that was initially used to treat prostate problems. Scientists discovered that as a bonus it also promoted hair growth in prostate patients, so they tested it as a baldness remedy. In clinical trials, 65 percent of men who used it stopped losing their hair within a year. Fifty-two percent of them got some hair growth within a year. Still, finasteride didn't do anything for 35 percent of men. Scientists speculate that it works by stopping the production of the DHT hormone.

Propecia is sold in the form of a pill, which he'd have to take every day. It's expensive, costing between $50 and $60 a month. Propecia can have some unpleasant side effects, such as impotence and a decrease in sex drive, but these have occurred in only 2 percent of the men who have used it and went away totally in men who stopped using it. Other reported side effects are allergic reactions, such as hives, swelling, itching, and rashes; chest pain; testicular pain; and ejaculation problems.

Pregnant women should *never* take finasteride or even touch the broken tablets of this drug because it can cause birth defects. Also, finasteride affects the results of a test to detect prostate cancer called the prostate-specific antigen (PSA) test. So if your husband takes Propecia and he's about to get a PSA test done, he should tell his doctor first. Finally, finasteride is forever. He can't stop taking it. If he does, all the hair that he grew while he used it will fall out.

Advise him to try minoxidil. Studies have shown that 2 percent minoxidil grew moderate amounts of hair in 25 percent of the men who used it. The newer "extra-strength" kind, which contains 5 percent minoxidil (marketed as Rogaine Extra Strength for Men), can grow 45 percent more hair for men than 2 percent minoxidil, according to studies conducted by the makers of Rogaine. He can get either formulation in most drugstores. Rogaine doesn't work for everyone, however. Hair growth will be light to moderate rather than luxuriant, and it takes at least 4 months of twice-a-day use to see results. Also, he has to keep using it, says Dr. Greene, or else any hair he's grown will fall out.

Suggest that he get some herbal help. According to James A. Duke, Ph.D., the world's foremost authority on healing herbs and author of *The Green Pharmacy*, saw palmetto can impede the production of the "bald hormone" DHT just like finasteride. Another professional who recommends the herb is Angela Christiano, Ph.D., professor of dermatology at Columbia University College of Physicians and Surgeons in New York City. She suggests taking 325 milligrams of the extract of the berry of the plant in capsule form once a day. Tell your husband to look for saw palmetto berry extract in health food stores.

Consider a hairpiece. A well-made hairpiece or hair weave "is the best and safest hair-replacement system there is right now," says Vaughn Acord, a senior hairstylist at Bumble and Bumble Hair Salon in New York City. A hairpiece consists of human or synthetic hair implanted into a fine nylon mesh and is attached to the scalp with glue, tape, or metal clips. By contrast, a hair weave involves sewing a wig into existing hair. Although a good hairpiece is expensive—it can cost thousands of dollars—it doesn't carry the risks of surgery, and it's virtually undetectable. "You'd be surprised at who's wearing hairpieces," says Acord.

Suggest he trying saving it with sage. Sage has had a long-standing reputation as a hair preserver. In the old days, people often used sage extract in hair rinses and shampoos. The herb allegedly had the ability to prevent hair loss and maintain color. Since this use of sage is unlikely to cause any harm, he can add a few teaspoons of sage tincture to his shampoo, suggests Dr. Duke.

Note: A tincture is a highly concentrated herbal liquid. It's made by soaking leaves in alcohol or glycerin—which extracts the herb's medicinal properties—for at least 6 weeks. Tinctures are sold in health food stores in small bottles with eyedroppers to give doses. Be sure to store them out of the reach of children.

Advise him to switch shampoos. If your husband's hair is thinning, he can try using a body-building or hair-repairing shampoo, suggests Dr. Greene. "These products often contain protein, which coats the hair and makes it appear thicker," he explains.

Have him try this restorative recipe. If he's up for it, he can make a hair oil that stimulates hair growth from the Ayurvedic herbs amla and ashwaganda, according to Partap Chauhan, an Ayurvedic physician in Haryana, India. Here's how. He should mix 1 ounce each of amla and ashwaganda herb (available through mail order) into a coarse powder (not a fine powder). Then he should combine the powder with 7 cups of water and soak overnight. The next day, he should boil the mixture until it's reduced by 75 percent. After that, he should strain it and add a small amount of sesame oil—approximately one-quarter the amount of the herb-water mixture. Then he should boil it again until everything evaporates and only the oil remains. Finally, he should let the oil cool, strain it, and bottle it. Some fragrance oils can be added at this time. He can massage the oil into his hair and scalp twice a week.

Encourage him to wear his hair short. "Men who are losing their hair tend to wear their hair the way they did when they were younger, to cling to a style that's just not working anymore," says Acord. "You have to face the problem and work with what you have." His recommendation is to go short, especially if the man has a receding hairline.

Suggest that he just accept it. Okay, if he's genetically predestined to lose his hair, there's not a lot he can do to prevent it. But he can prevent baldness from making him look or feel bad. He shouldn't shy away from baldness; he should embrace it and work with it. Perhaps he can grow facial hair; it'll offset the "dome effect." And if he's lost just about all his hair on top, he should consider shaving off the rest, suggests Acord. "I know a guy who shaved 15 years off his age when he shaved his head," he says. "He looks like a whole different guy."

Bursitis and Tendinitis

Trying to figure out whether your husband has a case of bursitis or of tendinitis requires a bit of detective work. Whether the culprit is a fluid-filled bursa or a wiry tendon, the first clue is in the pain. Is it sharp or dull?

Although bursitis and tendinitis are often lumped together, they are actually two distinct types of inflammation. A dull, persistent pain nagging at a joint could signal bursitis—swelling and inflammation of bursae, the small, fluid-filled sacs that help muscles and tendons glide smoothly and prevent them from becoming inflamed by friction from the underlying bone. If he has bursitis, the more he moves an afflicted

WHEN TO SEE THE DOCTOR

If he experiences increasing pain, swelling, weakness, or instability in any joint, he should consult a doctor to find out what's causing the problem.

joint, the more it hurts, says Andrew Cole, M.D., a physician in Seattle, Washington.

If he experiences a sharp pain triggered by movement, he may have tendinitis—inflammation of the tough, elastic fibrous tissue that connects muscles to bone. Like bursae, tendons generally become inflamed from repetitive motion, says Dr. Cole.

Tendons connect muscles to bone. When a muscle is contracted, it pulls on the tendon, which, in turn, moves the bone. Your husband may get tendinitis when he undertakes an activity that his tendons and muscles aren't accustomed to, such as throwing a Frisbee after a winter's layoff or playing baseball with the kids. Or it can come from repetitive motion, such as painting the house or computer mousing, says Alison Lee, M.D., a pain management specialist and acupuncturist with Barefoot Doctors, an acupuncture and natural-medicine resource center in Ann Arbor, Michigan. The bursa, which acts as a cushion between the bone and tendon, may become inflamed at the same time. He can also get recurrent bursitis from bone spurs, tiny but rough outgrowths that chafe and irritate the bursae, says Dr. Lee.

Rest is the first order of treatment for both bursitis and tendinitis. It's important, though, for your husband to see a doctor to find out which condition he has. Where bursitis responds better to moist heat, tendinitis generally is relieved by ice. These injuries take time, but they do heal on their own. In the meantime, he shouldn't repeat the offending activity. If he does, he'll get inflammation not only of the tendon but also of the sheath that houses the tendon. In the worst case, he could develop a long-lasting pain syndrome, says Dr. Lee.

Some Prescriptions for Your Pained "Patient"

Our experts suggest trying the following home treatments if your husband has bursitis or tendinitis.

Give him an ice massage. Tendinitis and bursitis pain generally are localized, so there's no need slap a big bag of ice over a large area. Instead, fill a paper cup with water, freeze it, peel off the upper edge to expose the ice, and then massage the ice up and down the tender area, says Jon Kluge, physical therapist, certified athletic trainer, and director of the Sports Injury Center in Waterloo, Iowa. Massage for 8 to 10 minutes until the skin is just reddened and numb to the touch.

Inhibit the inflammation. Your husband will get some pain relief and bring down the inflammation by taking an over-the-counter anti-inflammatory such as ibuprofen, following the package directions for dosage, says Kluge.

Treat him with boswellia. Boswellia, an extract from the frankincense tree, can relieve pain from chronic inflammatory conditions such as bursitis and tendinitis without causing unwanted side effects, says C. Leigh Broadhurst, Ph.D., a nutrition consultant and herbal researcher based in Clovery, Maryland. Research suggests that certain chemicals produced in this tree prevent the production of chemicals in our bodies that start the pain process. According to researchers, boswellic acid extract has been shown to prevent tissue breakdown and reduce the production of biochemicals that cause inflammation. Give your husband 400 to 500 milligrams of boswellia three times a day. As the pain lessens, give him the same dosage twice and then once a day, says Dr. Broadhurst. It's safe to take boswellia for 6 to 12 months. If his symptoms haven't improved by then, seek professional care.

Wrap it up. It's a good idea to give his sore tendon some support by wrapping it in an elastic bandage, says Dr. Lee. "The pressure of the bandage will hold down the swelling and probably make it feel better," she says. And the bandage will be a reminder that he's hurt, so he'll be more careful.

Apply some arnica. Arnica ointments and creams are available in health food stores and can be applied topically to the affected area, says Jill Stansbury, N.D., a naturopathic physician and chairperson of the botanical medicine department at the National College of Naturopathic

Medicine in Portland, Oregon. Rub arnica on the sore area two or three times a day. For best results when treating bursitis, cover the area with heat, such as a heating pad or hot water bottle, for as long as is comfortable after applying arnica. Arnica is thought to contain anti-inflammatory compounds.

Ease the pain with bromelain. Any type of inflammation heals faster with bromelain, says Jacqueline Jacques, N.D., a naturopathic physician in Portland, Oregon. An enzyme derived from the pineapple plant, bromelain helps us digest food when taken with meals. When taken on an empty stomach, it promotes circulation and reduces inflammation by inhibiting the release of inflammation-producing biochemicals called prostaglandins and thromboxanes. Patients who take bromelain report that they have less pain.

He won't get a healing dose of bromelain from a glass of pineapple juice. To get the right amount of the pineapple plant's healing enzyme, buy capsules of the standardized extract at a health food store. Have him take 500 milligrams 1 hour after meals three or four times a day. Bromelain strength is standardized in measurements called milk-clotting units (mcu) or gelatin-dissolving units (gdu), which indicate how much enzyme is needed to curdle milk or dissolve gelatin. Look for a product that has a strength between 1,200 and 2,400 mcu or between 720 and 1,440 gdu, says Dr. Jacques.

Bromelain, like other anti-inflammatory medications, is for acute injury. If he still has inflammation or pain after 2 to 3 weeks, consult a physician.

Suggest some stretches. Tendinitis is usually the result of tension in the muscles attached to a particular tendon, so you have to eliminate the tension in the muscle to relieve tendon pain, says James Waslaski, sports massage therapist at the Center for Pain Management and Clinical Sports Massage in Tampa, Florida. For example, advise him to try stretching his calf muscles if he has tendinitis in his Achilles tendon. Icing the inflamed and tight tendon will help the symptoms, but he needs to stretch regularly to address the underlying cause, says Waslaski.

Tell him to take manganese. When bursitis strikes, chronic inflammation can form waste products (oxidants) in the body. Dr. Lee recommends taking 50 to 100 milligrams per day of the mineral manganese in divided doses to help build up the body's antioxidant-fighting properties. Have him take this amount for 1 to 2 weeks, then cut back to 15 to

30 milligrams of manganese per day for up to a month if his pain persists. But after that, it's time to go back to an everyday-size dose of 2.5 to 5 milligrams of manganese per day, Dr. Lee says.

What to Do for a Chronic Condition

Here are some home remedies if he seems always to have pain.

Try tea. A gentle way to combat inflammation from chronic tendinitis and bursitis is to drink a tea made of ginger and sarsaparilla root, says David Winston, an herbalist in Washington, New Jersey.

"Ginger and sarsaparilla are both good systemic anti-inflammatory herbs," says Winston. "They're a good combination for chronic inflammation." For each 8-ounce mug of tea you'll need about 1 teaspoon of ground-up dried herbs, says Winston. Mix two parts sarsaparilla to one part ginger and steep for about 45 minutes. Give him three cups a day for several weeks, says Winston. Don't give him dried ginger without medical supervision if he has gallstones.

Oil him up. If your husband is prone to bursitis or tendinitis, keep a blend of the following oils on hand: St. John's wort, rosemary, juniper, eucalyptus, and chamomile. To make the blend, in a dark glass bottle mix 1 tablespoon of St. John's wort infused oil, 1 tablespoon of vegetable oil, 10 drops of rosemary essential oil, 6 drops of juniper essential oil, 5 drops of eucalyptus essential oil, and 4 drops of chamomile essential oil. Shake gently to mix. Rub the blend into the joint after you've applied a warm or cold compress. Use this blend three times a day to alleviate pain and swelling. It's safe to use this remedy indefinitely. The best St. John's wort oil is bright red, Dr. Stansbury says.

Give him curcumin. Curcumin, the powerful anti-inflammatory substance in the Indian herb turmeric, isn't a drug, but it can act like one, says Dr. Broadhurst. Although it has been used for thousands of years in India for cooking, dyeing, and medicinal uses, turmeric was largely overlooked in North America until the 1970s. When modern science finally took a closer look, the results were impressive. When compared to standard anti-inflammatory drugs, curcumin was found to be as effective or more effective in treating pain and inflammation. To relieve chronic pain and inflammation, give him 400 to 500 milligrams of extract three times a day. He can take turmeric for 6 to 12 months, Dr. Broadhurst adds.

Have him treat his tissues. Either of the botanical extracts grape seed or pine bark, when taken daily, will help strengthen and repair connective tissue between joints, which makes them especially helpful for tendinitis, says Dr. Jacques.

Packed with antioxidant activity 20 times more potent than that of vitamin C and 50 times greater than that of vitamin E, grape seed and pine bark extracts contain unique flavonols called proanthocyanidins. His body will quickly use these powerful antioxidants to heal inflamed tissues.

Grape seed and pine bark extract are extremely safe and nontoxic. Advise him to take a daily supplement of 30 to 60 milligrams of either one. At the dosages recommended here, they are safe to take indefinitely, says Dr. Jacques.

Get him simply to stop. If he's doing any activity that involves repetitive motion, he's prone to tendinitis, especially if he's not conditioned for the movement or hasn't warmed up adequately. Advise him that as soon as he feels pain in a specific area—an elbow, wrist, or knee—he should stop what he's doing because he's already doing damage, says Dr. Lee.

Pain is the body's signal to take it easy. It knows when enough is enough, and so should he.

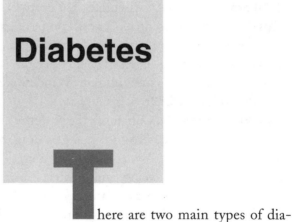

Diabetes

There are two main types of diabetes: type 1, or insulin-dependent diabetes mellitus; and type 2, or non-insulin-dependent diabetes mellitus. Type 1 accounts for 5 to 10 percent of diagnosed diabetes in the United States. Increased thirst and urination, constant hunger, weight loss, blurred vision, and extreme fatigue are all symptoms of type 1 diabetes. It develops most often in children and young adults but can appear at any age. A person with type 1 diabetes needs daily injections of insulin in order to live.

Type 2 diabetes accounts for 90 percent or more of diabetes cases. The symptoms for type 2 are similar to those of type 1, but they develop gradually and are less noticeable. Type 2 diabetes usually strikes people over age 40 and is most common after age 55. By then, other conditions are often thought to be responsible for the symptoms. If a man is over age 60 and needs to urinate frequently, he may think it's a prostate problem. Think again; it could be diabetes.

Both types of diabetes can be managed, but currently there is no cure for type 1 diabetes. People who inherit the potential for type 2 diabetes may be able to delay its onset and maintain normal blood glucose control by keeping active, maintaining a reasonable weight, and eating balanced meals throughout the day.

The Causes

Diabetes occurs because the pancreas, a large gland behind the stomach, produces no insulin (type 1) or the body cells don't produce enough insulin or don't respond to the insulin that is produced (type 2). Insulin is a hormone that moves glucose from our blood into our cells. Glucose is a simple sugar created by digestive juices and is the main

WHEN TO SEE THE DOCTOR

Contact your doctor if he has any symptoms of diabetes, including excessive thirst, frequent urination, unusual weight loss, or ravenous hunger. If he has already been diagnosed with diabetes, you both should work closely with your doctor when making any changes in his diet, exercise regimen, or nutritional and herbal supplement regimen. Even small changes can profoundly affect his blood sugar levels.

source of fuel for the body. In a person with diabetes, the glucose or blood sugar builds up in the bloodstream, spills into the urine, and passes out of the body, depriving the body of this vital fuel source. Type 1 diabetes is more common in Whites than in people of color, but African-Americans, Hispanics, and Native Americans and some Asian-Americans and Pacific Islanders are at greater risk for type 2.

Diabetes is a serious illness. It's estimated that diabetes costs the United States $98 billion annually in direct medical costs and in indirect costs such as lost wages, lost productivity, and premature death. Heart disease and stroke are two to four times more common in people with diabetes. It is the leading cause of new cases of blindness among people between ages 20 and 74. It can cause kidney and nerve disease, leading to kidney dialysis or transplantation and the amputation of lower limbs. Because men tend to be on their feet more and take care of their feet less, they tend to have more foot problems and amputations. People with diabetes have more frequent and more severe periodontal disease.

If all that doesn't scare your husband, maybe this will: Diabetes can rob men of their erections, or cause some loss of sensation so they'll need to be stimulated longer to get an erection. Sometimes these changes are irreversible. For men over age 50 with diabetes, the rates of impotence can be as high as 50 to 60 percent. Still, there are things you both can do at home to minimize the effects of diabetes.

Help Him Help Himself

Send him back to school. Diabetes school, that is. Men who have diabetes should learn all they can about the disease in order to manage it, says Frank Vinicor, M.D., director of the division of diabetes translation at the Centers for Disease Control and Prevention in Atlanta. Your husband should also learn to monitor his own blood sugar level at home and adjust his diet or insulin intake accordingly. "The doctor or nurse should become very much of a coach," says Dr. Vinicor. "People with diabetes are spending 99 percent of the time making decisions on their own."

Make him move. Exercise or less structured physical activity such as walking and gardening has a positive impact on blood sugar levels, says Dr. Vinicor. Being physically active helps people with type 2 diabetes lose weight, which is an important benefit because most people with type 2 diabetes are overweight. But it's also beneficial to those with type 1, who typically are of average weight or are thin, says Dr. Vinicor.

"The more fit a person is, the less insulin he needs to produce from his pancreas or get by injection," says Pat Schaaf, R.D., a research dietitian and diabetes educator at Stanford University's General Clinical Research Center. So try to encourage your husband to be more active. Although nagging him and playing the drill sergeant will probably get you nowhere, you could suggest that he try a favorite activity more often—bike riding, walking, hiking, or any other physical activity that he enjoys. Studies show that people stay more active doing things they enjoy, so think about what he likes before suggesting it to him. Or better yet, make it an activity you both will enjoy to get the added benefit of exercise for yourself and extra quality time for your relationship.

Encourage balance. People with diabetes are encouraged to eat balanced meals throughout the day for overall good nutrition, weight management, and control of blood sugar and fat levels, says Schaaf. What's not balanced eating? Skipping breakfast or lunch and overeating at dinner, or selecting foods from only one food group would be considered examples of unbalanced eating.

A person with diabetes should select a variety of foods from all food groups at every meal and throughout the day, Schaaf says. About 50 percent of each meal should be carbohydrates such as breads, cereals, rice, pasta, fruits, and vegetables. The rest should come from lean sources of protein—such as meat, poultry, fish, dry beans, eggs, and nuts—and from fat. Monounsaturated fats, such as olive oil and canola oil, and foods that contain them, such as olives, avocados, and nuts, are good sources of fat. For example, a balanced lunch could be a turkey sandwich on whole-grain bread with a couple slices of avocado and some lettuce and tomato with a glass of low-fat (less than 2 percent) or fat-free milk.

These are general guidelines. The exact percentages of carbohydrates, fats, and proteins need to be worked out on an individual basis with a dietitian. If your husband needs to lose weight to improve his blood glucose level, tell him not to eliminate meals or certain kinds of foods. He should just eat smaller portions, says Schaaf, especially at night, when most people overeat.

Get him some chromium. The mineral chromium may help regulate blood sugar levels, particularly if a person has a deficiency, says Dr. Vinicor. Deficiency is rare in the United States, but he could try a supplement of 200 micrograms a day. Still, before he tries any vitamin or mineral, you should check with his doctor, since it may affect the medication he's taking.

Herbal Helpers

Although herbs aren't substitutes for the fundamental changes in diet and lifestyle that he needs to make in order to control his diabetes, you can use herbs to help regulate his blood sugar. However, it is best to work with a practitioner who can develop a protocol specifically for him. Here are a few helpful herbs.

Make him bitter. Bitter melon is a traditional Asian remedy for diabetes. It is thought to help regulate blood sugar levels by slowing the absorption of glucose. According to Nancy Welliver, N.D., a naturopathic physician and director of the Institute for Medical Herbalism in Calistoga, California, studies suggest that bitter melon is most effective for type 2 diabetes and possibly early type 1. It's available in the United States at Asian markets. The recommended dose is 2 ounces of juice twice a day. You can make the juice by running the fruit through a juicer or by blending it with a little water until it is thin enough to drink. He can take bitter melon indefinitely at this dosage.

Have him try some ginseng. Known as a feel-good herb to boost vitality, Asian ginseng can help stabilize blood sugar levels of people with type 2 diabetes, says C. Leigh Broadhurst, Ph.D., a nutrition consultant and herbal researcher based in Clovery, Maryland. In a study in Finland, researchers found that a daily dose of 200 milligrams of ginseng for 8 weeks improved mood, diet, and activity, which reduced weight and helped lower blood sugar levels. Give him a daily dose of 200 milligrams in capsule form.

Help him Hindu-style. The leaves of *Gymnema sylvestre* (also known as gurmar) have been used in traditional Ayurvedic medicine from India as a treatment for diabetes, says Dr. Welliver. "It seems to enhance the production of insulin, possibly through the regeneration of beta cells of the pancreas," she says. That would make it appropriate for people with type 2 diabetes and even those with early type 1. The herb is safe to use on a regular basis, she says. Give him 400 milligrams in capsule form twice a day.

Add some spice to his life. The common spice cinnamon contains a phytochemical that helps people with type 1 or type 2 diabetes utilize blood sugar, says Dr. Broadhurst. In the past 10 years, researchers at the U.S. Department of Agriculture Beltsville Nutrient Requirements and Functions Laboratory in Maryland have tested 60 other medicinal and food plants looking for the same antidiabetes effect.

"Nothing has come close to the consistently excellent results of cinnamon," says Dr. Broadhurst. "Since the first report on cinnamon, hundreds of people have contacted the laboratory to say how cinnamon has helped them reduce their insulin or medication dosages." The recommended dose is 1 quart of cinnamon water every day. Seems like a lot, doesn't it? One way to make sure he gets the recommended dosage is to make a batch of this pleasant-tasting beverage and substitute it for part of his daily water intake. Add 3 tablespoons of cinnamon and 2 teaspoons of baking soda to 1 quart of boiling water. Reduce the temperature and simmer for 20 minutes, then strain the tea and store it in the refrigerator. He can drink it with breakfast, lunch, and dinner and easily consume a quart a day.

See if he'll try bilberry. French doctors have used bilberry since 1945 to prevent diabetic retinopathy. While the leaves of this European version of the blueberry lower blood sugar levels, the flavonoid-rich fruit has a potent antioxidant effect, which improves the circulation of blood in the eyes for those with both types of diabetes, says Dr. Welliver. Give him 80 milligrams of extract twice a day.

Flatulence

As unpleasant as it is, flatulence does serve a practical purpose: It's how the body gets rid of excess gas in the intestinal tract. The average person passes 1,500 milliliters of gas daily (about the amount of air in a half-inflated party balloon), released about 30 to 120 milliliters at a time. Flatus, the gas we pass via the rectum, is made of nitrogen, oxygen, carbon dioxide, hydrogen, methane, and trace amounts of other gases. Interestingly, the embarrassing odor that most of us can quickly identify as a "fart" is related to strong-smelling sulfur compounds that make up only 1 percent of flatus. Apart from its odor and embarrassing social consequences, flatulence itself is harmless and completely normal.

One common cause of flatulence is swallowed air, says Harris Clearfield, M.D., professor of medicine at Allegheny University of the Health Sciences–MCP Hahnemann School of Medicine in Philadelphia. People who chew gum or eat too quickly tend to gulp down a lot of air, which, of course, is made of gases. Most beers and sodas include lots of gases as well. Whatever the cause, gas builds up in the digestive tract. The body has to get rid of it either by belching or by passing it out the rectum.

The foods we eat, however, are often the more likely cause of flatulence, in particular fiber-rich foods such as broccoli, bran, and beans. Because these complex carbohydrates aren't fully digested in the small intestine, undigested bits travel to the colon, where they're fermented by bacteria, causing gas. For people who are lactose-intolerant, dairy products cause gas. Lactose intolerance is caused by a deficiency of lactase, an enzyme needed to break down the milk sugar lactose in the small intestine. Lactose is broken down by the bacteria that live in the colon, but gas is the unfortunate by-product.

Since flatulence is simply the body's way of ridding itself of gas, its presence doesn't usually signal a problem. Sometimes a problem with flatulence could simply be a "functional disorder," meaning that your husband's intestinal tract may not always function properly, leaving him uncomfortable but not at risk for serious disease.

Antigas Alternatives

Cure him with charcoal. Give him two activated charcoal capsules as needed. Purified and steamed, each bit of the porous activated charcoal helps trap intestinal gases in some people, says Roger Gebhard, M.D., professor of medicine at the University of Minnesota in Minneapolis.

Cultivate him. The active culture *Lactobacillus acidophilus* found in some yogurts—look for it on the label—not only digests the lactose in the yogurt but also may help to digest the lactose in other dairy products. To get the benefit, he needs to eat yogurt with acidophilus at the same meal with the other dairy products, says Dr. Gebhard.

Get him some aids. If cheese or milk products are chief offenders (and they are for some men), he doesn't necessarily have to give up pizza forever. Suggest that he try over-the-counter digestive aids such as Lactaid or Lactinex. They'll help digest lactose before it reaches the colon (where it ferments and causes gas), says Dr. Gebhard.

Eliminate it with enzymes. Beans, of course, are a gas giant among foods, but there's over-the-counter help for that, too. By dashing his food with the enzyme alpha-galactosidase (Beano), you can break down

WHEN TO SEE THE DOCTOR

If there's no apparent cause for his flatulence, if he can't trace it to a particular food, or if it stays with him for several weeks, have him get checked out by a doctor, who will want to rule out the possibility of any serious disorder.

the offending sugars in beans and avoid this unpleasant side effect of tasty dishes such as chili.

Give him papaya tablets. Papaya enzymes work by helping the body do the digestive tasks that it has trouble doing for itself, says Yvonne Tyson, M.D., a physician in Long Beach, California. The enzymes help break down foods that his gut may have trouble digesting, thus reducing the amount of gas that forms. You can buy papaya enzyme tablets in rolls like Tums or in a bottle. They come in different formulations, so check the package to see if the dose is appropriate for his symptoms. Give him one or two enzyme tablets after meals, or follow the package directions.

Suggest seeds instead. Fennel is classified as a carminative, says

recipe

ANTIGAS TEA

Perhaps your husband drinks coffee or tea on a regular basis already. Since he's used to having hot beverages over the course of the day, why not encourage him to drink something that can relieve excessive flatulence? This tea is packed with powerful carminatives, compounds that can blast that extra gas.

This particular mixture comes from Varro E. Tyler, Ph.D., Sc.D., distinguished professor of pharmacognosy at Purdue University in West Lafayette, Indiana. Have your husband drink it warm after every meal.

- 1   part dried chamomile
- 1   part dried peppermint
- 1   part dried valerian root
- 1   part caraway seeds
- 1   part aniseed

Combine the chamomile, peppermint, valerian, caraway, and anise in whatever amounts you choose. Many herbalists say that 1 ounce (28 grams) of herb can represent 1 part. To make a cup of tea, place 1 to 2 teaspoons of the mixture in a cup and add about 1 cup of boiling water. Steep for 10 minutes, then strain out the herbs.

Varro E. Tyler, Ph.D., Sc.D., distinguished professor of pharmacognosy at Purdue University in West Lafayette, Indiana. That means that it's a compound that expels gas and soothes the stomach. To get the gas out of his system, have him chew 1 teaspoon of fennel seeds after troublesome meals or simply after every meal if he's constantly plagued by gas. He should chew the seeds thoroughly before swallowing. You can find them at health food stores and well-stocked supermarkets.

Make him a cup of tea. Brew a tea with 1 to 2 teaspoons of anise or fennel seeds per cup of boiling water and steep for 10 minutes, suggests William Keller, Ph.D., chairman of the department of pharmaceutical sciences at Samford University in Birmingham, Alabama. Have him drink as much as he wants of this brew between meals, says Dr. Keller. Other gas-relieving teas, available ready-made in many supermarkets, include peppermint, ginger, and chamomile.

Preventive Measures

Tell him to swallow slowly. To avoid swallowing the excess air that could cause gas, advise him to try to slow down while he eats. If he does, he may be able to avoid flatulence in the first place, says Dr. Gebhard.

Recommend that he hold the cheese. Some adults who are lactose-intolerant experience some trouble digesting dairy products such as milk and cheese, says Dr. Clearfield. If you think your husband might be one of them, recommend to him that he limit the amount of dairy products he consumes, says Dr. Gebhard.

Advise him to say goodbye to gum. Gum chewing can lead to swallowing air and therefore to gastrointestinal distress, says Dr. Gebhard. The same goes for sucking on hard candies and the like. He should cut back on these candies and save his teeth while he avoids flatulence.

Have him be careful with carbonated drinks. Since drinking carbonated beverages can increase the amount of gas in his stomach, he should cut back on the amount of soda and beer he drinks, says Dr. Clearfield.

Gout

Gout has a long and distinguished hit list. Its many victims include King Henry VIII of England, Benjamin Franklin, the poet John Milton, and a 15th-century Florentine ruler so badly afflicted that he was nicknamed Piero the Gouty.

If your husband is in the midst of a gout flare-up, though, being in good company won't be of much comfort to him. Gout is a form of arthritis that starts when too much uric acid, one of the body's waste products, starts to collect in a joint, usually the big toe. Normally, this acid is excreted in urine, but when levels get too high, the excess can settle in the joints, forming needlelike crystals that cause swelling and pain. Although gout generally targets the toe or foot, it can affect other body parts, including the knee, the hand, the wrist, and even the ear. It may also be accompanied by chills, shivers, and a mild fever.

"The pain is excruciating," says Richard Brasington, M.D., director of clinical services in the division of rheumatology at Washington University School of Medicine in St. Louis. More than 1 million Americans have gout, and it's much more likely to affect men than women. In fact, three-quarters of those with gout are men between the ages of 45 and 50, says Doyt Conn, M.D., senior vice president of medical affairs for the Arthritis Foundation in Atlanta. "A gout sufferer is usually an overweight, hypertensive male who drinks too much," he adds.

For reasons that aren't yet completely clear to doctors, there are a few other things that can lead to gout attacks. "A person in the hospital who has suffered from an attack of gout in the past or is prone to gout is likely to suddenly suffer from a gout attack when admitted to the hospital for treatment or surgery," Dr. Conn says. "We think that the injury or surgery causes uric acid crystals to build up in the joint and then the stress of surgery somehow mobilizes the uric acid crystals in a painful way."

Gout attacks are acute (meaning that they come on suddenly and strongly and then the symptoms disappear), explains Dr. Brasington. But most people who have one episode will continue to get them over time. If there are more and more attacks, the pain will become chronic, he says.

"Even though gout has recognizable symptoms, only a doctor can diagnosis it," says Dr. Conn. "He'll take some liquid out of the joint, then put it under a microscope to see if there are uric crystals in it."

Fighting the Flare-Ups

Here are some ways you can offer relief to your husband if he suffers from gout.

Give him ibuprofen. Give him a prescription-strength dose of ibuprofen, says Dr. Brasington. "That means 800 milligrams four times a day," he says. You can try this for up to a week. The pain and redness should ease within a few hours, and he'll be completely better in a couple of days. Some people should not take such high doses of ibuprofen, so check with your doctor first. If your husband is currently taking blood thinners or has a heart condition or kidney disease, he should avoid high doses of ibuprofen, Dr. Brasington cautions.

Try a different anti-inflammatory. If ibuprofen doesn't help him, try giving him naproxen sodium (Aleve). It also helps relieve the pain and swelling. Give him up to five regular-strength tablets a day for up to a

WHEN TO SEE THE DOCTOR

If your husband has sudden swelling and tenderness in a joint, don't assume that it's gout. Have him see a doctor for a proper diagnosis. Even if he's had gout in the past and his physician has prescribed medication to take during an attack, he should consult his physician whenever he has a flare-up.

week, Dr. Brasington says. He should only take these higher doses if the doctor says that it's okay, he adds.

Apply ice. Wrap ice in a towel and place it on the painful joint for 20 minutes three times a day for several days, says Dr. Conn.

Have him drink lots of water. He should drink at least eight 8-ounce glasses of water a day to help flush the uric acid out of the kidneys, says Dr. Conn.

Put a compress on him. When gout attacks your husband, boil 2 quarts of water. Remove from the heat and grate a 2-inch piece of fresh ginger into the water. Cover and steep for 5 to 10 minutes. While the tea is still hot, but not so hot that you can't put your hand in it, soak a washcloth in the tea, wring it out, and apply it to his tender joint. Leave the cloth on until the heat dissipates, then immediately apply another cloth soaked in ice water. Leave the cold cloth on for 3 to 4 minutes, then reapply the hot cloth. Continue to alternate for about 15 minutes. As you're applying the treatment, keep the lid on the pot as much as possible so the tea stays hot.

Apply this hot/cold treatment every day until the swelling subsides, says Roy Upton, executive director of American Herbal Pharmacopeia, an herbal education foundation based in Santa Cruz, California. When using this treatment, always begin by applying the hot compress and end by applying the cold.

Defeat it with a duo. Bromelain, an enzyme found in pineapples, and quercetin, a bioflavonoid (a pigment in plants), are two natural remedies available in pill form at health food stores. Your husband should take 125 to 250 milligrams of each three times a day between meals when he experiences a flare-up, says Devra Krassner, N.D., a naturopathic physician from Portland, Maine. You can also add 1.8 grams of eicosapentaenoic acid (EPA) to this every day. EPA is a fatty acid found in foods.

Scientists have discovered that oils such as flaxseed oil and fish oils are rich in EPA (also known as omega-3 fatty acid), which is valued for its anti-inflammatory effects. Foods rich in EPA include green leafy vegetables, seeds (especially flaxseed), nuts, and grains. Some of the best seafood sources of EPA are anchovies, bluefin tuna, herring, mackerel, sardines, and all types of salmon except smoked. EPA is also available in pill and liquid form at health food stores.

Kill the pain with colchicum. "Colchicum is the homeopathic equivalent of colchicine, the prescription medicine that many Western doctors prescribe," Dr. Krassner says. "It may alleviate the acute pain of gout." Give him two or three pellets of the 12C or 30X potency two times a day until the pain subsides. If the pain continues for more than a week, a professional homeopath should be consulted. You can find this homeopathic remedy, which is specific to gout, in a well-stocked health food store.

Sting him a little. Apis, a homeopathic remedy made from bee venom, also is available at many health food stores. "Apis helps in conditions that mimic the symptoms of a bee sting, such as swelling, stinging pain, and heat," Dr. Krassner explains. Give him two or three pellets of a low potency, such as 12C or 30X, two or three times a day. If symptoms do not resolve in a week, a professional homeopath should be consulted, she adds.

Try giving him black cherry juice. Black cherry juice, which is available in health food stores as a concentrate, can help his body get rid of excess purines. Purines are substances in certain foods that can also cause gout in some people. The concentrated juice is very sweet, but you can dilute it with 8 ounces of water, says Jennifer Brett, N.D., a naturopathic physician in Stratford, Connecticut. It all depends on the extent of his sweet tooth. Give him 1 tablespoon of juice three times a day. This amount should be taken for acute gouty attacks until the pain subsides. For prevention, people generally take 1 tablespoon daily, she says.

Suggest taking horsetail to purge purines. The herb horsetail, a mild diuretic, also helps get rid of excess purines, Dr. Brett explains. Give him 60 drops of tincture per day or three 400- to 500-milligram capsules three or four times a day, or drink three cups of tea daily. Use these dosages for an acute attack until the pain and swelling subside. To make horsetail tea, use 1 tablespoon of loose dried herb for each cup of hot water. Steep for 10 to 20 minutes and strain before drinking.

To prevent attacks, give him two or three 400- to 500-milligram capsules or 20 drops of tincture a day. If he's taking capsules, remember that freshness is extremely important, Dr. Brett says. Check the date information on the container before buying.

Note: A tincture is a highly concentrated herbal liquid. It's made by soaking leaves in alcohol or glycerin—which extracts the herb's medicinal properties—for at least 6 weeks. Tinctures are sold in health food stores in small bottles with eyedroppers to give doses. Be sure to store them out of the reach of children.

Give him some celery seed. Celery seed is another cleansing herb, which means that it helps the body rid itself of wastes, including excess uric acid. Simply add 1 teaspoon of dried celery seed to 8 ounces of water and bring to a boil. Boil for 3 to 5 minutes, then steep for another 5 minutes. Dr. Brett doesn't recommend this as a preventive treatment because of the taste. She also cautions that since you'd need copious amounts of the spice to get the benefit of one cup of tea, simply adding celery seed to food during cooking probably isn't a good idea for treating gout. Have him drink a cup of tea once a day until the pain and swelling subside.

Stopping It Before It Starts

Advise him to watch how much meat he eats. Foods that are high in purine lead to high uric acid levels in the body. "Most people with gout eat a lot of meat, which is high in purines," Dr. Conn says.

Ask him to avoid alcohol. "Alcohol reduces the body's ability to get rid of uric acid," Dr. Conn says. "It's very important to avoid alcohol to possibly get rid of gout long-term."

Encourage him to lose weight little by little. Carrying too much weight can cause uric acid levels to build up, Dr. Conn says. "However, it's not advisable to go on a crash diet," he says. "Slow and steady weight loss not only will be more effective, it also will help keep gout from flaring up." (For tips on weight loss, see Abdominal Fat on page 161 and Overweight on page 445. Although the tips in the latter chapter are in the section for women, men can also use them effectively.)

Have him avoid aspirin. Low doses of aspirin may increase blood uric acid. If your husband is on a low-dose aspirin therapy for heart disease, you should talk to his doctor about the risk of getting gout. "It isn't an automatic cause-and-effect relationship," says Dr. Conn, "but it's a possible side effect to keep in mind."

Heart Disease

The number one killer of men, heart disease claims more lives each year than the next eight leading causes of death combined. The disease progresses as clogged, narrowed arteries fail to deliver enough blood to the heart, slowly suffocating the muscle. Though chest pain alerts some men early, nearly half of the men who die suddenly of heart disease have no previous symptoms.

Heart disease is the end result of a long chain of events. The chain starts with a diet high in fatty, protein-rich foods; low in fruits and vegetables; and low in vitamins. Eating this way raises the levels of low-density-lipoprotein (LDL, or "bad") cholesterol and triglycerides (fatty substances that can irritate the lining of artery walls) circulating in the blood. It also increases levels of a molecule called homocysteine, which can damage arteries, encourage plaque growth, and promote clotting. Though researchers are still unraveling exactly how LDL, triglycerides, and homocysteine interact, they suspect that the substances embed themselves in the artery walls, irritating and injuring them. The immune system then tries to repair the damage by pasting over the injured sections. Such repair work results in hardened plaque along the artery wall. The plaque increases over time, narrowing the artery and restricting bloodflow. Sometimes sections of the plaque completely block bloodflow, causing a heart attack.

Heart Helpers

Now you know how the enemy operates. Here are some practical suggestions from experts to help your husband keep his heart healthy or fight heart disease if he already has it.

Give him a couple of beers a day. This is probably the one tip in this book he'll start using right away. It seems like crazy advice, but according to studies, two bottles of dark beer a day offer the amount of anticlotting, vitamin-like flavonoids that may help keep his arteries clear. Flavonoids are found in hops—the ingredient that gives beer its bitter taste. Some paler, hoppy beers such as India Pale Ale may have just as many flavonoids as darker beers, but no one has tested them to find out, says John D. Folts, Ph.D., professor of medicine and director of the coronary thrombosis laboratory at the University of Wisconsin Medical School in Madison.

India Pale Ale aside, the brewing process usually filters much of the flavonoids from paler beers. So he'd have to drink much more Budweiser to get the same effect he'd get from a dark beer like Guinness. The problem is that drinking too much beer or other types of alcohol can raise the blood pressure. So make sure you explain to him that although he can enjoy this "medicine" to keep heart disease at bay, he needs to limit himself to two 12-ounce dark beers a day and nothing more.

Juice him. Drinking one 12-ounce glass of purple grape juice will slow the level of platelet activity in the blood within a few hours. If we regularly consume something that slows down platelet activity, it should reduce the risk of a heart attack, says Dr. Folts. Other grape products such as red wine do the same. Daily intake of grape juice would probably be best, says Dr. Folts.

Go with an old health standby—fruits and vegetables. Fruits and vegetables contain numerous substances that counteract the artery-clog-

WHEN TO SEE THE DOCTOR

If you or your husband suspects that he has heart disease, consult a physician. If he has any symptoms of a heart attack—chest pain, nausea, radiating pain to the jaw or arm—take him immediately to the emergency room, advises Kilmer McCully, M.D., pathologist at the Department of Veterans Affairs Medical Center in Providence, Rhode Island.

ging process. Scientists have yet to isolate all of the anticlogging fruits and vegetables, though they suspect that grapes, apples, and onions may top the list. Produce is naturally high in fiber, a substance that may block cholesterol and triglycerides from making their way into the arteries. Encourage him to eat five to seven servings of produce every day, Dr. Folts says. You can work them into breakfast, when you make his lunch, and when you cook dinner. Any whole fruit or vegetable, a half-cup of chopped produce, an 8-ounce glass of fruit juice, and a cup of leafy greens each count as one serving.

Teach him how to handle stress. Stress damages the arteries, makes the blood clot, and may even raise blood pressure. He probably can't eliminate stress, but he can change his reaction to it. For instance, take the typical commute. "Certainly, you need to be alert and aware to avoid an accident," says Michael Babyak, Ph.D., professor of medical psychology at Duke University Medical Center in Durham, North Carolina. "But you can learn to expect what happens during the commute. Sometimes people are going to cut you off. Sometimes you're going to sit in traffic. Sitting behind the steering wheel clenching your fists and stewing isn't going to change anything."

Instead, advise him to try and focus his mind on something else—for instance, what he feels like eating for lunch. Also, adds Dr. Babyak, stressed people should pay attention to breathing and muscle tension. Tell him to "slow his breathing down and relax his muscles."

Make sure he eats fish. Eating a lot of fish may reverse and prevent heart disease by inhibiting clotting and lowering levels of triglycerides, says William S. Harris, Ph.D., professor of medicine at the University of Missouri in Kansas City.

Fish's heart-healing properties probably come from high amounts of omega-3 fatty acids, an oil mostly found in fattier fish such as mackerel, salmon, and herring. Studies have yet to determine how much fish oil does the trick, Dr. Harris says. But it'd be better for him to eat at least three 3-ounce fish servings a week, Dr. Harris says. Keep in mind that shellfish and whitefish are not good sources of omega-3 fatty acids. He'll need fatty fish to keep his arteries clear.

Encourage him to exercise. Regular exercise can help keep the arteries clear and decrease the risk of heart disease. And he doesn't have to spend thousands of dollars on a posh health club membership to get the benefits. Taking a quick walk for 20 minutes a day can make a huge difference, experts say. Stair climbing, moderate sports, and even gardening are all good ways to get regular exercise. "Diet is the most important factor in reducing the risk of heart disease, but exercise complements it by controlling weight gain, lowering homocysteine levels, and raising high-density-lipoprotein (HDL, or 'good') cholesterol levels," says Kilmer McCully, M.D., pathologist at the Department of Veterans Affairs Medical Center in Providence, Rhode Island.

Suggest tea instead of coffee. Drinking a lot of coffee—nine or more cups a day—can raise levels of homocysteine. On the other hand, drinking any kind of tea can lower homocysteine levels because tea contains folate, says Dr. McCully.

In addition to lowering homocysteine levels, drinking four to five cups of green or black tea a day can provide the arteries with protective flavonoids to help keep cholesterol from sticking to the sides, Dr. Folts says. Tea has approximately half the caffeine content of coffee. So if he usually drinks two cups of coffee a day, four cups of tea will keep him just as alert.

Cut the fat out of your kitchen. The American Heart Association recommends limiting fat intake to less than 30 percent of daily calories. Some evidence, however, suggests that the less fat—particularly animal fat—the better. For the past 20 years, Dean Ornish, M.D., president and director of the nonprofit Preventive Medicine Research Institute in Sausalito, California, has studied how fat and heart disease interact. He recommends limiting fat intake to 10 percent of the daily calories consumed.

"Several studies have shown that the majority of people with coronary heart disease who only make moderate changes in their diet and lifestyle (including lowering their fat content to 30 percent) show worsening of their coronary artery disease. They get worse more slowly than if they made no changes, but they still get worse. On the other hand, our studies indicate that if you reduce fat and cholesterol much further, when combined with other lifestyle changes, you are likely to see a reversal in the progression of coronary artery disease," says Dr. Ornish.

To cut fat, replace high-fat foods—such as milk, cheese, and mayonnaise—with their low-fat counterparts. Instead of beef, cook more chicken and turkey. And if you do buy beef, buy cuts such as round and top round, which are lower in fat. When cooking, bake foods instead of frying them. Try to avoid using vegetable or corn oils and use no-stick olive oil or canola oil cooking sprays; these two oils are rich in mono-unsaturated fat, which is heart-healthy. Also, read those food labels. Check to see how much fat foods have. If possible, try to keep your husband's fat intake between 55 and 80 grams a day. Obviously, you can't watch him all the time, but if you're label-conscious—and can train him to be—you'll have a good shot at keeping him within this range. While all these changes won't ensure that your husband only gets 10 to 30 percent of his calories from fat, they will at least help him reduce his fat intake significantly and take better care of his heart.

Let him have that peanut butter and jelly sandwich. Peanut butter may actually be good for the heart. It turns out that peanut butter is rich in vitamin E, a powerful antioxidant that prevents LDL cholesterol from embedding in the walls of the arteries. "LDL particles carry cholesterol around your arteries," explains Lawrence Kushi, Sc.D., associate professor of public health, nutrition, and epidemiology at the University of Minnesota School of Public Health in Minneapolis. "If LDL particles get oxidized, they can damage the arteries a lot easier. Vitamin E helps prevent oxidation."

Eating more nuts and vegetable oils will boost vitamin E levels, Dr. Kushi says. True, both sources also contain a bunch of fat. But the fat found in nuts and vegetable oils does not clog arteries as does the type of fat found in animal products.

Another way to get enough vitamin E is with supplements. Dr. Kushi recommends 200 IU taken daily.

Fortify him with folate. The body needs three B vitamins—folate, B_6, and B_{12}—to activate important enzymes responsible for breaking down and disposing of excessive levels of homocysteine. Without those vitamins, the homocysteine levels rise, damaging the arteries and causing plaque growth and clotting.

He probably gets plenty of B_{12} from his normal diet. But folate and B_6 are another story. Men should be sure to get the Daily Value of 400 micrograms of folate, says Dr. McCully. And they should shoot for 3.5 milligrams of B_6 daily, almost double the Daily Value. Good sources of folate include green leafy vegetables, orange juice, and beans. Good sources of B_6 include bananas, nuts, grains, and fish.

Hemorrhoids

Once upon a time, when the Philistines met the Israelites on the battlefield, they got more than they bargained for. Although they defeated the Israelites, they still suffered casualties. It turns out that after the Philistines won the battle described in the Book of Samuel, they celebrated by taking the Ark of the Covenant, a sacred chest representing the presence of God among the Israelites. Little did they know how much this displeased God. Their celebrations were cut short when the heavy hand of the Lord smote them all with hemorrhoids.

Perhaps your husband can empathize with the Philistines. Sometimes, hemorrhoids can make him feel like a great power has taken hold of his hinder parts. There's pain when he moves his bowels, and often he may find bright red blood in the toilet. In the worst cases, bleeding can continue slowly throughout the day.

Hemorrhoids occur when the many veins in the rectum become stretched, swollen, and inflamed. Basically, they're like the varicose veins that you see on people's legs, except that they're in a far more sensitive spot. And the rich supply of nerves around the rectum lets you know clearly that hemorrhoids are there. In some cases, such as with large or chronic hemorrhoids, conventional medical intervention may include removing them surgically.

There are two types of hemorrhoids: internal and external. Internal hemorrhoids are inside the anus. Typical symptoms are blood covering a stool, on toilet paper, or in the toilet bowl. You can't see or feel internal hemorrhoids except in the case of a protruding or prolapsed hemorrhoid, which can push through the anal opening and cause a dull ache, itch, or bleeding. External hemorrhoids may include painful swelling or a hard lump around the anus that occurs when a blood clot forms. If irritated, they can itch and bleed.

Common causes of hemorrhoids are constipation; excessive straining, rubbing, or cleaning around the anus; obesity; and lifting heavy objects. Standing or sitting for long periods can cause flare-ups. There may also be a hereditary factor.

Fortunately, hemorrhoids aren't a serious problem. "Hemorrhoids never turn to cancer," says James Surrell, M.D., a colorectal surgeon at the Ferguson Clinic in Grand Rapids, Michigan. "They're more of a nuisance." Dr. Surrell emphasizes, however, that whenever there is rectal bleeding, it should be evaluated by a doctor. Rectal bleeding is always abnormal, he says; it could be a symptom of colorectal cancer or other serious problems.

Nuisance Neutralizers

Here's how Mom's Medicine can help if your husband suffers from hemorrhoids.

Tell him to soak for a while. Taking warm baths for 10 to 15 minutes several times a day relaxes the sphincter muscle and allows protruding hemorrhoids to recede back into places less painful, says Lester Rosen, M.D., professor of clinical surgery at the Milton S. Hershey Medical Center in Hershey, Pennsylvania.

Advise him to try cortisone cream. Over-the-counter topical steroid creams containing cortisone can help relieve itching but should be used

WHEN TO SEE THE DOCTOR

If home remedies simply don't work or the hemorrhoids worsen over a period of several weeks, get your husband to the doctor. There are simple outpatient procedures that can get rid of the worst cases. Although it's common with hemorrhoids to see bright red blood on the toilet paper or on stool, it is best to have any rectal bleeding evaluated by the doctor.

only for a few weeks, says Dr. Rosen. They can thin the skin, making it more susceptible to cracking and bleeding if used excessively, he cautions. Your husband can go back to using them several months later.

Recommend that he fiber up. Over-the-counter fiber supplements and stool softeners containing psyllium and methylcellulose can be effective when taken with a meal, Dr. Rosen says. Two examples of fiber supplements are Metamucil, which contains psyllium, and Citrucel, which contains methylcellulose. Dr. Rosen recommends taking them with breakfast or lunch to relieve constipation and excessive straining, which can lead to hemorrhoids. Taking these kinds of supplements every day would be a good habit for anyone who has experienced constipation problems in the past, he advises.

Also, it's important for your husband to get more fiber in his diet. Fiber-rich foods such as fruits, vegetables, seeds, nuts, and legumes can soften stools and make them easier to pass, says Dr. Rosen. He recommends at least 20 grams of fiber per day. Your husband will get about 2 grams of fiber per serving from each of the foods listed above, and a serving of an all-bran type cereal would account for another 5 to 10 grams, Dr. Rosen says. You and your husband should check the nutrients listing on the food package to get the exact amounts. Dr. Rosen suggests slowly building up fiber intake. Too much too fast can cause bloating and cramps.

Make sure he gets his fluids. Fluids help move what we've eaten through the digestive tract and soften stools, says Eric G. Weiss, M.D., staff colorectal surgeon and director of surgical endoscopy at Cleveland Clinic Florida in Fort Lauderdale. He recommends that your husband drink eight to ten 10-ounce glasses of alcohol-free, caffeine-free fluids a day to help him stay regular and avoid painful hemorrhoids. Beverages containing alcohol and caffeine act as diuretics, causing him to lose fluids, so he should avoid drinking too much of them.

Encourage him to exercise. Regular exercise helps maintain bowel regularity, Dr. Rosen says. So guys with hemorrhoids should walk a mile or two, bike, or do some kind of aerobic activity every day. "Walking and exercise will help tone the abdominal muscles," he says. "That usually makes for more regular people."

Soothe the irritation with witch hazel. Soaking a piece of toilet paper or cotton in witch hazel and applying it to the affected area works for some people, Dr. Rosen says. "Some people say that it burns; others say that it's soothing," he says. "If someone has very irritated hemorrhoids that are open and bleeding, witch hazel doesn't usually work well. With hemorrhoids that are pushing out and are a little irritated and itching, witch hazel works." As long as it soothes, he can apply it several times a day.

Consider comfrey to speed healing. Comfrey is rich in allantoin, an anti-inflammatory agent that promotes healing, says Connie Catellani, M.D., medical director of the Miro Center for Integrative Medicine in Evanston, Illinois. Comfrey also contains mucilage, which soothes the irritation associated with hemorrhoids. At the pharmacy or at a health food store, look for a topical balm made with comfrey, she suggests. Apply it as needed. Alternatively, your husband can moisten powdered comfrey with a little bit of vegetable oil and apply it with a cotton ball or his fingers, as long as they're clean. He can then leave it on until the next time he bathes.

Tell him that A-L-O-E can spell relief. Applying an aloe gel can supply hemorrhoid relief, says Andrew Weil, M.D., director of the program in integrative medicine at the University of Arizona in Tucson. Your husband should use a pure gel, with no additives, which can be found in most drugstores. He can apply a small amount several times a day.

Encourage him to switch to a new reading room. If your husband likes to read in the bathroom for long periods, he should stop. With the legs open and knees up, this position can cause slippage of hemorrhoids, says David Beck, M.D., chairman of the department of colorectal surgery at the Ochsner Clinic in New Orleans.

That's not all. "People who sit on the hopper and strain a lot and push and just can't go are better off getting off," says Dr. Rosen. "I think if you don't go within 10 minutes, you probably should leave and try again later."

Tell him he should be wary of dairy. Dairy products such as cheese, chocolate, ice cream, and milk can make people constipated, causing straining on the toilet that can aggravate hemorrhoids, says Dr. Rosen.

High Blood Pressure

One in three American men has high blood pressure, which can prematurely wear out the heart as well as damage artery walls. When blood surges through vessels, it erodes material from the artery walls, much the same way a river slowly erodes its bed. Immune cells rush in to repair the damage, leaving a thick, hard paste behind. This clogs the arteries (as can high-fat foods), forcing the heart to beat harder to squeeze blood through a narrower opening, causing further damage.

Blood pressure is measured with two numbers: systolic (the high number) and diastolic (the low number). The systolic pressure measures how hard the heart must beat to pump blood through the body. The diastolic measures the pressure when the heart relaxes between contractions. A pressure reading of 120/80 is considered optimal, and 140/90 is viewed as high.

The two most common causes of high blood pressure are age and narrowed arteries. As we get older, our arteries naturally get more ridged, making our hearts beat harder. Also, years of high-fat foods increase levels of blood cholesterol, which irritate the artery lining, resulting in plaque buildup. Drugs such as nicotine can also constrict arteries. The less room blood has to flow through, the more the heart has to push to move the blood along. "If the heart has to pump through pipes the size of the Hudson River, it doesn't have to push much to get the blood out. But if the heart has to push blood through something the size of the lead in a pencil, it's going to push pretty hard," says Peter M. Abel, M.D., director of cardiovascular disease and prevention at the Cardiovascular Institute of the South in Morgan City, Louisiana. Stress also can make blood pressure soar by dumping heart-stimulating hormones into your system.

Though do-it-yourself machines at drugstores can give you an approximate measure of your blood pressure, the only way to get an accurate reading is to see a health professional. Because high blood pressure can cause stroke and heart attack, your husband should consult a doctor. Once he hits 140/90, serious health problems such as stroke or heart attack become likely, Dr. Abel says.

Pressure Control

Here are some ways you can help your husband control his blood pressure.

Tell him to shake a leg. Exercise relaxes and dilates the blood vessels, creating less resistance for the heart to push against. After exercise, the blood vessels are wide open. If your husband wants some low blood pressure numbers, have him take his blood pressure right after he exercises, says Dr Abel. Consistent exercise can also permanently lower blood pressure. Tell him he needs to get his heart pumping for a half-hour to an hour three to five times a week.

Advise him to lose weight to lower pressure. The heart is like a pump that's designed to keep a medium-size home stocked with liquid. Being overweight is like hooking that pump up to a condominium complex instead of a medium-size home. "Fat is alive. Fat is very vascular. It needs blood. So having extra fat makes the heart do extra work," Dr. Abel says. To quickly estimate your husband's healthy weight, grab a calculator. Multiply his weight in pounds by 700, divide that number by his height in inches, then divide again by his height. If the answer is 25 or above, he's overweight. Dropping just 10 percent of those pounds will do his blood pressure some serious good.

WHEN TO SEE THE DOCTOR

Your husband should have his blood pressure checked by a doctor or other health professional at least once every 2 years. If it's higher than 140/90, the doctor will probably want to monitor it more often.

Make sure he eats his fruits and vegetables. Researchers have long suspected that nutrients found in both fruits and vegetables—such as magnesium, fiber, and potassium—could lower blood pressure. The problem is that supplement pills that provide the nutrients typically do not reduce blood pressure. The only exception is potassium supplements. In one study, instead of supplements, researchers fed people foods naturally high in these nutrients. In the people with high blood pressure, systolic blood pressure dropped 7.2 points and diastolic blood pressure dropped 2.8. "We don't know if it is the potassium, magnesium, or fiber. What we can say is that fruits and vegetables can be beneficial even in persons with lower levels of blood pressure," says Lawrence Appel, M.D., a study coauthor and professor of medicine at Johns Hopkins University School of Medicine in Baltimore.

To get the same benefit, says Dr. Appel, your husband will need to work into his diet 8 to 10 daily servings of fruits and vegetables, which is more than double the national average and three servings more than the minimum government recommendation. Any whole fruit or vegetable, a half-cup of chopped produce, an 8-ounce glass of fruit juice, or a cup of leafy greens all count as one serving.

Advise him to get his daily doses of dairy. People who ate 8 to 10 daily servings of vegetables saw even larger blood pressure drops when they improved their diet in other ways. This diet provided two to three servings of low-fat dairy products a day. (A cup of fat-free milk or yogurt equals one serving.) A diet this low in fat and rich in dairy products further reduced blood pressure by an additional 4.1 points systolic and 2.6 points diastolic. He should stick with low-fat foods and eat and drink dairy products rather than calcium supplements.

Play it safe with salt. You probably have read about various studies on sodium restriction that produced conflicting results. The truth is that some people are salt-sensitive. Doctors really have no sure way of figuring out who is. So stay on the safe side by banning the shaker from the table and having him cut back on high-salt foods such as canned soups, Dr. Abel says.

Say goodbye to aspartame. This artificial sweetener can cause mood swings, which can raise blood pressure. Also, each time we drink a diet soda laced with aspartame, the amino acids phenylamine and aspartic acid are dumped into the blood. This is what causes the fluctuations in our blood sugar levels. If your husband abuses aspartame (drinking six to eight diet sodas a day), he can eventually become prone to insulin resistance, a condition that can lead to even higher blood pressure, says Stephen T. Sinatra, M.D., director of the New England Heart Center in Manchester, Connecticut.

Encourage him to get some of this kitchen cure. "Garlic is a good example of something that's common in the diet and also helpful as a botanical medicine," says George Milowe, M.D., a holistic physician in Saratoga Springs, New York. "Studies have shown that it actually lowers blood pressure."

If his blood pressure is at an acceptable level and you want to keep it that way, have him eat a clove of garlic every day—preferably raw—alone or as flavoring in some other dish. That will definitely help, says Robert Rountree, M.D., a holistic physician at the Helios Health Center in Boulder, Colorado. "If he already has high blood pressure, though, he needs something more potent," he says.

He can get that potency by taking four to six 600-milligram capsules or tablets a day in divided doses. Although that sounds like a simple suggestion, things can get a little confusing, because what's actually in those tablets or capsules depends on a wide array of processing methods. And the array of arguments about which process is best is just as wide.

Dr. Rountree recommends cutting through the controversy by finding a garlic product that's standardized for allicin, the beneficial natural constituent of garlic. It may be in the form of substances that convert to allicin in the body, so your husband will need to measure his dose in "allicin potential." Dr. Rountree suggests taking capsules that provide 8,000 micrograms of allicin potential daily. He'll probably need to keep taking this dosage for at least a month before seeing results. It's safe to take garlic indefinitely.

Consider hawthorn. The leaves, berries, and flowers of the hawthorn tree get standing ovations for their cardiovascular health benefits. Does that include helping to lower elevated blood pressure? You bet. "Hawthorn is one of the most commonly used herbs for hypertension," says Ian Bier, N.D., Ph.D., a naturopathic physician in Portsmouth, New Hampshire. "It's very powerful, yet very gentle. It takes a while, but it works." Actually, hawthorn works a lot like conventionally prescribed medications, but it does so naturally and without side effects. For high blood pressure, look for hawthorn standardized for a specific flavonoid (a natural plant nutrient) known as vitexin, Dr. Rountree says.

Your husband should take two 500-milligram capsules or 1 teaspoon of tincture three times a day. The liquid extract of hawthorn in tincture form is not as potent as capsules, he says, but if your husband prefers that form, put a teaspoon in some water and have him drink it three times a day.

If he has been diagnosed with high blood pressure or other cardio-vascular condition, he should not take hawthorn regularly for more than a few weeks without medical supervision. He should also have his blood pressure checked at least every 2 weeks. When it starts to come down, he should take one 500-milligram capsule or ½ teaspoon of tincture three times a day, then reduce it to twice a day.

Note: A tincture is a highly concentrated herbal liquid. It's made by soaking leaves in alcohol or glycerin—which extracts the herb's medic-inal properties—for at least 6 weeks. Tinctures are sold in health food stores in small bottles with eyedroppers to give doses. Be sure to store them out of the reach of children.

Suggest he try an oriental option. There's an all-star lineup of ori-ental mushrooms that natural and holistic physicians prescribe for lots of things. The best one for high blood pressure is reishi. "I recommend reishi a lot for blood pressure, both as a tonic (long-term preventive) and as a medicinal," Dr. Rountree says. "It's a direct blood pressure reducer, it's very safe, and it has all kinds of other benefits, too."

Have your husband take 2,000 to 4,000 milligrams daily in capsule form. You can get reishi capsules at health food stores or by mail order. Dr. Rountree suggests finding them in concentrations that are strong enough to let him take 2 to 4 grams (2,000 to 4,000 milligrams) daily without having to swallow too many capsules. It's safe to take this dose forever.

Try motherwort to take off some pressure points. Traditional Chi-nese Medicine uses the flowering herb motherwort extensively for con-trolling blood pressure. "It has a calming effect and also directly lowers blood pressure," Dr. Rountree says. Motherwort is easily found in health food stores as a tincture. A typical dose, according to Dr. Rountree, is two to three dropperfuls a day on an ongoing basis. You can mix it with a glass of water or have him drink it straight.

Give him a combination of cures. Ginkgo is best known as a brain herb, but it has cardiovascular benefits as well, including mild blood-pressure-lowering effects. "Ginkgo dilates the peripheral vessels, and anything that does that will automatically bring the pressure down by giving the blood more room to move through," Dr. Bier says. "I would definitely throw it into a formula with hawthorn." Dr. Bier recommends making your own formula from the tinctures, using twice as much hawthorn as ginkgo. Just buy a 1-ounce bottle of ginkgo and a 2-ounce bottle of hawthorn and pour the two together. Mix the resulting formula in a little water and give him a teaspoon of this tincture three times a day.

High Cholesterol

A fatlike substance that circulates in the blood, cholesterol is deposited in and irritates artery walls, causing plaque buildup. Once enough plaque accumulates, clots form more easily, blocking bloodflow and potentially causing heart attack or stroke. Not all cholesterol is created equal. Low-density lipoprotein (LDL) is the villain responsible for artery damage. High-density lipoprotein (HDL) is considered good because it carries cholesterol from the different organs to the liver for excretion from the body. The lower the LDL and the higher the HDL, the better.

Our bodies are capable of making all the cholesterol we need. (Yes, some cholesterol is needed to manufacture hormones.) So when we eat cholesterol-raising foods and live a cholesterol-raising lifestyle, we end up with far more cholesterol in our blood than our bodies could ever use, says James Cleeman, M.D., coordinator of the National Cholesterol Education Program in Bethesda, Maryland. The excess builds up in the arteries. Among the factors we can control, saturated fat is the worst cholesterol-raiser, closely followed by dietary cholesterol, inactivity, and being overweight.

Genetic makeup may also predispose a person to high blood cholesterol. Some people are born with fewer or less efficient LDL receptors than others. That means that their bodies can't remove excess LDL from their circulatory systems as well as they should. Some of these people can still lower their levels with diet and lifestyle changes, but they must be especially vigilant, Dr. Cleeman says. Others have to add medication to their diet and lifestyle regimens to lower cholesterol levels sufficiently.

"If somebody has high blood cholesterol when they're a teenager or when they're in their twenties, they'll have a higher risk of heart attack 30 to 40 years later," Dr. Cleeman says. "They should lower their levels as soon as possible. Otherwise, they'll end up in middle age, when, although cholesterol lowering is still worthwhile, it won't reduce the risk as much—or, at worst, it may literally be too late." So advise your husband to get his cholesterol checked at least once every 5 years.

The diet and lifestyle tips in this chapter will be your first resort in helping your husband lower his cholesterol levels. But if his LDL levels stay above 190 milligrams per deciliter despite your best efforts, you should talk to the doctor about cholesterol-lowering medication, even if he has no other heart disease risk factors, says Dr. Cleeman. If he does have two or more risk factors, consider medication if his levels stay above the 160 mark. And if he has heart disease or artery blockages, consider medication whenever his LDL levels are at the 130 mark or above. If he's younger than 35, his LDL levels should be 220 or higher before taking medication to reduce the risk of long-term side effects.

Resources for Reducing Cholesterol

Give him some garlic. It doesn't matter whether it's raw, pickled, fried, sautéed, or made into a pill; garlic's organosulfur compounds lower cholesterol levels, says Stephen Warshafsky, M.D., professor of medicine at New York Medical College in Valhalla, New York. The more garlic he eats, the better. Eating a half-clove to a whole clove a day can lower cholesterol levels 5 to 10 percent in just 3 months. And eating 10 cloves a day can lower levels 21 percent over the same period. That said,

Key Heart-Healthy Changes

High blood cholesterol is just one of many heart attack risk factors. In descending order, here's how much a man can lower his risk of heart attack by lowering cholesterol and making other dietary and lifestyle changes, according to Peter M. Abel, M.D., director of cardiovascular disease and prevention at the Cardiovascular Institute of the South in Morgan City, Louisiana.

- Stop smoking: Risk drops 50 to 70 percent

- Exercise: Risk drops 45 percent

- Maintain an ideal weight: Risk drops 35 to 55 percent

- Take an aspirin a day: Risk drops 33 percent

- Consume one alcoholic drink a day: Risk drops 25 to 45 percent (Excessive alcohol consumption, however, increases your heart disease risk, says Dr. Abel.)

- Lower cholesterol levels 1 percent: Risk drops 2 to 3 percent

- Lower blood pressure 1 point: Risk drops 2 to 3 percent

garlic breath is not the best thing in the world for your love life. But if he takes enteric-coated garlic capsules, he'll be able to get garlic's cholesterol-reducing benefit and keep his kissing privileges.

Feed him fiber. In the body, soluble fiber forms a protective gel that keeps cholesterol from getting absorbed in the intestine, Dr. Cleeman explains. Eating 10 grams of soluble fiber a day (a cup of cooked oat bran, one orange, a cup of navy beans, and one baked potato) can lower blood cholesterol levels by 5 to 10 percent, he says.

Serve him some soy. Eating 20 to 25 grams of soy protein each day can lower blood cholesterol levels by up to 10 percent, according to one study. To get soy's cholesterol-lowering effect, you don't have to force-feed him tofu, says Carla Green, R.D., a research dietitian at the University of Kentucky in Lexington. Instead, try the following methods to make sure he gets more soy in his diet.

- Suggest he try various types of soy milk with his cereal (some taste better than others).

- Substitute half of the white flour in baked goods with soy flour.

- Mix textured soy protein, which you can find in health food stores, with tomato sauce.

- Hide tofu in other recipes, such as stir-fries, soups, and pasta casseroles. For instance, make a tofu mousse by pureeing a box of tofu with ¾ cup of chocolate chips and ½ teaspoon of vanilla.

For 20 to 25 grams, he'll need to drink a cup of soy milk, have a couple of soy muffins, and eat some tofu stir-fry for dinner, says Green.

Spice up his meals. Chiles contain the oil capsaicin, which can keep LDL cholesterol from sticking to the sides of the arteries, says Stephen T. Sinatra, M.D., director of the New England Heart Center in Manchester, Connecticut. "A little goes a long way," he warns. Add some ground red pepper and other pepper spices to your husband's favorite foods and watch his cholesterol numbers fall.

Try to get him going. Exercise raises levels of the good HDL cholesterol, which shuttles artery-clogging LDL cholesterol out of arteries, says Peter Wilson, M.D., director of laboratories at the Framingham Heart Study in Massachusetts. There's some controversy about the most beneficial level of exercise intensity.

The best data come from runners. In a large study at Georgetown University in Washington, D.C., men who jogged between 11 and 14 miles a week had higher levels of HDL (11 percent) than those who didn't exercise. If jogging's not for him, suggest that he walk 2 miles or more a day, suggests Dr. Sinatra.

Help him fight fat. Although saturated fats found in meat and whole-milk dairy products raise cholesterol levels, other types of fat (such as the unsaturated fats of olive oil, soybean oil, corn oil, and nuts) don't seem to clog the arteries, Dr. Cleeman says. But such fats are still high in calories. So if he's overweight, which also contributes to high blood cholesterol, he should consume these oils and nuts in moderation. His goal should be to keep his saturated fat intake to 8 to 10 percent of his total daily calories. If he already has heart disease, he should keep it below 7 percent.

You can help him cut his saturated fat levels by using leaner cuts of meat and dairy products made from fat-free or low-fat (1 percent) milk. Also, try to limit his intake of meat, poultry, and fish to 6 ounces or less a day—roughly the size of two decks of cards. Of course, since men generally love meat, this is easier said than done. What you could try is a Chinese trick for meat control, which is mixing in veggies or legumes (such as beans) with meat dishes, making sure that there are more veggies (which are filling) than meat on the plate.

Another tip for helping your husband eat less saturated fat: When you're shopping, read the ingredients lists of baked goods. Lots of them have unhealthy fats such as coconut, palm, or palm kernel oils. Avoid those products in favor of ones that don't contain these fats.

Also, don't overlook the obvious when studying labels: See how much cholesterol a food has before you buy it. After all, you don't have to be a doctor to know that the cholesterol he eats will raise the level of cholesterol in his blood. Keep in mind that most labels list nutrient amounts per serving, so you'll have to do a little math in some cases to make sure he doesn't end up getting a ton of cholesterol because he ate too many servings of the food. He should try to keep his cholesterol intake at around 300 milligrams a day.

Have him take this reducing resin. Guggul's name sounds like baby talk, but the small guggul tree from India yields a gummy resin that lowers LDL cholesterol, raises HDL cholesterol, and reduces overall cholesterol. "I've seen it dramatically lower cholesterol," says Ralph T. Golan, M.D., a holistic general practitioner in Seattle. "I've had patients whose cholesterol levels have come down as much as 20 percent with guggul."

Also called gugulipid (which sounds even more like baby talk), the powdered extract is available in capsule form and is usually standardized for an active constituent called guggulsterone. Give your husband three 500-milligram capsules daily with meals, which should get him a daily total of 75 milligrams of guggulsterone. Once he's able to optimize his cholesterol through diet, exercise, and other lifestyle changes, he won't need to continue taking guggul, says Dr. Golan.

Get some hawthorn. Hawthorn's the best herb there is for the heart, which is too often the victim when cholesterol accumulates in the bloodstream. That by itself is enough reason to give him hawthorn if he has high cholesterol. But here's another one: "There's also some research that shows that hawthorn lowers cholesterol," says George Milowe, M.D., a holistic physician in Saratoga Springs, New York.

Give your husband 2,000 milligrams daily in capsule form or 1 teaspoon of tincture two to four times a day. Hawthorn is best when it's standardized for a flavonoid called vitexin. If you prefer the liquid extract, Dr. Milowe suggests a 1:5 (1 part hawthorn to 5 parts alcohol) tincture. Your husband can take hawthorn indefinitely, but if he has any type of cardiovascular condition, talk to your physician before starting, advises Dr. Milowe.

Note: A tincture is a highly concentrated herbal liquid. It's made by soaking leaves in alcohol or glycerin—which extracts the herb's medicinal properties—for at least 6 weeks. Tinctures are sold in health food stores in small bottles with eyedroppers to give doses. Be sure to store them out of the reach of children.

Protect his liver as well. Natural healers often concentrate on the connection between blood cholesterol and the liver. "A neglected liver can really elevate cholesterol," says Pamela Sky Jeanne, R.N., N.D., a naturopathic family physician in Gresham, Oregon. "Your digestive system may not be eliminating the cholesterol, or your liver may be overproducing it." That's where dandelion root can help. Although there's no direct evidence linking dandelion to reduced cholesterol levels, there's no doubt that it's a great herb for the liver, according to naturopathic doctors. It's easy to find, but make sure the tincture is made from the root, says Dr. Jeanne. Use the bottle's dropper to fill a teaspoon, put the tincture in a small amount of water, and have him drink it. Give him 1 teaspoon of tincture three times a day. It's best to administer dandelion for about 2 months and then stop for about 2 weeks, says Dr. Jeanne. He can then take it for another 2 months and continue cycling until his cholesterol is lowered.

Impotence

Ten million to 30 million men in America are believed to have a total inability to have an erection, an inconsistent ability to do so, or an ability to maintain only brief erections. These conditions are often called erectile dysfunction. About 10 to 20 percent of cases are due to psychological factors such as stress, anxiety, guilt, low self-esteem, depression, or fear of sexual failure. Between the ages of 20 and 40, psychological causes are more common, says Neil Baum, M.D., professor of urology at Tulane University Medical School in New Orleans.

After age 50, it's most often a physical problem. Diseases and disorders—including diabetes, kidney disease, chronic alcoholism, vascular disease, and especially atherosclerosis (hardening of the arteries)—account for about 70 percent of cases of impotence. Other causes include prostate, bladder, and rectal surgery; pelvic and spinal cord injuries; drugs to treat high blood pressure; antihistamines, antidepressants, tranquilizers, and appetite suppressants; and long-term use of alcohol, marijuana, and other intoxicants. Excessive tobacco use can also block penile arteries.

While impotence may be a symptom of a serious disease such as diabetes, its psychological impact also is significant. A guy's manhood is defined in part by his, well, manhood. If he can't get an erection, he often feels like less than a whole man, says Dr. Baum. He may well become discouraged and depressed. As his wife, you are also affected, says Dr. Baum. You won't be sexually fulfilled and may wonder if your husband is cheating on you. "His wife thinks that he's giving at the office," says Dr. Baum. "It creates a lot of anxiety and tension and marital discord." For men who find that they are failing in the bedroom more than they are succeeding, Dr. Baum suggests that they visit a physician. One or two doctor visits can often identify whether it is a physical or a psychological problem, he says. For psychological impotence, a referral is then made to a therapist, who meets with the man and his partner to resolve any emotional or marital conflict, Dr. Baum explains.

Potency Promoters

Do it first thing. You should try making love early in the morning, says Dr. Baum. A man's testosterone level is higher in the morning than at night, and chances are he'll be less fatigued, he says.

Play nice . . . and slow. Rather than focusing on vaginal penetration, try leisurely, gentle foreplay, advises Dr. Baum. This promotes intimacy while removing the pressure to perform, and if he gets and sustains an erection, then maybe you'll want to make love the next time, he says.

Advise him to quit smoking. Smoking can narrow blood vessels, preventing sufficient blood from surging into his penis when he's aroused and denying him an erection, says Dr. Baum.

Close the bar. Alcohol is a sedative that actually makes getting an erection more difficult, says Dr. Baum. "Alcohol stimulates the desire but inhibits the performance," he says.

Tell him that being in shape can help. Obesity can impair a man's ability to have an erection, says Dr. Baum. A healthy lifestyle helps maintain healthy erections. Obesity often is a precursor of that erection-killer, diabetes—yet another reason to take care of the situation, says Dr. Baum. He adds that regular exercise will also maintain the general health of the blood vessels. (For more information, see the chapters Abdominal Fat on page 161 and Overweight on page 445. Although the

WHEN TO SEE THE DOCTOR

All men have occasional erection problems. If he has difficulty over a period of months, however, have it checked out. It could be a sign of a serious health condition such as diabetes or high blood pressure.

tips in the latter chapter are in the section for women, men can also use them effectively.)

Try to help him relax. "A lot of guys don't realize it, but they get a lot of stress from work and elsewhere," says David Schwartz, M.D., a urologist in Alexandria, Virginia, who treats men with impotence. "If you get stressed enough, that will turn off erections."

Use vitamin E. A study done by Suresh Sikka, Ph.D., professor of urology at the Tulane University School of Medicine in New Orleans, found that impotent men with diabetes had significantly lower levels of vitamin E in their plasma than either men with diabetes who were potent or a control group. Vitamin E is an antioxidant that can help stave off damage to red blood cells, which is common in men with diabetes, says Dr. Sikka. He recommends 400 to 800 IU of vitamin E combined with 500 milligrams of vitamin C daily as a preventive measure. If you are considering giving this amount of vitamin E to your husband, discuss it with the doctor first.

Give him ginkgo to get things going. Ginkgo is widely used in Europe for all sorts of circulatory problems. It increases blood and oxygen flow to the extremities and penis, exactly what is needed for a powerful erection, says Steven Margolis, M.D., an alternative family physician in Sterling Heights, Michigan. In one study, 60 men with erectile dysfunction who didn't respond to injection treatments with a prescription medication were given 60 milligrams of ginkgo daily for 12 to 18 months. After 6 months, 50 percent of the men who took the ginkgo reported that they had regained potency. Dr. Margolis advises taking ginkgo phytosome, which is absorbed better. Your husband should take an 80-milligram capsule twice a day.

Suggest he try another potent plant. Asian ginseng (also called panax or Chinese ginseng) is a traditional Chinese virility tonic that has been shown in several studies to boost sexual activity. The effect builds over time, which means that he'll have to take it for a few months before seeing the benefits.

The recommended dose is capsules providing 15 percent ginsenosides daily. "Have him check the label to make sure he knows how many ginsenosides are in each capsule," says Steven Rissman, N.D., a naturopathic physician at American WholeHealth in Littleton, Colorado. "If it's a 100-milligram capsule but contains only 5 percent ginsenosides, he'll know he has to take three capsules a day."

Buy this Brazilian solution. Also known as potency wood, muira puama, which is derived from a Brazilian shrub, has a long history as an herbal treatment for impotence. "In my experience, this ingredient is particularly effective, with no notable side effects," says Dr. Margolis. A landmark study at the Institute of Sexology in Paris found that 51 percent of men who had difficulty attaining or maintaining erections reported some improvement after receiving a daily dose of muira puama for 2 weeks. Have him take capsules containing 300 milligrams once a day.

If his prostate is a problem, try this plant. Saw palmetto is best known as a treatment for prostate troubles, but it can also have a positive impact on erections. The reason? An enlarged prostate can impair bloodflow, thus interfering with sexual performance. In addition, having an enlarged prostate can necessitate getting up several times during the night to urinate, and fatigue can play a role in impotence. By returning the prostate to its normal size, saw palmetto may eliminate these erection obstacles. "Research shows that saw palmetto has revitalizing effects for the prostate and possibly throughout the entire urinary system," says Dr. Rissman. The recommended dose is two 160-milligram capsules daily.

Inhibited Sexual Desire

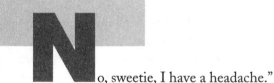

o, sweetie, I have a headache."
How many times have we seen women use that excuse on TV or in movies, as if a lack of sexual desire were just a women's problem? The fact is that many men also have this problem. There are several causes, including depression, illness, side effects of medications, a childhood

trauma such as being a victim of sexual abuse, fatigue from work or family responsibilities, hormonal changes, or boredom with one's partner.

"It can be a major problem if the desire for sexual activity from one partner is significantly greater than the desire of the other partner," says Robert Hawkins Jr., Ph.D., professor of health sciences at the State University of New York at Stony Brook. "A lot of us males feel as if we're expected to be ready to go anytime, anywhere. When we're not, we run a risk of some self-esteem damage." On the other hand, if a guy only feels like having sex once a month and so does his partner, he doesn't have a problem.

Ideas to Inspire Him

Encourage him to try to find out the cause. If a man always has had inhibited sexual desire, he should think about what may have caused this or talk to somebody about it, advises Martin Goldberg, M.D., clinical professor of psychiatry at the University of Pennsylvania School of Medicine in Philadelphia. "It helps to know," he says. "Knowing is part of the cure."

View sex as an adventure. Neither men nor women should see sex as an obligation, a relationship requirement, or work, advises Dr. Goldberg. "That's about the most self-defeating and negative thing that can happen," he says. "It does happen an awful lot." He suggests that we should view sex as part of loving someone and having fun, and as a chance to be physically expressive and creative.

Break the routine. You should add some new elements to your lovemaking repertoire, such as fantasizing more, watching an adult video together, or playing sexual games together, suggests Dr. Hawkins.

Make an appointment. It doesn't sound too romantic, but couples frazzled by the demands of careers and children should schedule private time together, says Dr. Hawkins. If they don't, they may discover that 2 or 3 weeks have whizzed by without their having been alone, he says. That time to themselves doesn't necessarily have to culminate in intercourse. "What you do in that interaction has to be determined by the needs of the couple," Dr. Hawkins says.

Stimulate him with smells. Certain smells have been found to increase bloodflow to the penis, says Alan R. Hirsch, M.D., a psychiatrist and neurological director of the Smell and Taste Treatment and Research Foundation in Chicago. In one study, Dr. Hirsch found that a combination of pumpkin pie and lavender elicited a 40 percent increase in penile bloodflow. Second place went to a cross between black licorice and doughnuts. (Maybe it's not a coincidence that doughnuts make Homer Simpson drool.) Try serving pumpkin pie as a dessert or drizzling some drops of lavender essential oil on your sheets; you can buy essential oils in health food stores. Dr. Hirsch speculates that these aromas work because they provoke a certain kind of nostalgia, so another option is to recreate an especially pleasurable lovemaking session from the past with scented candles, incense, or potpourri.

Try some love, European-style. *Tribulus terrestris*, a little-known

Did You Know . . . ?

When the authors of *Sex in America* took the sexual pulse of the nation, one of the findings that surprised them was how infrequently most of us make love.

Roughly 2 out of 10 men said they had sex only a few times in the previous year, and 14 percent reported none at all. Another 37 percent of men said they had sex a few times a month, while 26 percent reported getting intimate two or three times a week. A mere 8 percent said they had sex four or more times a week.

Apparently, it is feast or famine for guys between the ages of 18 and 24. They were the most likely to have had no sex at all, but they also were the age group most often having sex four or more times a week. And contrary to the stereotypes about swinging bachelors, married guys and those living with women had sex more often than the men who did not live with women.

herb from eastern Europe, shows exciting potential as a treatment for low sex drive in men, says Steven Margolis, M.D., an alternative family physician in Sterling Heights, Michigan. It works primarily by stimulating the body's natural production of testosterone, and it appears to increase sexual desire and maximize bloodflow to the penis. He should take one 250-milligram capsule each day.

Get him going with damiana. Damiana leaves appear to benefit mainly the female libido, says Dr. Margolis, but the herb can have benefits for both sexes. For one thing, it appears to be a mild antidepressant, which would be helpful for both women and men if the lack of sex drive has an emotional component, says Steven Rissman, N.D., a naturopathic physician at American WholeHealth in Littleton, Colorado. In addition, experts speculate that damiana causes mild inflammation of the urethra, thus increasing penile sensitivity for men. You both can take 2 to 4 milliliters of tincture or drink one cup of tea daily.

Suggest trying this wood. Muira puama, also known as potency wood, is derived from a tropical Brazilian plant and has a long history in South America as a male libido booster. In a study done at the Institute of Sexology in Paris, 62 percent of male subjects with low sex drive reported improvement after taking muira puama daily for 2 weeks. "It's very effective," Dr. Margolis says. "And there are no side effects." Give him a 300-milligram tablet once a day.

Work out. Generally, the more fit people are, the better they feel about themselves. The better people feel about themselves, the more sexually aroused they are apt to be, says Dr. Hawkins. Does this mean you and your hubby should start marathon training? Not unless you're into that. For most couples, a good way to put this tip into practice is to do physical activities you enjoy together. You can join a gym together, walk, hike, bicycle . . . whatever you like that gets you moving. You'll benefit not only from the exercise but from being together—which should lead to being together in other ways.

Kidney Stones

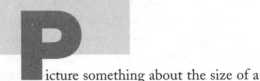

Picture something about the size of a sesame seed trying to pass through a tube as thin as a strand of spaghetti. Now imagine the smooth seed sprouting jagged spurs and becoming lodged in the tube. That's what happens in a typical kidney stone attack, says Jean L. Fourcroy, M.D., Ph.D., editor of the *Women in Urology* newsletter.

A kidney stone is formed from crystals that separate from urine and build up in the inner surfaces of the kidney. If the crystals remain small enough, they will travel through the urinary tract and be excreted without your husband even being aware that they existed. But when one of the nasty larger nuggets is finally excreted, the first clue is intense pain. As the jagged stone makes its way inch by agonizing inch through the ureter—the tube that passes urine from the kidneys to the bladder—dozens of needlelike protrusions slowly rake through the soft tissue, generating pain that radiates from the upper back to the lower abdomen and groin.

Seventy to 80 percent of stones are composed primarily of calcium oxalate. Oxalate is an acid that all people make and that also is found in plants, says Linda Massey, R.D., Ph.D., professor of food science at Washington State University in Spokane. They can range from the size of a tiny speck of sand to (ouch!) that of a dime or marble. Generally, though, as long as it's smaller than a pea—and 80 percent of stones are—doctors will let your husband's body pass the stone on its own. When stones are larger than 8 to 10 millimeters, however, they are usually too large to be passed. Often, they remain in the kidneys, where they can cause infection.

A kidney stone may produce such severe pain that it causes significant loss of work time. In addition, kidney stones also can cause infections and bleeding; if untreated, irreparable damage may be caused to the kidneys, says E. Douglas Whitehead, M.D., professor of urology at the Albert Einstein College of Medicine of Yeshiva University in New York City. If your husband has had two or more stones or if he is feeling the awful pain associated with kidney stones, he ought to see a urologist for tests that can determine why he's forming stones and what sorts of medications or changes in diet or lifestyle can prevent future episodes, says Dr. Whitehead.

Nonetheless, your husband doesn't have to accept future agony as inevitable. There's a lot he can do to prevent attacks. First, though, be sure to find out from your doctor what kinds of kidney stones he has or is prone to, since different types of stones are treated differently. The preventive measures and remedies we offer here are relevant mainly to the most common types of stones—those formed from calcium phosphate or calcium oxalate.

How He Can Avoid Them in the First Place

Tell him to drink lots of water. He should drink at least eight 8-ounce glasses of water spread out over the course of the day, every day, not just when he's having a kidney stone attack. "That's about twice as much as most people drink," says Dr. Massey. All that water dilutes the chemicals in his urine so that calcium and oxalate—the two main components of most kidney stones—can't get together, Dr. Massey says. "It works," she says. "People say, 'It's inconvenient because I have to go to the bath-

WHEN TO SEE THE DOCTOR

Contact the doctor if your husband develops symptoms of kidney stones, which include pain that radiates from the upper back to the lower abdomen and groin, frequent urination, pus and blood in the urine, and sometimes chills and fever.

room so often.' Well, which is worse: the pain or going to the bath-room?"

Have him get his calcium. It wasn't too long ago that doctors were telling people with kidney stones to restrict their calcium intake. Since then, they've learned that calcium binds to oxalate, preventing it from forming stones, says Dr. Massey. She recommends including some high-calcium food, such as a glass of milk or a slice of cheese, with every meal, every day.

Encourage him to drink fruit juices. Beverages rich in citric acid, such as orange juice and lemonade, inhibit calcium stone formation, says Dr. Massey. A 6-ounce glass of orange juice with each meal, or a 10-ounce serving of lemonade a couple of times a day, every day, should be effective, she says. An extra benefit is that some orange juices are forti-fied with calcium.

Give him dandelion tea to help get rid of kidney stones. During the acute phase of an attack, to pass the stone as quickly as possible, doctors recommend drinking copious amounts of water. Instead of plain water, Silena Heron, N.D., a naturopathic physician and professor at South-west College of Naturopathic Medicine and Health Sciences in Tempe, Arizona, recommends dandelion leaf or goldenrod tea. Dandelion and other diuretic herbs increase urine output by stimulating blood circula-tion through the kidneys. This action helps flush the stone from his system faster. Unlike diuretic drugs, which can deplete the body of potassium, dandelion leaf is one of the best plant sources of this crucial mineral. A cup of cooked dandelion greens contains as much potassium as a small banana.

If you can't find dandelion leaf tea in your local health food store, you can substitute goldenrod tea, suggests Dr. Heron. Along with its diuretic properties, goldenrod helps repair the inflammation caused by the pas-sage of the stone. To make either tea, add 2 teaspoons of dried herb to 1 cup of boiling water and steep for 15 minutes.

Brew teas to repair and soothe his urinary tract. The urinary tract is lined with mucous membranes to protect it from irritation and in-flammation. As a kidney stone passes through, it strips away this pro-tective layer. He can help replace it by drinking tea made from marshmallow root or corn silk, says Orest Pelechaty, O.M.D., a doctor of oriental medicine in Short Hills, New Jersey. The slimy texture of the tea helps by assisting the mucous membranes. Marshmallow is a good source of mucilage, large sugar molecules that produce a sticky, jellylike mass when they soak up water. The silica content of corn silk will aid in the repair of the urinary tract tissues. It's probably easier to find good-quality marshmallow than corn silk, says Dr. Heron. "Corn silk is one herb that is best used in fresh form, and it should be carefully collected so that you're using only the green or yellowish parts. Most commercially available corn silk is of a low quality," she says. To collect your own, buy organic corn on the cob and keep the silk as you husk the ears. Trim away any dried-up or brown pieces of silk.

To make the most soothing tea from marshmallow root, simmer the herb for several minutes in a pan of water. "Use 2 ounces of herb to 1 quart of water and boil for 5 to 10 minutes," says Dr. Pelechaty. "Corn silk is best steeped using 1 ounce of material to 1 pint of water," he continues. "Let it stand and cool for 5 minutes so it thickens." Have him drink one cup of tea three times a day before meals.

Give him saw palmetto. Better known for its benefits in treating prostate problems, saw palmetto also relaxes the ureter, making it easier for both men and women to pass kidney stones.

"Saw palmetto is also believed to reduce the pressure on the neck of the bladder," says Dr. Heron. She feels it's key because of its general tonic effect on the entire urinary tract. Give your husband two 160-milligram capsules of extract daily or ½ teaspoon of tincture three times a day for as long as needed.

Note: A tincture is a highly concentrated herbal liquid. It's made by soaking leaves in alcohol or glycerin—which extracts the herb's medicinal properties—for at least 6 weeks. Tinctures are sold in health food stores in small bottles with eyedroppers to give doses. Be sure to store them out of the reach of children.

Try giving him cranberry to stop future attacks. Preliminary research suggests that cranberry juice may help reduce the amount of calcium in the urine, says Amy Howell, Ph.D., a researcher at the Blueberry and Cranberry Research Center of Rutgers University in Chatsworth, New Jersey. In a study of people with calcium-containing kidney stones, cranberry was shown to reduce the amount of ionized calcium in the urine by 50 percent. Less calcium in the urine means that there may be less risk of forming new stones. Cranberry juice also has a very cleansing effect on the urinary tract. Have him drink 16 ounces of juice every day.

Watch Out for These Foods

Certain foods may promote kidney stone formation in people who are susceptible, but researchers don't think that any particular food causes stones to develop in people who are not susceptible. If your husband is among those who are prone to calcium oxalate stones, Linda Massey, R.D., Ph.D., professor of food science at Washington State University in Spokane, says to avoid or limit the following foods, which are rich in oxalates.

Black tea
Spinach
Rhubarb
Beets—the roots and the leaves
Chocolate, especially concentrated chocolate, such as that in a candy bar (chocolate flavoring isn't too bad)
Wheat bran, particularly the concentrated form used to enrich food, such as bran muffins
Nuts, especially peanuts
Berries, including strawberries, raspberries, and gooseberries

Tell him to cool it with the caffeine. He should keep caffeine use, especially coffee, at moderate levels, advises Dr. Massey. Caffeine increases urinary calcium, which ups the risk of forming a calcium-containing kidney stone. She suggests no more than two cups of coffee a day.

Advise him to watch out for salt, another stone-maker. Salt consumption should be watched for the same reason that caffeine should be, says Dr. Massey. It's harder to do so, she says, because salt is included in many processed foods and consumers may be unaware of it unless they read food labels. Dr. Massey recommends keeping salt intake under 2,400 milligrams per day.

Make sure he gets plenty of fluids. Men who are what doctors call stone-formers need to be especially diligent about drinking plenty of fluids when they do any form of exercise, says Dr. Whitehead. He recommends drinking fluids before, during, and after exercise, and drinking past the point at which thirst is quenched.

Premature Ejaculation

Here the basic problem is that your husband is ejaculating during intercourse more quickly than you (and he) would like. The length of time varies from couple to couple, says Robert Birch, Ph.D., a sex therapist in Columbus, Ohio. The average man ejaculates perhaps as soon as 2 minutes after penetration. "I see guys who go 12 minutes and think they ought to be able to go an hour. It all depends on expectations," Dr. Birch says. He prefers the term *rapid ejaculation* rather than *premature ejaculation*, which has a more negative connotation.

There are several causes. Some men are just really excitable. "They're in an altered state of consciousness" during sex, says Dr. Birch. Others are overly anxious. And some men may just have unusually sensitive penises, he says. Premature or rapid ejaculation isn't limited to young guys, either. "I'm seeing a 72-year-old man who is a rapid ejaculator even on the second episode in the same evening," says Dr. Birch.

This can be a pretty devastating problem if you believe that the only way you can have an orgasm is via vaginal stimulation. If he ejaculates quickly, you may feel he is depriving you of an orgasm, and naturally, hard feelings may ensue.

How You Can Help Improve His Endurance

Start, then stop, then start, then . . . you get the idea. There are many techniques a man can use to learn ejaculatory control, says Roger Crenshaw, M.D., a psychotherapist and sex therapist in La Jolla, California. But the most common and effective is the simple "start-stop" method. The bonus of this method is that you can do it together, even make a game of it. Or if he's embarrassed, urge him to do it on his own and then surprise you with his progress. The idea is to stimulate the penis manually, almost to the point of ejaculation, and then stop. After he regains his composure, repeat the process—several times. Over time, he can learn to tolerate longer and longer periods of sexual stimulation. Eventually, switch from manual stimulation to intercourse, doing the same thing—lots of starting and stopping—until both of you are ready for the grand explosion.

Consider masturbation. If a guy who ejaculates quickly isn't having sex as often as he would prefer, then he should masturbate, says Dr. Birch. "One of the things that will lead to superexcitability is deprivation," he says. "A man needs to keep track of frequency and fill in any gaps."

Switch positions. By stopping and switching positions every so often, you're helping to moderate the amount of stimulation he's getting, which will help you prolong intercourse, says Dr. Birch. Ultimately, though, the idea is to find positions that better enable him to postpone ejaculation. For many men, lying passively on their backs with their partners on top does the trick, says Dr. Birch. He should relax and let you do the thrusting. Not only will he be less apt to pull the trigger too quickly, but you can move in ways that provide the most stimulation of your clitoris, says Dr. Birch.

Squeeze him. When he's nearing ejaculation, he should withdraw and you should gently but firmly squeeze the tip of his penis, where it meets the glans or head of the organ, between your thumb and first finger, advises Neil Baum, M.D., professor of urology at Tulane University Medical School in New Orleans. When your husband has regained control, resume intercourse. If he is about to climax too quickly again, squeeze him again. "It requires a very cooperative partner to help do it," says Dr. Baum. Of course, he can always do the squeezing himself, too.

Try to use a condom for control. Many men find that they last longer if they wear condoms, says Dr. Birch. If this is why he is going to wear a condom, make sure it is one that is not lubricated, he says. Those that are lubricated are warm and slippery, and you both know how that sensation affects him.

Have him work out. We don't mean weights or aerobic exercise this time. Kegel exercises, which strengthen the pelvic muscles, can help pump more blood to the penis and provide more ejaculatory control, says Dr. Baum. He should contract the muscles he uses to hold in urine or to stop the flow for 3 to 5 seconds and then relax. Dr. Baum recommends doing a set of 10, four or five times a day.

Tighten up. Some guys wear constriction bands, commonly called cock rings, at the base of their penises, says Dr. Birch. It doesn't delay ejaculation, but it keeps him from going soft after he does climax by trapping all that blood in the penis that made him erect in the first place. He should never wear one for longer than 30 minutes, Dr. Birch warns. He also advises that your husband avoid using a constriction band when he's drinking because he might fall asleep with it on. Depriving his penis of blood and oxygen for any length of time can prove disastrous, he adds. He suggests using adjustable rings that are easily removable.

Suggest he slow down his breathing. Breathing exercises may help him maintain some measure of control, says Marty Klein, Ph.D., a sex therapist in Palo Alto, California. He suggests that your husband deliberately slow down his breathing during sex so that it's deep and relaxing (it'll take some effort, we know). This breathing technique will reduce anxiety and help delay ejaculation.

Consider a cream. Some men apply desensitizing creams to the penis in order to delay ejaculation. Dr. Birch doesn't recommend them because they are simply not very effective. It's hard to tell how much to use, he adds, and there is a good chance that the cream will rub off on you, desensitizing you as well (definitely not the goal you want). But if he does decide to go this route, Dr. Birch adds, he should look for a penis desensitization cream—preferably with Novocain—that has specific instructions for penile application, and he should follow the directions carefully.

Tell him to stop peeking. Men are notoriously visual in sexual matters, so he should keep his eyes closed during at least part of intercourse, advises Dr. Birch. Let's say you're in the woman-on-top position that Dr. Birch recommends. The sight of your breasts bobbing may quickly bring on a tidal wave of lustful feelings and—uh-oh!—he's to the point of no return. When he feels that he's under control, he can try opening his eyes again, says Dr. Birch.

Play around for a while. In reality, the majority of women don't have orgasms through intercourse, so if he feels he has to prove that he can give you an orgasm through penetration, he may be setting himself up for failure.

Instead, turn your attention to foreplay and afterplay techniques that satisfy you both. Taking the emphasis off of intercourse and thrusting may, in the long run, improve the intercourse, says Judith Seifer, Ph.D., a sex therapist and associate clinical professor at Wright State University in Dayton, Ohio.

Do it again. Most men have more self-control the second time around, so take advantage of his refractory period (the time when his erection begins to fade after an orgasm).

"After you've had sex, get up, go to the bathroom if you need to, get some water, come back to bed, and cuddle," says Dr. Seifer. "Then try again in 20 minutes. It will probably last longer the next time."

Set realistic expectations. Anything more than 10 minutes of vaginal penetration and thrusting is going to make one, if not both, of you uncomfortable, says Dr. Crenshaw. Let your husband know that you aren't expecting him to last all night.

"Most men have enough control so they can postpone their orgasms for a few minutes," Dr. Crenshaw says. "Ask your partner to slow down while you're starting to come in order to pace himself to you a little more. Tell him exactly what it is you're looking for in terms of time and technique."

Consider medication. Not long after the drug Prozac became available to treat depression, a side effect caught the attention of researchers: Prozac seemed to delay orgasm. Today, the class of selective serotonin reuptake inhibitor (SSRI) antidepressants that includes such common prescription drugs as fluoxetine (Prozac) and sertraline (Zoloft) is being prescribed for more serious premature ejaculation cases—usually when physiology is to blame, says Gerald Hoke, M.D., chief of urology at Harlem Hospital Center in New York City. "You take the pill 4 hours before intercourse," he explains.

The only downers? Having to plan when you're going to have sex and drowsiness afterward (a common side effect of antidepressants). Then again, don't most men get drowsy after sex anyway?

Prostate Problems

Nothing is certain but death and taxes. And, for men, prostate problems.

It's not really a question of if his prostate gland will start acting up; it's more a matter of when, says Steven L. Bratman, M.D., medical director for Prima Health Publishing in Fort Collins, Colorado.

The walnut-size prostate gland's job is to manufacture globs of milky fluid for sperm to surf through. About 90 percent of ejaculate is prostate fluid. The prostate secretes and stores the fluid during sexual arousal. As a man approaches climax, the fluid is pumped into the urethra, where it mixes with sperm from the testicles. At climax, the mixture spurts out of the penis.

It's a small but important job. Prostate fluid insulates and protects sperm from the hostile environment they encounter once they exit the penis and begin searching for an egg to fertilize.

And, researchers say, it appears as though prostate fluid carries flowers and talks sweetly to a woman's cervix. It somehow coaxes the cervix to relax, open up, and pay no mind to the flotilla of sperm rapidly approaching.

WHEN TO SEE THE DOCTOR

If he has difficulty getting his urine flow started and then has only a dribbling stream, plus the sensation that his bladder is still partly full even after he's done, have him see a doctor right away. These symptoms, along with a need to get up often during the night to urinate and occasional abdominal pain, can be signs of BPH. But prostate cancer can cause similar symptoms, and so can prostatitis (an infection), so he needs to have a doctor's diagnosis.

Unfortunately, it also secretly breeds cancer. Prostate cancer is the chart-topping cancer among men over age 50. One in 8 men will develop prostate cancer, and 1 in 20 of them will die of it. By age 100, all men have it. Overall, it's the second leading killer cancer in men. Sometimes it's a virulent cancer that runs by night, without lights and in perfect silence, then launches surprise attacks that take out some of the best and brightest. But usually, it develops slowly. Cancer caught early can be stopped cold 91 percent of the time. If discovered after spreading, it can be treated . . . for a while. The object of this game is to snag it early.

Your husband also needs to maintain a healthy lifestyle. Here are some general tips for preventing cancer and keeping his prostate from acting up.

Checkmate cancer with checkups. Every man should have a digital/rectal exam every 2 years beginning at age 40, as well as a prostate-specific antigen (PSA) test every 2 years beginning at age 50, switching to every year at age 60.

To perform the digital/rectal exam, the doctor slips on a glove, lubricates his finger, and feels as much of the prostate as possible through the rectum wall, probing for lumps, growths, hardening, and more. The PSA test is a blood test. It finds cancer that the digital/rectal exam misses. He shouldn't delay testing until he's 50 if he urinates blood, has a hard time urinating, or is in a high-risk group.

Get him exercising. Men in good shape have less prostate trouble, plain and simple. So make sure he gets exercise.

Suggest he urinate frequently. When the bladder is overfull, it's relatively easy for urine to back up into the prostate. When that happens, his irritated prostate will let him know. So tell him not to hold it in. In particular, he should "always empty his bladder before doing any exercise or lifting," says E. David Crawford, M.D., chairman of the division of urology at the University of Colorado Health Sciences Center in Denver. It's easy to irritate the prostate with urine during exercise.

Get him off his butt. Now you have another reason (and one he can't argue with) to make him get up when he's sitting around doing nothing on weekends. Sitting squishes the prostate, which is under enough pressure already. So he should get up and get going. You'll surely find something to keep him busy.

Make love. Here's a prostatic therapy you'll probably both enjoy. Doctors say regular ejaculation keeps the prostate from getting stagnant and inflamed from congestion. Truck drivers, motorcycle cops, bicycle riders, and others whose genitalia are subjected to constant vibration are particularly prone to congestion. The vibration apparently teases the prostate into secreting fluid. It becomes engorged when there is no release. So make sure he takes his, uh, medicine on a regular basis.

Help him win the fat war. A diet high in fatty foods seems to irritate the prostate and increase cancer risk. Saturated fat seems particularly troublesome. The best meals for prostate health are low in fat and cholesterol and big on vegetables, whole grains, leafy greens, and fiber. Foods high in vitamins A, C, and E are particularly healthy for the prostate. Good sources of vitamin A include carrots, squash, pumpkin, sweet potatoes, apricots, cantaloupe, and dark green, leafy veggies such as spinach, kale, and broccoli. For vitamin C, give him citrus fruits and juices, strawberries, peppers (both red and green), broccoli, tomatoes, melons, brussels sprouts, and cauliflower. He can get vitamin E from wheat germ, peanut butter, almonds, sunflower seeds, shrimp, vegetable oils, and green, leafy vegetables.

Prevent Prostate Enlargement, Naturally

Besides cancer, another common prostate-related problem is prostate enlargement. By age 45, 10 to 15 percent of men have enlarged prostates, a condition known medically as benign prostatic hyperplasia (BPH). For men over age 60, it's 50 percent, and if a man makes it past age 80, the number rises to 90 percent or more, adds Dr. Bratman.

When the prostate enlarges, it pinches the urethra. That leads to the symptoms of BPH, which include difficulty getting the urine flow going, a dribbling stream when it does start, and a feeling that the bladder is still partly full even after finishing. It also causes men to get up often during the night to stand in frustration over the toilet. Occasionally, there's some abdominal pain.

Conventional medicine treats BPH in one of two ways. The first is surgery, in which a portion of the gland is removed to open the urethra. The second treatment is with a prescription medication such as finasteride (Proscar). Surgery works, but it's invasive, and recovery takes a while, says Donald R. Counts, M.D., an Austin, Texas, physician who combines conventional medicine and proven alternative treatments in his practice.

Prescription medication will allow him to avoid surgery but is less effective in some cases. Plus, there can be some troubling side effects with either surgery or medication, such as a decreased interest in sex, ejaculatory problems, and erection difficulties.

To strengthen his protection against BPH, there are a variety of natural supplements that may be helpful. However, if your husband is experiencing any BPH symptoms, he should visit the doctor immediately for proper diagnosis and treatment. If his symptoms are mild or moderate, he can talk to a practitioner of alternative medicine to find out which of the following supplements might be right for him. Before he takes these supplements, though, he should discuss them with his doctor to make sure that they won't interfere with any other medications that he may already be taking.

Here are nature's top choices for prostate enlargement.

Try saw palmetto. There's been a lot of hubbub over this extract from the berry of the saw palmetto tree—and for good reason, says Dr. Bratman, since it usually works. No one knows for sure how it works, although one theory is that it prevents the prostate from converting testosterone, the male hormone, into a related hormone that stimulates cell production. Whatever the mechanism, though, evidence shows that saw palmetto can actually shrink a growing prostate. Give him 160 milligrams in capsule form twice daily. Look for a standardized extract that contains 85 to 95 percent fatty acids and sterols.

Be advised, however: Saw palmetto, like other herbs and even prescription drugs, is not a permanent cure. He has to take it on an ongoing basis. The good news is that in studies, saw palmetto has been associated with milder side effects than finasteride. In his practice, Dr. Counts has found that the herb is as effective as the prescription drug, but without the side effects.

Encourage him to try this remedy. Nettle root also works to shrink the prostate. "Nettle has all the same possibilities as saw palmetto," explains Dr. Bratman.

He should take 200 to 400 milligrams of dried root extract in capsule form three times a day on an ongoing basis. Be sure to look for root extract. Capsules of dried leaves are also available, but they contain very different compounds and are used for treating conditions such as allergies.

Buy this beneficial bark. Pygeum is an extract from the bark of an African tree. "It is extremely well researched, and it's effective," says Dr. Bratman. Give him capsules supplying 50 to 100 milligrams twice a day on an ongoing basis.

If he has tried a couple of herbal remedies and hasn't had much luck, he shouldn't give up quite yet, says Dr. Counts. Sometimes, herbs can work better in combination than they do alone. Saw palmetto and pygeum are good examples. Look for a brand that combines the two herbs (Solaray and Jarrow are two), he recommends. The capsule should have about 320 milligrams of saw palmetto and 100 or so milligrams of pygeum.

Suggest a seedy solution. Pumpkin seeds were once used as a traditional remedy for BPH in countries such as Bulgaria, Turkey, and Ukraine. Now, they're used globally, says Tim Hagney, N.D., a naturopathic physician in Anchorage. Pumpkin seeds have multiple actions. They provide essential fatty acids, which have an anti-inflammatory effect and can help relieve the symptoms of a swelling prostate, says Dr. Hagney. They also seem to confound the mechanism that turns testosterone into a prostate-enlarging hormone. On top of that, they are rich in zinc, a mineral that promotes a healthy prostate. One problem, though, is that the fatty acids are fragile and easily destroyed by heat and even light. Grind fresh raw seeds and sprinkle them over his cereal and other foods.

If he prefers the taste of roasted seeds, look for some that are already roasted or roast them yourself in the oven. To do this, spread the seeds on a shallow pan and slide the pan into a 350°F oven for 5 minutes, or until the seeds are very lightly browned. "When they're roasted, they're pretty good," says Dr. Hagney. "They taste a lot like sunflower seeds, and he will still get the benefits of the zinc in them, since heat doesn't affect it." Have him eat 5 grams (about 1 tablespoon) of seeds a day.

Give him pollen for a pesky prostate. Once upon a time, grass pollen was available only through mail-order companies. Now, with increasing demand, it's available in some health food stores and drugstores, says Dr. Bratman.

Usually, the tablets contain rye pollen, but sometimes the pollen can come from other grasses, such as timothy or corn. Bear that in mind and don't give him these pollens if he has allergies to grasses. Otherwise, this herb may work well for him if none of the others seems to help. "That's the good thing about all of these herbs that are used to treat BPH," says Dr. Bratman. "If you don't get results with one, you can try another. They're all quite safe and take about the same amount of time—1 to 3 months—before you see an improvement in BPH symptoms." Give him 25 to 40 milligrams in tablet form three times a day.

Recommend that he zap it with zinc. Some alternative practitioners believe that zinc is the most important mineral for preventing and treating BPH. "The prostate has one of the highest concentrations of zinc of any tissue in the body. It's abundant in semen and in the thin, milky fluid that the prostate gland secretes in the urethra just before ejaculation to prevent infections," says Thomas Kruzel, N.D., a naturopathic physician in Portland, Oregon.

In one study, zinc was shown to reduce the size of the prostate, and it alleviated symptoms in most men who were taking it. A laboratory study found that zinc could inhibit the activity of a critical enzyme that converts the male hormone testosterone to dihydrotestosterone (DHT). What's more, other laboratory studies have shown that zinc influences a hormone that helps control the production of DHT. By helping to lower the production of that growth factor hormone, even indirectly, zinc does the prostate a favor.

If your husband has BPH, he should consult the doctor for the appropriate zinc dosage. Doses higher than 20 milligrams daily should be taken only with medical supervision. Depending on the severity of his condition, the doctor may prescribe up to 60 milligrams a day. At that level, give him the zinc in divided doses, says Ian Bier, N.D., a naturopathic physician in Portsmouth, New Hampshire.

Advise adding acids to his anti-BPH arsenal. Some naturopaths believe that men who supplement their diets with fatty acids can reverse BPH and kiss irritating symptoms goodbye.

The human body can make all but two fatty acids. Those two must come from plant food and are known as essential fatty acids. In our bodies, they act as components of substances called prostaglandins, the regulators of inflammation, pain, and swelling. One, linoleic acid, is an omega-6 fatty acid, while the other, alpha-linolenic acid, belongs to the omega-3 group. "Essential fatty acids can inhibit cell growth in the prostate, therefore stopping its growth. They rebalance the appropriate fatty acid ratios in the gland," says Dr. Bier.

These fatty acids, especially omega-3's, are essential in helping to promote healthy cell growth and function. They also help prevent up to 60 illnesses, including prostate disease, says Dr. Kruzel.

The richest source of omega-3's is flaxseed oil, and some naturopaths recommend 1 tablespoon a day if he's trying to control or prevent a prostate problem. Dr. Kruzel has some concern, however, that flaxseed oil may increase testosterone levels in the body and that not everyone can metabolize the oil properly to reap the benefits. He suggests having your husband take 1,000 to 2,000 milligrams of fish oil daily for 1 to 2 weeks if he is being treated for BPH.

For maintaining prostate health rather than treating BPH, the recommended dose is 500 to 1,000 milligrams, Dr. Kruzel says. Check with your doctor before deciding to take fish-oil capsules.

Consider other alleviating acids. The combination of the amino acids alanine, glutamic acid, and glycine has been shown in some studies to relieve many symptoms of BPH. "There are many amino acids that are present in the prostate gland, but these three, in particular, are key in developing and maintaining prostate health," says Dr. Kruzel. In one study, 45 men were given this supplement combination. At the end of the study, researchers saw a reduction in nighttime bathroom visits in 95 percent of the participants. Eighty-one percent said they didn't have the urge to urinate as often, and 73 percent made fewer daily trips to the bathroom.

For symptom relief, Dr. Kruzel suggests taking combination products that contain herbs and vitamins as well as 50 milligrams each of alanine and glycine and between 50 and 100 milligrams of glutamic acid. He suggests taking two capsules twice a day for 10 to 14 days and then reducing the dose to one capsule once or twice a day as a maintenance dose.

Your husband may need to get this specific formula from a holistic practitioner, but similar products are available commercially. Dr. Kruzel recommends that your husband talk to his doctor before he begins taking these amino acids.

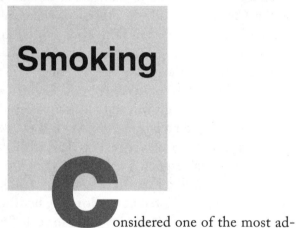

Smoking

Considered one of the most addictive substances in the world, nicotine keeps more than 47 million Americans puffing away on cigarette after cigarette. Only about 23 percent of smokers are able to quit. If your husband has to smoke every day, if he smokes his first cigarette within 10 minutes of waking up, or if he experiences withdrawal symptoms when he tries to quit smoking, then he is addicted to nicotine.

When a smoker drags on a cigarette, the drug travels to the brain and triggers a release of neurotransmitters—chemicals that transport messages from the brain to the body—that makes him feel good. But after a while, the brain becomes dependent on nicotine to release these feel-good substances. Eventually, he needs more nicotine to get the same pleasurable effects. And if he doesn't get his drug, the brain goes into withdrawal, causing him to feel irritable and downright ill.

Cigarette smoking has been associated with almost every serious disease in the human body. Lung cancer and heart disease are the biggest two, but smoking has also been linked to pancreatic cancer, dementia, colon cancer, and stroke. In a study at the Royal Free Hospital School of Medicine in London, researchers followed 7,735 middle-aged men for 15 years. Only 42 percent of those who smoked could expect to live to age 73, compared to 78 percent of those who were nonsmokers.

A Deadly Mix He Must Avoid

If your husband is using a nicotine patch with or without bupropion, he must not smoke. It can cause a heart attack on the spot. "Nicotine can constrict the blood vessels feeding the heart muscle, and may cause irregular heartbeats, so too much nicotine can lead to a heart attack," explains Paul Roberts, R.Ph., pharmacist at Kaiser Permanente in Santa Rosa, California, who teaches smoking cessation. Signs of too much nicotine include blurred vision, nausea, drooling, vomiting, and headaches. "A person who wears a patch, and smokes, and suffers these symptoms should dial 911 immediately, remove the patch—and of course put the cigarette out," says Roberts.

If your husband gets these symptoms and he's not smoking, the patch may be too strong for him. He should remove it and call the doctor. "Never cut the patch to decrease dosage," says Roberts. "The nicotine can leak out the cut end, which can be very dangerous. He can fold part of the patch back if he wants. The strength of the patch is dependent on the surface contact with the skin."

Smokers also report having more problems with sleeping disorders and impotence than nonsmokers.

If your husband tries the following strategies to quit smoking but can't kick the habit, he should seek help, says Douglas E. Jorenby, Ph.D., professor of psychology at the University of Wisconsin in Madison. Many hospitals and clinics offer smoking-cessation programs, where he can learn coping skills and hang out with other would-be ex-smokers who know exactly what he's going through.

Or you can make an appointment with your own doctor, who can offer your husband some prescriptions to help him fight his addiction. One option to ask about is an antidepressant called Zyban, Dr. Jorenby suggests. Although it contains no nicotine, it was approved by the FDA to be used as a smoking-cessation medication after studies showed that it helps smokers kick the habit, he says.

Helping Your Guy to Quit

Of course, the role of Mom's Medicine is pretty limited when it comes to smoking. You can't make your husband quit if he doesn't want to. And smoking is not like a bruise you can ice that will heal in a couple of days. Quitting is a long, hard battle, and almost no one is successful the first time he tries to do it. However, if he does want to stub out his smokes for good, you can offer him support and the following expert strategies.

Advise him to set a quit date. He can pick a special milestone like his birthday or an upcoming holiday to be the first day of the rest of his smoke-free life. That way, he's not always saying he'll quit someday . . . a day that may never come. By picking a date, he'll also give himself time to prepare for the trying times ahead. "People actually do better when you give them time to prepare. Look 1 or 2 weeks down the road," says Dr. Jorenby.

Suggest he go cold turkey. It's not the most effective way to quit: Only 5 out of every 100 who go cold turkey successfully kick the habit. But giving up cigarettes all at once, as opposed to gradually weaning yourself off them, is the *cheapest* way to quit. And it just may work for him, says Dr. Jorenby. "If one has never tried to quit before, going cold turkey is a great way to start. If it works, it's cheap and doesn't need a lot of resources," he says.

Get him ready for the cravings. No matter what method he uses to quit, he's going to be hit from time to time with an urge to smoke. The best way to beat these urges is to have a line of defense ready, Dr. Jorenby says. First, your husband should figure out when and where he's most likely to be hit by an urge to smoke. Classics include right after he awakens, while he's driving, and after meals. Then, he should think about what he's going to do when he gets that urge: drink a tall glass of water; take a few deep, relaxing breaths; chew a piece of gum; or whatever it takes to distract him from his desire for a cigarette.

"Urges can be pretty strong when they hit, but they don't last long. Within a few minutes, the urge is going to pass regardless of whether one has smoked. Having a distraction ready allows one to resist the urge and let it pass," Dr. Jorenby says.

Toss it all. The night before his quit date, help him throw out all his packs of cigarettes and clean out the ashtrays. That butt that looks disgusting right now when he has a fresh pack is going to look a whole lot more attractive as soon as he tries to quit, Dr. Jorenby says. He should also search any places where he may have cigarettes hidden, such as closets or desk drawers, and places where he may have inadvertently left a pack. You both should search high and low for all cigarettes and throw them out.

He may have put a coat away last fall with a pack in it and never thought about it. But if he stumbles upon it in a couple of months, it's going to be a big temptation for him. Don't leave any cigarettes around.

Suggest trying a patch. If going cold turkey fails, your husband can give one of the many over-the-counter nicotine patches (such as Nicoderm) a try, Dr. Jorenby says. Or he can try nicotine gum, such as Nicorette, which does the same thing as the patch. Most drugstores carry these easy-to-use products, and he won't need a prescription.

Try another medicine. If he's tried to quit a dozen times already, without permanent success, he may want to consider bupropion, a prescription antidepressant approved as a smoking cessation aid and sold under the brand name Zyban.

One study found that almost twice as many smokers who used bupropion were able to abstain from tobacco compared with those who used either the nicotine patch or a placebo. (A nicotine patch delivers enough nicotine through the skin to reduce withdrawal symptoms and help wean the wearer off inhaled smoke that damages heart and lungs.)

"Bupropion tends to decrease the severity of withdrawal symptoms," says Myra Muramoto, M.D., professor of family and community medicine at the University of Arizona in Tucson. It does this by affecting the mood-regulating chemicals in the brain. An additional benefit is that it suppresses the weight gain usually associated with quitting smoking.

Although bupropion does have some potential side effects—most notably insomnia and headaches—these generally go away soon after people stop taking it. (The drug treatment is usually about 9 weeks.)

Suggest that he improve his mood naturally. Many people who smoke may also be slightly depressed, says William Page-Echols, D.O., osteopathic doctor at Full Spectrum Family Medicine in East Lansing, Michigan. Smoking, he says, may be a sign of self-medication. "Nicotine clearly affects mood, and people who smoke are using it to manipulate their mood. It makes sense that herbs could be used in the same way to help a person quit." While there isn't any scientific research to prove it, Dr. Page-Echols believes that the effects of the herb St. John's wort are similar enough to those of the prescription mood-elevator bupropion to help smokers quit herbally. "I've had great success using it with my patients," he says. "It's less expensive, and there are fewer effects to worry about."

Give your husband 300 milligrams of standardized extract in capsule form three times a day, for a total of 900 milligrams. The actual number of capsules he'll have to take will depend on the formula you buy. He should start taking the herb 2 full weeks before his chosen quit date, says Dr. Page-Echols. This will give the St. John's wort time to build up in his body, making quitting easier than it would be without it. Once he's smoke-free, he can continue to take the herb for 3 to 4 months. After that, he can stop by gradually reducing his dose.

Keep him away from bars for a while. "If I had a dollar for every one of my patients who has relapsed in a bar, I'd be wealthy and retired by now," Dr. Jorenby says.

Cigarettes and a drink go hand in hand. And bars are filled with smoke and even more smokers, putting his willpower to a Herculean test. Advise him to avoid the temptation for at least a few weeks, if not longer, says Ken Leonard, Ph.D., senior research scientist and clinical psychologist at the Research Institute on Addictions in Buffalo. When he's kicked the habit and can cope with the sights, smells, and easy availability of cigarettes, then he can take his seat at the bar.

Urge him to make a quit list. He should think about why he wants to quit. Maybe he wants to see his grandchildren grow up, or he wants to run a race, or he just wants to breathe freer and feel healthier again. Then, he should write it down on a piece of paper or an index card and stick it in his wallet. The next time he feels close to taking a puff, he should take the list out and remind himself why he wants to quit. When a smoker is in the middle of one of those big urges, it's not always obvious to him why he decided to quit. Remembering what he stands to gain by quitting is critical, Dr. Jorenby says.

Give him this to counterattack the cravings. Tell him to take one dropper of a blend of tinctures of the herbs Siberian ginseng, licorice, oatstraw, and lobelia whenever cravings come on. "Herbs that are commonly used for countering addiction are basically adrenal-supporting in nature," explains Nancy Welliver, N.D., a naturopathic physician and director of the Institute of Medical Herbalism in Calistoga, California.

Each adrenal gland (we have two) is a small, triangle-shaped organ that's attached to the top of a kidney. These complex little nuggets are responsible for releasing hormones that go on to stimulate other organs, affecting heart rate, metabolism, circulation, and digestion. Herbalists believe that boosting adrenal gland function is important for recovery from chronic stressors such as nicotine addiction.

Get one 2-ounce bottle each of Siberian ginseng, licorice, and oatstraw tinctures and a 1-ounce bottle of lobelia tincture from the health food store. If he has high blood pressure, substitute 1 ounce of lemon balm and 1 ounce of hawthorn for the licorice, since licorice may exacerbate high blood pressure. Empty the contents of the four bottles into a large measuring cup or a bowl with a pour spout. Set the empty bottles aside. Gently stir the liquid to blend the tinctures well, then use a small funnel to refill the bottles with your new craving-calming tincture.

When a cigarette craving hits him, all he has to do is squeeze one dropper of the mixture into half a glass of water and sip. If water's not available, he can take the tincture by putting it directly under his tongue, says Dr. Welliver, but he should be prepared for a potent taste. He can take this blend up to 10 times a day. If he feels the need to take it more often, he can mix half a dropper with an even smaller amount of water and take it up to 20 times a day. After the first couple of weeks, he should start decreasing the amount of lobelia and increasing the amount of Siberian ginseng. Generally, he can take this mixture for anywhere from 2 weeks to 2 months.

Note: A tincture is a highly concentrated herbal liquid. It's made by soaking leaves in alcohol or glycerin—which extracts the herb's medicinal properties—for at least 6 weeks. Tinctures are sold in health food stores in small bottles with eyedroppers to give doses. Be sure to store them out of the reach of children.

Remind him that just breathing can be beneficial. When a craving hits, he should slowly breathe in, then breathe out. This technique can calm him down and help fight the temptation to grab a cigarette. "It's a relaxation skill and can help him cope with urges caused by stress," Dr. Jorenby says. So instead of reaching for a cigarette the next time he's stressed out, he should sit back, relax, and breathe deeply until the urge passes.

Kill cravings with orange juice. Starting the day with orange juice may be a good way to deter the craving for a morning cigarette, Dr. Jorenby says. The combination of most citrus juices and tobacco makes for an awfully unpleasant taste in the mouth. Many patients have told Dr. Jorenby that even the thought of a cigarette after a glass of orange juice makes them sick. Advise him to carry some citrus juice around with him and take a swig when he feels an urge coming on. But he shouldn't use orange juice as a deterrent if he uses nicotine gum, Dr. Jorenby warns. The citrus changes the chemicals in the mouth and will inhibit the effectiveness of the gum. He should wait to use the gum at least 20 minutes after drinking a glass of citrus juice or any acidic beverage, such as coffee or cola drinks.

Advise him to get some aerobic antismoking aid. Getting some exercise may help quell his urges before they start. A study at the University of Wisconsin Medical School found that ex-smokers who got regular aerobic exercise said that their cravings for cigarettes were less severe than those in ex-smokers who didn't exercise, Dr. Jorenby says. And there's an even bigger plus, he adds: Regular exercise reduces stress and may help keep off the pounds that many people gain when they try to quit.

Snoring

If necessity is the mother of invention, then a cure for snoring must be one of the most needed remedies around. There are at least 140 antisnoring devices registered with the U.S. Patent and Trademark Office. Although none of them work any better than simply staying awake, inventors keep on trying. That certainly says a lot about the difficulty encountered when you try to silence a snorer.

During sleep, the muscles in the throat relax, the tongue slips back a bit, and the airway narrows. Usually, that's not a problem. But if the opening is so constricted that the sleeper has to draw hard to breathe, the airflow vibrates the soft tissues of the palate. This giant sucking sound is akin to wind howling down a narrow canyon, says Neil Kavey, M.D., director of the Sleep Disorders Center at Columbia-Presbyterian Medical Center in New York City.

There also may be an obstruction blocking the free flow of air through the back of the throat and the nose. That respiratory roadblock can be put in place by many things, including flabby throat muscles, a double chin, or even a misshapen soft palate.

Allergies are another major cause of snoring, says Connie Catellani, M.D., medical director of the Miro Center for Integrative Medicine in Evanston, Illinois. That's because food allergies as well as hay fever can cause chronically swollen nasal passages and draining sinuses. These problems—no matter what the cause—are a sure source of snores. If your husband's snoring is allergy-related, you'll need to figure out what he's allergic to and he'll need to do his best to avoid it, says Dr. Catellani.

We all snore sometimes: when we're extremely tired or lying on our backs, or after an evening of beer drinking with our friends. But if your husband snores every night, loudly enough that you complain or a business associate refuses to share a motel room with him on the road, he may have a problem, says Dr. Kavey.

The warning signals to watch for are restless sleep (tossing and turning) and extreme daytime sleepiness, says William Finley, Ph.D., director of the Sleep Disorders Center at St. Mary's Medical Center in Knoxville, Tennessee. Heavy snorers often experience apneas (Greek for "without breath"), complete blockages of the airway that literally choke off their wind. He may struggle for breath and wake up frequently at night, although he may not be aware of these nocturnal arousals, says Dr. Finley.

"Apneas are a real health risk, associated with heart problems, high blood pressure, stroke, and automobile accidents caused by falling asleep while driving," says Dr. Finley. "And many heavy snorers who now only have partial blockage of their airways will eventually progress to full-blown apneas." Even if he doesn't have sleep apnea, loud snoring may damage the muscles in his throat, according to a study by Swedish researchers.

WHEN TO SEE THE DOCTOR

Snoring can be seriously disruptive to family life, disturbing the sleep of others and sparking resentment. If your husband's snoring is affecting your relationship, that is reason enough for him to visit the doctor, but snoring can threaten physical health as well. If he snores, awakens unrefreshed, and often feels sleepy during the day, he may have sleep apnea. Apnea is a potentially serious condition in which loud snoring alternates with periods of completely obstructed breathing. If you suspect that your husband's snoring may be related to this condition, have him see the doctor for an evaluation.

Noise Neutralizers

Tilt him. If he snores in bed but not on the recliner, it could be the tilt of his body that's causing the problem. When he's sprawled out flat on a bed, gravity is more likely to pull his tongue down into the airway, says Dr. Kavey.

Try tilting your bed by placing bricks or phone book–size blocks under the headboard. Or he can put an extra pillow under his head. That angle may make his airway fall just a little differently and smooth out the airflow.

Tell him to suspend the smoking and slow down on the booze. A night on the town makes for noisy sleep. Smoking swells throat tissues and narrows the airway, while alcohol so relaxes the neck muscles that it makes a partial collapse of the airway more likely at night, says John Galgon, M.D., medical director of the Sleep Disorders Clinic at Lehigh Valley Hospital in Allentown, Pennsylvania.

Your husband shouldn't drink in the evening before bed, and—for many health reasons—he should quit smoking, Dr. Galgon says. "Smokers almost always have inflamed, swollen throat tissues."

Stick 'em. Sleep doctors call them external nasal dilators, but you may know them as those fancy pieces of tape that football players wear on their noses. "Dilators open a normally narrow portion of the nose," explains Dr. Finley. "They increase airflow, and for some folks, that's all that's needed." Nasal dilators such as Breathe Right are available at drugstores. However, they won't help men with true apnea, because the disorder stems from problems in the throat and breath control, not the nose.

Make him an antiallergy tea. Nettle is sometimes called stinging nettle because of its bristly, spiny leaves. Herbalists consider this mineral-rich plant helpful for various ailments, but it's particularly good for easing the respiratory inflammation brought on by allergies, says Steven Rissman, N.D., a naturopathic physician at American WholeHealth in Littleton, Colorado. Give him nettle as a tea. To make it, pour 1 cup of boiling water over 1 tablespoon of dried nettle leaf, cover and steep for 5 minutes, then strain the tea into a mug. If he has allergies, start with one cup a day for the first few days, since nettle may worsen symptoms. After that, he can drink up to three cups a day. Just be sure to make one of them a nightcap, in order to get the best nose-clearing effects while he sleeps.

Have him spray his nose. If he wakes up in the morning with dry mouth, the problem may be in his nose, not his throat, Dr. Galgon says. Many snorers have deviated septums, chronic congestion, postnasal drip, or nasal polyps that force them to breathe through their mouths. He should try to clear a path through his plugged nose with an over-the-counter nasal spray or allergy medication. These sprays can be effective but may be addictive, so advise him not to use them more than three times a day or for more than 3 days, advises Dr. Galgon.

Tell him to try an herbal rinse. Oak bark is an astringent herb that contains water-soluble chemical compounds called tannins. Tannins can protect inflamed mucous membranes in the throat and nose and will help dry up secretions that can contribute to snoring. To get these effects, an infusion of oak bark is often recommended as a gargle and nasal rinse, says Dr. Rissman.

If you can't find oak bark, an infusion made with Oregon grape root works pretty much the same way. Besides being an astringent, this herb also possesses an antimicrobial effect, says Dr. Rissman, which is helpful if there is any infection brewing inside your inflamed sinuses.

To make a strong infusion, start with 2 tablespoons of either dried herb and cover with 1 cup of boiling water. Steep for up to 15 minutes, then strain the liquid into a small cup or bowl that has a pour spout. Wait until the infusion cools to room temperature before using it.

Gargling is the easy part: He simply needs to take a small mouthful of the liquid, tilt his head back, and gurgle away before spitting the liquid out. Rinsing his nasal passages (nasal lavage) is a little trickier, but it's also the most effective part of the treatment for snoring. He should form a cup with the palm of one hand and fill it with about 2 table-spoons of infusion. Keeping his head upright, he should bring his hand up to one nostril while pressing the other nostril closed. Then he should gently sniff the liquid into his nose, then release it through his mouth. He may sputter at first, but have him keep trying. Once he gets the hang of it, nasal lavage will actually feel good as it frees his nostrils and sinuses of congestion.

Advise him to work this problem out. When the muscles of the upper airway lose their tone and strength from aging or inactivity, they may be more likely to sag during sleep, says Dr. Finley.

How British Women Keep Their Husbands from Snoring

Imagine trying to sleep in the middle of rush hour in London. That's essentially what Julie Switzer did for more than 30 years. At 92 decibels, her husband Melvyn's snoring was equivalent to heavy traffic or thunder—so loud that he made it into *The Guinness Book of World Records*.

People sent the Switzers remedies from around the world, but nothing seemed to work—until they tried homeopathic drops containing wild yam (*Dioscorea villosa*) and common ginger (*Zingiber officiale*). Melvyn stopped snoring, at last.

The remedy the Switzers used—called Y-Snore Anti-snoring Nose Drops—is just one of various strategies that can help put an end to snoring, says Toni Bark, M.D., medical director of the Center for the Healing Arts in Glencoe, Illinois. Luckily, it's available at pharmacies in the United States.

Vigorous aerobic exercise and physical fitness may put the tone and tautness back in his upper airway muscles. Aerobic exercise activates muscles that dilate the upper airway so that he can take in more air, which may also strengthen upper airway muscles.

For overweight people, weight reduction often leads to marked improvement of snoring by removing fat from the walls of the upper airway, says Dr. Finley. "Physically fit people, such as runners, rarely appear at the sleep center complaining of loud snoring or breathing pauses while they sleep," he says.

For most of us, aerobic exercise such as brisk walking, jogging, or playing basketball for 30 to 40 minutes three or four times a week will lead to improved physical fitness. He should choose a form of exercise he really enjoys doing because if he doesn't, he's unlikely to stay with it long enough to tone up sagging muscles and to lose weight, says Dr. Finley. As an added bonus, being physically fit is associated with better, more restful sleep, he adds.

Tell him to turn over. He's most likely to snore when sleeping on his back. He can stay off his back by stuffing Styrofoam peanuts (packing material) into a sock and then sewing the sock onto the back of a tight-fitting night shirt, Dr. Kavey says. Each time he turns onto his back, he'll be prodded by the Styrofoam and forced to turn onto his side, says Dr. Kavey. "Some people recommend several tennis balls, but those get heavy."

Consider an antisnoring device. Retainer-style mouthpieces that pull the jaw forward can be fitted by a dentist who specializes in this treatment. If he wakes up tired and with headaches and he knows that he snores heavily, he should ask his doctor to refer him to an accredited sleep center. The staff there can assess his condition, and most often they will prescribe a ventilator with mask known as CPAP (for continuous positive airway pressure) to keep his airways open and his sleep snore-free.

Suggest he drop pounds. Most snorers are overweight guys with big necks. If he's carrying extra pounds around the middle, then he probably has fat deposits in the back of his throat, which narrow the space behind his tongue. When he's asleep, his throat muscles relax and narrow that space even more, causing him to snore, says Dr. Galgon. If your husband wants to stop snoring, he should try losing some weight. "Just 25 to 30 pounds can make a difference for some patients," says Dr. Galgon. (For more information on how to lose weight, see Abdominal Fat on page 161 and Overweight on page 445. Although the latter is in the women's section, men will be able to use the tips given there.)

Sports Addiction

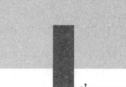

It's normal for a guy to like sports. Maybe he meets his friends in a bar every Sunday to watch the games during football season. Or perhaps he faithfully forks over $49.95 for every big pay-per-view fight. Or it could be that the first thing he does in the morning is to turn on ESPN's SportsCenter.

But when your husband knows his favorite players' batting averages down to their last at-bats but forgets your daughter's birthday every year or if sports dominate his life to the point where it's virtually all that he watches and thinks about—negatively affecting the family, his job, and your social life—he's probably a sports addict.

What is it with guys and this obsession with sports? "Men get a lot of vicarious enjoyment from watching competitive sports," says Shirley Glass, Ph.D., a clinical psychologist and marital therapist in the Baltimore area. "Most men are more nostalgic and sentimental about playing and watching sports than women are."

Another reason is male bonding. Put a guy in a roomful of other guys he has never met and all someone has to say is "Who do you like for the NBA title this year?" The next thing you know, they're talking as though they have known each other for years. "It's tremendous bonding. When men get together, they have an immediate conversation. Men are more comfortable talking about those things," says Leonard Jason, Ph.D., professor of clinical and community psychology at DePaul University in Chicago. But in order to keep up with the other guys, you also have to be right on top of the latest stats, scores, and deals, leading some men to become compulsive. And, like other addictions, sports can be a way to avoid dealing with other problems.

Although this may seem like a minor problem, it's something you—and he—shouldn't ignore. At the least, it can make him a bore. At its worst, sports addiction has brought many a couple to the marriage therapist's office. "I have had women threaten divorce," says Robert Pasick, Ph.D., a clinical psychologist at the Ann Arbor Center for the Family in Michigan.

In extreme cases, men can become so obsessed with sports that it can cause them to avoid problems in their own lives, says Merrill J. Melnick, Ph.D., sport sociologist and professor of physical education and sport at the State University of New York at Brockport. "It's like a sweaty Land of Oz for them," he says. If sports obsession interferes with your daily routine or takes precedence over your family or work responsibilities, you may need professional help, says Dr. Melnick.

Assistance for Addicts . . . and Sports Widows

Try it. Striking the right balance between time apart and time with a sports zombie is easier if you like sports. If you can enjoy the occasional baseball game, the World Series is that much easier on your relationship.

This strategy worked for Diana Adile Kirschner, Ph.D., a psychologist in Gwynedd Valley, Pennsylvania. When her husband started training for a triathlon, she decided to start exercising more as well. They ran and biked together. Though an injury tempered his interest, hers is still going strong.

Of course, it helps if your sports zombie gives sports that interest you a try. You're a tennis devotee? He might become one, too.

Focus on the players' personalities. If you can't get interested in the complexities of the game he loves, maybe you can get interested in the personalities.

"Read the sports page and get to know who the players are," Dr. Glass says. "Women are more relationally oriented. If you know stories about the players, you're likely to be more interested."

A few years ago, one woman dealt with her husband's die-hard enthusiasm for the New England Patriots by taking an interest in the coaching style of Bill Parcells and how he handled the team's promising star quarterback, Drew Bledsoe, idolized by her mate. As a new manager herself, the woman was interested in finding out more about how Parcells's coaching style translated into results on the football field.

Similarly, if you know he's competitive, pick a rival team and follow its performance. It's worth the effort just to see his reaction when you report on the other team's relative standings.

Try to find out what's missing. According to the Indian discipline of Ayurveda, sports addiction is similar to an affliction called vigil, or staying up late. If a person practices vigil, he doesn't want to retire at bedtime because he feels that he hasn't gotten satisfaction out of his day. In men with sports addiction, perhaps their work life, home life, or even spiritual life isn't what they want it to be, says Jay L. Glaser, M.D., medical director of the Maharishi Ayur-Veda Medical Center in Lancaster, Massachusetts. So they turn to sports to live vicariously through others, he suggests.

Tell him to think about what may be bothering him. Is his work not satisfying? Is he unhappy with his body? His spirituality? Then, instead of watching sports, ask him to focus all of his attention on making that part of his life better, Dr. Glaser says. "One of the most important teachings in Ayurvedic medicine is that whatever we put our attention on is what grows in our lives," Dr. Glaser says.

Suggest that he be selective. A compromise that may please both of you is if he watches only the most important sports events, such as the World Series, the Super Bowl, and the Final Four college basketball tournament. Negotiate with him to get him to skim the TV guide beforehand to decide which event he really wants to see during the week, says Philip Levendusky, Ph.D., clinical psychologist at McLean Hospital in Belmont, Massachusetts. Propose to him that he pick the ones he really wants to watch—perhaps a sports news show for an hour each night or a few big games each week—and plan to watch them. Then, he can watch only those programs that he decided were the most important, recommends Dr. Levendusky. Make it clear up front that as soon as the show is over, he'll turn off the TV or change the channel so he won't get sucked into another sporting event, he says.

Ask him to take a break. Suggest that he take a week off from sports. That's right—no football, no SportsCenter, no *Sports Illustrated*—for at least a week. Explain to him that this isn't going to cause him to keel over from massive withdrawal. What it will do is force him to find something else to do with his life, Dr. Pasick says. "A lot of times, people just fall back on watching sports because they don't have anything else to do and they get stuck there," he says. He can pass his sports time reading a good book, going to the movies, catching a show, or just getting out of the house. Or he could do something completely new and crazy, like spend the day at the park with you and the kids.

Have him suit up. Although the company softball tournament may not be as exciting as the World Series, it is a great way to enjoy sports, socialize, and get fit at the same time, says Joel H. Fish, Ph.D., director of the Center for Sport Psychology in Philadelphia. If you and your kids go to cheer him on, then you could have a nice family day together.

Air your grievances. If his sports appetite is so voracious that there's negligible time left for fun together, you need to talk, says Dr. Kirschner. "If you feel hurt, the danger is that you'll allow yourself to drift away in a sea of resentment until there's real distance between you," she says.

Negotiate for equal (or nearly equal) time. "The ideal thing is to try to create a contract with your partner," Dr. Kirschner says. "You might say, 'I'm willing to support your watching this or playing that, but in return, I want you to do something for me.'" You could agree to make snacks for him and his buddies while they watch the Sunday night game, if he, in turn, agrees to cook you a special dinner on Saturday night. Or you might decide to spend every other Sunday doing something together and allow him the remaining Sundays with the Dallas Cowboys.

Have him relive his childhood. You may think, "He does that already, every day," but hear us out on this one. For many men, sports evoke happy childhood memories: playing stickball with the neighborhood kids, tossing a football with Dad, going to their first major-league game. But he should dig deeper and remember the other things he enjoyed when he was a kid. Maybe he built model airplanes, worked in a wood shop, or rode his bike all the time. "As men fade into sports addiction, they often drop hobbies they used to like," Dr. Pasick says. Suggest to him that he pick up some of his old hobbies and rekindle some other fond memories of his youth.

Enjoy your time alone. Do whatever interests you while your partner indulges his yen for sports, suggests Irene Deitch, Ph.D., a professor of psychology at the College of Staten Island in New York. "The notion of a woman being helpless and at the mercy of the man, who has to devote all his time to making her happy, is a sexist concept," says Dr. Deitch, who finishes the *New York Times* while her husband watches sports. "We want to move away from a 'dependency notion' to an empowering concept."

Sprains

Ligaments connect bones and cartilage with each other, like hinges on gates, allowing a wide range of motion in knees, ankles, elbows, shoulders, and wrists. But the flexible connective tissue can only bend and move so much. When those ligaments give way, you've suffered a sprain.

If you take a thin rope and pull on it hard enough, the fibers in the rope start to tear. Keep pulling on the rope, and eventually the fibers may break completely. That's what happens during a sprain: Pressure pulls on the ligaments, causing them to tear or rip apart. The ligament rupture brings about swelling, pain, and instability of the joint.

Orthopedic surgeons grade sprains in three categories: Grade one is a small tear; grade two, a larger partial tear; and grade three, a complete tear. No matter what the degree, the treatment remains the same—just wait. "Even a complete tear will heal on its own," says Quinter Burnett, M.D., an orthopedic surgeon with the Western Michigan University athletic department in Kalamazoo. Scar tissue eventually reconnects the torn ligaments. If the swelling is severe, see a doctor and get an x-ray to rule out a fracture, says Dr. Burnett.

Sprain Solvers

Here are some ways you can help your husband when he comes home limping from a tough game of basketball or anything else that can cause a sprain.

Make him rest. Using a sprained ligament can turn a partial tear into a full one. He should rest the sprained area immediately and try not to use the joint for a few days, says Dr. Burnett.

Ice him. Place an ice pack wrapped in a thin towel on the sprain for

15 to 20 minutes, Dr. Burnett says. The ice reduces the swelling by contracting the blood vessels.

Reapply the ice pack every few hours for 36 hours, says Kevin Pugh, M.D., professor of orthopedics at the University of Kentucky in Lexington.

Wrap him up. Use an Ace bandage or any piece of material that applies moderate pressure, recommends Dr. Pugh. After the initial 36 hours, use the bandage to keep the swelling down while he's up and about. The pressure shuts down the bloodflow from the damaged blood vessels and decreases the swelling.

Tell him to raise it. When ligaments are torn, blood can pool in the broken vessels, causing swelling and bruising. By elevating the injured area, he'll slow down the bloodflow to it. Have him lie down on the ground and prop up the injured part, if possible above the level of his heart, Dr. Burnett says.

Don't let him rest for too long. He should try to keep the injured joint immobile for a few days after the sprain. But sprains actually heal faster when the joint is used, Dr. Burnett says. So after a few days, let him get up and around a bit . . . but slowly. He should let the pain guide him. If it hurts a lot and he can't use the joint, he should rest for a few more days. But if he can withstand some pressure with minimal pain, he should use the joint, but with care, Dr. Burnett says.

Apply comfrey. Although hard to find, leaves of the comfrey plant can soothe a bruised, swollen sprain, says Eve Campanelli, Ph.D., a holistic family practitioner in Beverly Hills, California. Look in homeopathic stores for the leaves, or try to grow them in your garden. Crush

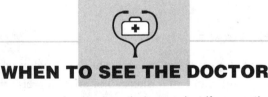

WHEN TO SEE THE DOCTOR

In most cases, sprains heal on their own, but if you notice that he has increasing pain, swelling, weakness, or instability, have him see a physician.

AN HERBAL SPRAIN HEALER

This warming homemade liniment promotes circulation and helps heal strains, sprains, and bruises. "After you put it on, you're going to feel better," says Phoebe Reeve, an herbalist in Winchester, Virginia. She is a big fan of using everyday herbs to make home remedies.

The vitamin E in this formula helps keep the oil from oxidizing and going rancid. You can apply this mixture to sore areas as often as needed, either warmed or at room temperature.

4	ounces safflower or canola oil (or any other fresh vegetable oil)
2	tablespoons dried peppermint leaves or 4 tablespoons fresh, chopped
1	piece (2" long) fresh ginger, coarsely chopped
8–10	cloves
1	capsule vitamin E liquid

Put the vegetable oil, peppermint, ginger, cloves, and vitamin E in a wide-mouth glass jar and shake to mix. Place the jar on a sunny windowsill or in a warm, dry place for 7 to 10 days to let the herbs infuse the oil. Shake the jar occasionally. Then strain, rebottle, and keep refrigerated.

If you want to speed the process, heat the vegetable oil over low heat, then add the peppermint, ginger, and cloves and simmer very gently for 20 minutes to 1 hour. Let cool before adding the vitamin E, then strain, rebottle, and refrigerate.

a fistful of them, then place the crushed leaves around the sprain and keep them in place with a bandage overnight, Dr. Campanelli says. If tinctures are more your speed, give him one dose of homeopathic comfrey tincture or the pellet form, as the label recommends, every 15 minutes during the first hour after a sprain, she advises. After the first hour, continue with the dose recommended on the bottle three times a day until the sprain heals. You can find the remedy in health or homeopathic stores. Don't use comfrey on broken skin. Also, avoid using it for prolonged periods or if his skin is sensitive; it may trigger an allergic reaction.

Note: A tincture is a highly concentrated herbal liquid. It's made by soaking leaves in alcohol or glycerin—which extracts the herb's medicinal properties—for at least 6 weeks. Tinctures are sold in health food stores in small bottles with eyedroppers to give doses. Make sure to store them out of the reach of children.

Put some arnica on him. Arnica reduces swelling, bruising, and pain, says Andrea D. Sullivan, Ph.D., a naturopath at the Center for Natural Healing/Sullivan and Associates in Washington, D.C. You can buy arnica cream at most health and homeopathic stores. Apply the cream to the sprained area as soon as possible. It should be applied three or four times a day for 5 days, says Dr. Sullivan. Do not use arnica on open wounds or broken skin. Also, it can cause allergic dermatitis if used on sensitive skin or for a prolonged period.

Preventive Measures

Have him band together. This quick and simple exercise won't completely prevent him from suffering another sprained ankle, but it may decrease the chances. He should find a 6-inch rubber loop or piece of tubing or purchase flex bands at a sporting goods store. While sitting with his feet together, he should wrap the tubing around the balls of both feet, Dr. Burnett says. Then he should bend his knees slightly. Keeping his heels together, he should slowly rotate his feet apart and then bring them back together. Dr. Burnett advises repeating this 10 to 20 times. This exercise can be done daily, or at least 3 days a week. It strengthens the muscles around the ankle joint, giving the ligaments better protection the next time they take a hit, Dr. Burnett says.

Encourage him to protect the joint. For 1 to 2 weeks after the sprain, he should wear a protective bandage, such as an Ace bandage, around the sprain. Wrap it snugly, but not so tightly that it causes swelling. Other products such as air and lace braces also protect the sprained body part. After a few weeks, he can start wearing the bandage only when he plays sports or puts extra force on the injured joint. He should keep that up for 2 to 3 months, Dr. Burnett says.

Encourage him to stretch. When he jumps right into an athletic activity without warming up, the ligaments may just snap, says Michael Bemben, Ph.D., professor of exercise science at the University of Oklahoma in Norman. Instead, he should begin with a slow 5-minute jog, or ride his bike to the company softball game. Then, once he has increased his body temperature, he should take a few minutes to stretch his muscles. The increased body temperature warms up the muscles and ligaments, allowing them to stretch more easily and making them less likely to get injured.

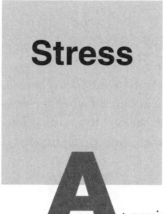

Stress

At precisely the moment you need a clear head, steady hands, or a deep voice, stress makes you feel jittery, sweaty, and confused. More than half of all people admit to feeling stressed, though only 9 percent of men seek professional help.

Stress is a biological response designed to sharpen the senses and heighten alertness during life-threatening situations. When the brain perceives imminent danger, it signals the body to secrete stress hormones, which speed up the heart rate, breathing, and sweating, later leaving us feeling exhausted. When human worries were primal, such as avoiding being eaten by sharks, this stress response was a very good thing, indeed. But in these more civilized times, when the most dangerous sharks wear three-piece suits and carry cellular phones, it can be destructive.

The brain misinterprets relatively benign events—an encounter with an angry boss or wife, a looming deadline—as life-threatening and triggers the stress response. It usually can be traced back to a thought: My wife is going to kill me. I'm gonna lose my job.

"Stress is all in the mind," says Peggy Kileff, M.S., a wellness consultant at Methodist Hospital's Institute for Preventive Medicine in Houston. "You always have a thought before you have a feeling."

However, stress is more than a nuisance. Stress can be deadly. Chronic stress raises levels of hormones in the body that can damage blood vessels, raise cholesterol, spike blood pressure, impair immunity, and generally make us feel wiped out, says Michael Babyak, Ph.D., professor of medical psychology at Duke University Medical Center in Durham, North Carolina. Also, we usually don't take good care of our health when stressed. We eat lots of junk, don't get enough sleep, and blow off our workouts.

Soothing Suggestions and Relaxing Remedies

If you notice that your husband is very stressed out, give him the following tips. (Or use them yourself when the world gets on your nerves.)

Advise him to think "heavy" thoughts. "Sensations of heaviness are relaxing for people," Kileff says. So tell him to take a short break and sit

WHEN TO SEE THE DOCTOR

If your husband is constantly experiencing headaches, bowel or bladder problems, tension and pain in his neck or lower back, heart palpitations, irritability, or depression, he should see a doctor, says Michael Babyak, Ph.D., professor of medical psychology at Duke University Medical Center in Durham, North Carolina. Everyone gets these symptoms occasionally, but if they become chronic, that's when it is time to take action.

The same applies if he's under so much stress that it's keeping him up night after night or interfering with his ability to work or with his relationships.

or lie down for 5 minutes. He should imagine that his body weighs 600 pounds and feel that weight press into the floor. The more he allows his body to plaster itself to the floor, the more stress will sink away.

Tell him to stop and think. Sometimes, evaluating the situation helps control stress. He should ask himself if stress will help him achieve anything useful, such as sprinting to rescue a loved one from an oncoming car. If not, then he should try to slow down his breathing and be aware of his heart rate and level of muscle tension, says Dr. Babyak.

Then your husband should take 10 to 15 minutes to pace his breathing and let his mind and body relax. He'll be soothing and slowing himself down by repeating a cue word or visualizing a pleasant place. For this to be effective, he has to do this exercise *before* he gets stressed. While visualizing himself in a quiet, restful place, he should relax his muscles and slow his breathing. Also, he should use a cue word, such as "peace," while doing this. That way, when stress hits, he can repeat his cue word and his previously trained body will already know how to relax, explains Dr. Babyak.

Have him try an old trick: breathing slow and easy. To slow his breathing, he'll have to pay attention to his breath, which means that he can't pay attention to all the other things that made him feel stressed out to begin with. Slow breathing also helps him physically feel relaxed. To do this technique, he should inhale deep into his belly for a count of four. Then he should slowly exhale for another count of four. "We inhale and exhale thousands of times a day, so we have lots of chances to practice slow breathing," Kileff says. Whenever he's stuck at a traffic light, on hold, or waiting for the elevator, he should practice, she recommends.

Offer him the oatstraw option. For a remedy that is mild enough for everyday use but plenty strong to help him deal with intense stress, try giving him a tea made from oatstraw, says Susun S. Weed, an herbalist from Woodstock, New York. To make the tea, put 1 ounce (by weight) of dry oatstraw in a quart jar and fill it with boiling water. Screw on the lid and let it steep overnight or for at least 4 hours before straining off the liquid. "I drink one to four cups a day to strengthen my nerves and relieve stress. The only side effect," says Weed, "is increased libido." (Not a bad side effect, huh?) Oatstraw is available in health food stores.

Consider another helpful herb. "When I am acutely stressed, I use tincture of flowering motherwort," Weed says. It's important to use a tincture of motherwort prepared from fresh (not dry) plants—the label will indicate this. A dose of 15 to 20 drops in about a half-cup of liquid promptly relieves symptoms of stress. "If I don't feel better in 5 minutes, I take another dose," says Weed. "Motherwort brings the calm of sitting in your mother's lap. No matter how hard life gets, it helps me cope."

Note: A tincture is a highly concentrated herbal liquid. It's made by soaking leaves in alcohol or glycerin—which extracts the herb's medicinal properties—for at least 6 weeks. Tinctures are sold in health food stores in small bottles with eyedroppers to give doses. Be sure to store them out of the reach of children.

Have him go back to the root. Ginseng is noted for helping those under stress. It won't necessarily calm, but it does help with the physical effects that accompany stress, says Weed. She prefers the American ginseng root, at least 5 years old, dried or in a tincture. When your husband is stressed out, give him either a hunk of dried root to chew that's "the size of the last joint closest to the tip of the little finger" or a dropperful of the tincture (according to the instructions on the bottle), recommends Weed. Ginseng is available at health food stores and drugstores.

Calm him with some chamomile. Calming and exceptionally safe, chamomile is a good choice for stressed-out people, says Anne Cowper, a medical herbalist in Morisset, Australia. To brew a calming cup of chamomile tea, stop at a health food store and buy some dried chamomile flowers that are yellow and white, she says. (If they're straw-colored, they're too old.) Add 2 teaspoons of bulk flowers or 1 teaspoon of finely ground flowers to a mug, pour in 8 ounces of boiling water, cover, steep for 15 minutes, and strain. Have him drink one cup of tea three times daily.

Try this quick, calming combo. The common herbal combination of valerian, passionflower, and skullcap, found in many health food stores, can help him relax, too, says George Milowe, M.D., a holistic physician in Saratoga Springs, New York. Passionflower is a popular stress remedy throughout Europe; Romanian shops even carry tension-easing passionflower chewing gum. Both skullcap (a member of the mint family) and valerian have been shown to have mild sedative effects as well.

Give him two droppers of the mixed tincture in ½ cup of water three times daily. Be sure to dilute this remedy as recommended, since many tinctures contain alcohol that may be hard on the stomach if they are not diluted.

Get him to relax with kava. A popular stress remedy in Germany, kava contains active ingredients called kavalactones that act like muscle relaxants. Give him 200 milligrams of root extract in capsule form three times a day or 1 teaspoon of tincture twice daily. If you buy capsules, look for a product that contains 30 percent kavalactones. In a 1:5 tincture form, give him no more than 1 teaspoon twice a day. He can take kava as needed during periods of high stress, but he shouldn't take it for long periods of time.

Tell him to do nothing. If he sets aside some time each day to do absolutely nothing and let his mind wander, his mind will eventually take him to various worries. But this isn't a bad thing. "He has to put himself in a situation where he's relaxed, so he can view these things with a clear head. Usually, he'll realize that the problem isn't as big as he thought," says Andrew Yiannakis, Ph.D., professor of leisure, tourism, and sport at the University of Connecticut in Storrs.

Now, you don't want him to use this tip to get out of what he has to do around the house, so tell him he should do it in the morning. It turns out that morning is the best time of day to do nothing. Advise him to wake up a bit earlier than usual and sit in a comfortable chair while he leisurely drinks his morning coffee (or preferably tea, if you can get him to switch), Dr. Yiannakis suggests. That way he'll have time both to decompress from stress *and* clean out the garage later on.

Make him move his body. When we exercise, our heart rate quickens, our blood pressure jumps, our breathing speeds up, and we sweat. When we feel stressed out, our heart rate quickens, our blood pressure jumps, our breathing speeds up, and we sweat. Sound familiar? "Exercise is like a fire drill," Kileff says. "People who exercise seem to handle stress better." Any exercise is better than no exercise. So, even if you can only get him to take a walk around the block once in a while, he'll still do himself some good. But let him know that the more strenuously he exercises, the more relaxed he'll feel, says Kileff. Advise him to aim for a 30- to 45-minute workout three times a week.

Whatever exercise he does should be something he enjoys. And if he picks a team sport, remind him not to be overly competitive, or he'll raise his stress level all over again. "The goal of playing should be to enjoy the process," says Dr. Yiannakis. "People who are outcome-oriented want to win. People who are interested in doing the activity because it is fun are less concerned with competition and winning."

Changing his mindset won't be easy. He'll have to consistently remember to go easy on himself when he makes a mistake, so if you can, go out to watch him and encourage him if he decides to play for his company's softball team or a local soccer team. He should allow a month to adjust to this new way of playing. If, at the end of the month, he still plays to win and can't play for fun, he should probably try switching to a less competitive activity such as hiking, dancing, or stationary cycling.

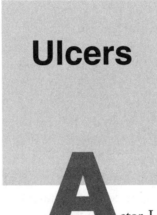

Ulcers

ctor Lorne Greene, perhaps best known for his role as the widower Ben Cartwright on the television show *Bonanza*, was hospitalized in 1987 for surgery on a perforated ulcer. He developed pneumonia and never recovered. Sadly for fans of the popular actor, doctors didn't know then what they know now. For Greene, ulcers were no bonanza. Indirectly, the disease killed him.

In the year Greene died, no one had ever heard of *Helicobacter pylori*. It wasn't until several years later that Australian doctors found the bacteria in the stomach lining of many people with peptic ulcers and were able to identify it as the cause. Until then, it was believed that ulcers were caused by stress and poor diet.

Antibiotics that target *H. pylori* have changed the way doctors tackle ulcers. In the process, they have saved lives and allowed many more people to go through their days without the burning, stabbing pain that marks this disorder.

Nevertheless, says Mark J. S. Miller, Ph.D., professor of pediatrics and physiology at Albany Medical College in New York, as helpful as antibiotics have been in the fight against ulcers, they aren't a cure-all.

H. pylori is becoming increasingly resistant to some of the antibiotics used to treat it. And even if antibiotics do work, you can still be reinfected.

What's more, for 30 percent of the people with peptic ulcers, bacteria aren't the cause. For them, ulcers are more likely to be associated with long-term use of caustic nonsteroidal anti-inflammatory drugs, such as aspirin, that they take for other conditions such as headaches, says Dr. Miller.

Although ulcers aren't necessarily serious, ulcer pain is notorious for awakening its sufferers in the middle of the night. The discomfort is episodic, however. It lasts for a couple of days or weeks and then goes away, but it always returns. Ulcers sometimes grow so large or do so much damage that they produce bleeding as well as lots of scarring. If your husband sees blood in his stool (it looks black) or has severe stomach pain and a high fever, then he should see a doctor, says David Peura, M.D., a gastroenterologist and professor of medicine at the University of Virginia Health Sciences Center in Charlottesville.

"Most ulcers will heal on their own," Dr. Peura says. "But only antibiotics can get rid of the underlying problem, which is the presence of *H. pylori*. If you don't take care of that, there's a good chance that you'll have another ulcer." So if your husband has an ulcer, he should ask his doctor to test for *H. pylori*.

Getting rid of the *H. pylori* bacteria involves a 2-week series of three medications. However, there are many other ways to combat the actual pain and discomfort of an ulcer attack.

WHEN TO SEE THE DOCTOR

If home remedies don't work within 2 weeks, and he has sustained abdominal pain and burning, have a doctor check him out. Ulcers can turn into stomach cancer in some cases. If he experiences abdominal pain or chronic indigestion during or after meals, have him see the doctor immediately.

Antiulcer Assistance

Give him antacids. For quick relief from stomach pain that you think may be an ulcer, give him antacids, says David Rooney, M.D., a family physician with Southern Chester County Family Practice Associates in Oxford, Pennsylvania. (Follow the directions on the label.)

"Antacids can help him wait out the 'telling time.' If the pain goes away in 2 weeks and doesn't return, then he probably didn't have an ulcer. If you find that he has to keep taking the medicine after 2 weeks, suspect an ulcer and have him see his doctor," Dr. Rooney advises.

"There's no major difference among the antacids you'll see on your drugstore shelf," says Dr. Rooney. "Buy whatever is on sale."

Watch his diet. Certain foods may trigger his ulcer. In fact, one of the leading candidates—milk—was for a long time widely considered a home remedy. "Milk isn't good for ulcers because the proteins in it stimulate the secretion of stomach acid," Dr. Peura says. "We generally tell people to simply see which foods bother them and then to avoid those foods."

In fact, food allergies can exacerbate ulcer symptoms, and milk is a leading allergen. Other allergens include corn and wheat. It's better for him to eat whole grains lower in gluten, such as brown rice, millet, or buckwheat, advises Priscilla Skerry, N.D., a naturopathic physician and homeopath in Portland, Maine.

Advise him to snack. Food can be either part of the problem or part of the solution. It's up to him. If he has late-night discomfort, a snack of bread or crackers can serve as a good sponge for stomach acid and bring temporary relief, says Thomas Gossel, Ph.D., professor of pharmacology at Ohio Northern University in Ada.

Encourage relaxation. Although studies relating ulcers to stress are inconclusive, it is certain that stress can aggravate ulcers, says Dr. Skerry. (It's not the stress so much as the reaction to it that causes the problem.)

Whether through exercise, relaxation techniques, or meditation, he should take time each day to de-stress his life. His stomach will thank him.

Give him some cabbage juice. Drinking 1 liter of fresh, raw cabbage juice throughout the day may help, Dr. Skerry says. Cabbage is high in glutamine, a nonessential amino acid. "Glutamine helps the healthy stomach cells regenerate and stimulates the production of mucin, which protects the stomach lining," Dr. Skerry says.

To make it, slice and then juice or blend an ordinary green cabbage, says Dr. Skerry. "It's not bad tasting," she says.

Consider a homeopathic option. Arsenicum album is one homeopathic remedy available in health food stores that can help the burning pain and anxiety that often accompany an ulcer. Give him three 30X or 30C pellets when the symptoms are acute, advises Dr. Skerry. "You can repeat that in a half-hour if you need to, but if the symptoms don't ease within an hour, then discontinue its use because this isn't the right remedy."

Give him cat's claw. Once falsely promoted as a cure for cancer, cat's claw has been at the center of some highly promising laboratory research on ulcers that Dr. Miller and another colleague are conducting at Albany Medical College, he says.

Cat's claw works in a number of ways against ulcers. First, it is a powerful anti-inflammatory that calms the ulcerated tissue by preventing the immune system's attack on the stomach lining. Its second action relates to the development of stomach cancer down the road. Although it's not well-known, stomach cancer is one of the top cancer killers in the world. Research suggests that cat's claw actually inhibits the toxic effects of compounds thought to be involved in gene mutations in the stomach that can lead to cancer.

To get the benefits of cat's claw, you need to know how it's manufactured. The recommended dosage, which is 300 milligrams in capsule form twice a day with meals, is for cat's claw that has been atomized, or ground exceptionally finely. If the herb has only been pulverized, a less refined form, you'll need to increase the dosage to 1,500 milligrams twice daily with meals. The reason for this is that fewer of the active compounds are digested with the cruder form, says Dr. Miller. The best form is freeze-dried, in which 3,000 milligrams of micropulverized cat's claw is concentrated into a single 90-milligram tablet, he says. To tell which form you have, check the label or break open a capsule and pour the powdered herb into a glass of water. If most of it settles to the bottom without dissolving, it was pulverized, and you should give him the higher dose, says Dr. Miller.

Give him two cloves of garlic a day. Garlic has strong antibiotic properties, says James S. Sensenig, N.D., a naturopathic physician and professor at the University of Bridgeport College of Naturopathic Medicine in Connecticut. Research bears this out. Scientists at the Fred

ANTIULCER FRUIT COCKTAIL

In his book The Green Pharmacy, *James A. Duke, Ph.D., an herbalist and ethnobotanist in Fulton, Maryland, gives a delicious home remedy for ulcer disease. Every ingredient in this fruit/herb cocktail contains large amounts of soothing, antiulcer compounds. (Try to be especially generous with the ginger, since it has 11 antiulcer compounds concentrated in one humble spice.) If only all medicine tasted like this!*

Bananas
Pineapple
Blueberries
Ground cinnamon
Ground ginger
Ground cloves
Honey (optional)

Cut up the bananas and pineapple; the amounts and proportions will vary according to the number of servings and which fruits you like best. Put them in a serving bowl and add the blueberries. Season to taste with the spices and sweeten with the honey (if you wish).

Hutchinson Cancer Research Center in Seattle exposed *H. pylori* to garlic and found that the herb consistently knocked the bacteria dead. And the bacteria showed no ability to become resistant to garlic, as they do to antibiotics.

Now for the taste: Eating raw garlic isn't a pleasant experience for most people. No problem. Mash or crush the cloves as smoothly as you can, then spread them on dry toast or crackers. "That masks the strong taste. It's actually pretty good," says Dr. Sensenig.

Make him some chamomile tea. It's believed that chamomile's healing properties come from three sources—volatile oils, which are anti-inflammatory; flavonoids, which are antispasmodic; and mucilages, which soothe irritation of the mucous membrane in the stomach. To make a tea from chamomile flowers, buy some of the dried herb. Cover 1 teaspoon with 1 cup of hot water and steep for 5 to 10 minutes, then let it cool slightly. Have him slowly drink one cup of tea three or four times daily.

Give him licorice. Licorice contains flavonoids that can reduce the inflammation of an ulcer, says Dr. Sensenig. Deglycyrrhizinated licorice, or DGL, is a modified form of licorice root that contains no glycyrrhizic acid, a compound that can raise blood pressure and deplete potassium stores in the body. DGL lozenges have no such side effects, and they're a relatively pleasant way to get the medicine to go down. Buy the chewable kind and have him chew them slowly, holding the compound in his mouth for at least a minute before swallowing in order to absorb more of the active ingredients and reap all of its benefits. Have him chew one or two DGL lozenges four to six times daily, or take one or two 400-milligram capsules before each meal.

Prevention Tactics

Tell him he should quit smoking. Here's another reason for him to give up smoking, but this one has nothing to do with the health of his lungs. "Smoking depletes the saliva, which is our own internal antacid," Dr. Peura explains. Without healthy saliva, stomach acid can't neutralize the foods that irritate it. Smoking also stimulates acid, which can aggravate ulcer pain and slow healing, adds Dr. Peura.

Be careful with aspirin. Many men take one aspirin a day to fight heart disease, and that's good. But about 1 percent of all regular aspirin users end up with problem ulcers.

He should only take a daily dose of aspirin or other painkillers under the care of a physician, who should be checking for signs of an ulcer. "The worry isn't so much that the medication will cause an ulcer but that it will cause an ulcer to bleed, which can be very serious," says Dr. Peura.

If he needs to take a painkiller, have him use acetaminophen instead, suggests Dr. Peura. It provides relief without irritating the stomach.

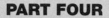

PART FOUR

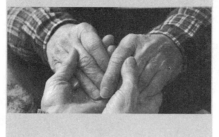

Mom's Medicine for Older Folks

Arthritis

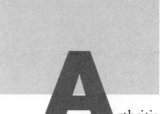rthritis is basically a packaging problem. The joints, remarkable and elaborate hinges, are cushioned by cartilage. They're held together with various other tissues, including muscles and tendons. Lubrication is in the form of an oily substance called synovial fluid, which is released by the synovial lining of the joints.

If your relative has osteoarthritis, the kind that most frequently coincides with aging, the cartilage around his joints starts to thin down or disappear. That's not his fault. What's more, it's not always preventable either. Overuse may be the root of the problem. "It is caused by years of wear and tear or overuse of the joints," says Arnold Katz, M.D., a rheumatologist at the Overland Park Regional Medical Center in Kansas. Obesity may contribute to the development of osteoarthritis in weight-bearing joints.

The runner-up, rheumatoid arthritis, is far less common, more mysterious, and equally pain-producing. Rheumatoid arthritis is an inflammatory disease. With some people, the onset begins between the ages of 30 and 40, but more often it starts when people are between the ages of 40 and 60. For reasons that aren't fully understood, the body's immune system attacks the joints, which start to suffer dire consequences.

For osteoarthritis, there are many tactics that can help hold off pain and maintain mobility. Some of these strategies might help people with rheumatoid arthritis as well. It all hinges on staying active, Dr. Katz emphasizes.

Keep him moving. To keep arthritis pain at bay, your loved one should start exercising, says Dale L. Anderson, M.D., a doctor from Minneapolis and an expert in pain relief. "Folks who are suffering from osteoarthritis must stay active; otherwise, the already-affected joints will get weaker, and the people's overall aerobic capacity will drop," he says.

If your relative is over 60, he should start with low-impact aerobic activities such as 20-minute walks or exercises in a swimming pool at least three or four times per week, says William Pesanelli, a physical therapist and director of rehabilitation services at Boston University. Any aerobic exercise program should be matched to physical capacity. "If a person has been inactive for a period of time, then we're not suggesting that he go out and try to run the Boston Marathon. Instead, he should start with something like a 5-minute walk a couple of times per week, and then slowly start to increase the distance as he feels more comfortable," he says.

Counteract it with a hot-pepper cream. Capsaicin cream, made from the active ingredient in hot peppers, has been shown in studies to ease arthritis pain when used regularly, according to Jeffrey R. Lisse, M.D., professor of medicine at the University of Texas Medical Branch at Galveston. You can buy this cream over the counter. Follow instructions on the label, wash your hands thoroughly after application, and keep this stuff away from your relative's eyes and other mucous membranes. It can really burn. And, of course, keep it out of the reach of children.

Help him lighten up. Arthritis gets worse more rapidly in overweight individuals, according to Dr. Anderson. If a person loses 5 to 10 pounds, it considerably lightens the load on all of the weight-bearing joints—

WHEN TO SEE THE DOCTOR

If any of the joints in your relative's body appear red or swollen or if tenderness in them persists for several weeks, you should take him to see a doctor, suggests Robert Swezey, M.D., medical director of the Arthritis and Back Pain Center in Santa Monica, California. Also, be sure to schedule an appointment if your loved one's hands are bright red and swollen and he can't grab things properly. Whatever you do, don't put off seeing a doctor if your relative is in pain. "An early, accurate diagnosis will help immensely," he says.

hips, knees, ankles, and feet, he says. (For more information on weight loss, see the Overweight chapter on page 445.)

Suggest a change of scenery. Walking is always recommended, but it's important to not get into a rut. "If a person walks the same exact path every day, then he's landing on the same part of the foot each and every day and putting stress on the knees and hips the exact same way every day," says Dr. Anderson. For the sake of maintaining interest as well as exercise, recommend that your loved one seek out new terrain like hills, fields, and pathways as well as flat roads or sidewalks.

Encourage him to walk, not march. Dr. Anderson believes that there are two types of walkers in this world: soft walkers and hard walkers. Soft walkers glide across a room like Gene Kelly and don't put their heels, ankles, feet, or knees through much stress. Hard walkers are in the habit of hitting the ground with their heels or the soles of their feet.

If your relative suffers from arthritis and is a hard walker, have him try out a softer, more gliding style. He should try to *place* his feet when walking, rather than *plunk* them. Or he can imagine that he's gliding on a layer of air or has puppetlike strings attached to his head and shoulders that straighten him up. Upon doing this, your relative will feel as though he's walking on air, and it will save serious wear and tear on the weight-bearing joints, promises Dr. Anderson.

Fill him with fish. Serve up more salmon or other cold-water fish such as herring and sardines if your loved one has rheumatoid arthritis, says Dr. Katz. That's because these fish are high in omega-3 fatty acids, a type of fat that actually eases the aches and swelling of an arthritic joint.

Ask for alternative oils. If your loved one doesn't like fish, Dr. Katz recommends a visit to the nearest health food store. Look for either evening primrose oil, flaxseed oil, or fish oil. All contain the same omega-3 fatty acids found in cold-water fish. If you give your relative 1 teaspoon of any of these each day, it may lightly ease some of the inflammatory aspects of arthritis, Dr. Katz says. If you decide to give him capsules, follow the manufacturer's instructions on the label.

Get some glucosamine. Some studies suggest that glucosamine sulfate, a nutritional supplement, may build cartilage and slow the progression of the disease. According to Walter Crinnion, N.D., a naturopathic physician in Kirkland, Washington, 500 milligrams of glucosamine sulfate taken three times a day before meals "works great" among his patients who suffer from osteoarthritis. But your relative shouldn't expect to be pain-free right away. This is a slow, natural process of rebuilding a damaged body part.

Dr. Crinnion advises his patients to take 1,500 milligrams daily of the supplement for about 6 months, and then lower the dosage to between 500 and 1,000 milligrams daily, according to how their bodies feel. If your relative doesn't feel relief at a maintenance dose of 500 milligrams, increase it to 1,000 milligrams daily, he suggests. And here's a consumer tip from Dr. Crinnion: Make sure that the label says glucosamine *sulfate*. "There are other forms of glucosamine being sold, and they don't work as well," he says.

Treat it with a tree. Boswellia, an extract from the frankincense tree, may hold the key to relieving pain from arthritis without undesirable side effects, says C. Leigh Broadhurst, Ph.D., a nutrition consultant and herbal researcher based in Clovery, Maryland. Inside the fragrant tree are chemicals called boswellic acids. Research suggests that these acids interrupt inflammation early on by preventing the production of biochemicals in the body that start the pain process. In other words, instead of trying to stop the train when it's barreling down the track at 100 miles an hour, boswellia cuts the engines while it's still pulling out of the station.

The bark of this tree, which is grown on the dry hills of India, is cut to collect the aromatic gum resin that's used to make a standardized extract. The extract has been shown to improve blood supply to the joints and prevent the breakdown of tissues caused by all types of arthritis. To ease chronic pain, your relative should take 450 milligrams in capsule form four times a day. It's safe to take boswellia for arthritis indefinitely.

Buy some turmeric. Curcumin, the powerful anti-inflammatory substance in turmeric, isn't a drug, but it can act like one, says Dr. Broadhurst. "If my fate were such that I could have only one medicinal plant, it would be turmeric," she says. Although it has been used for thousands of years in India for cooking, dyeing, and medicinal uses, turmeric was largely overlooked in North America until the 1970s. When modern science finally took a closer look, the results were impressive.

When compared to the popular anti-inflammatory drug phenylbutazone (Butazolidin) in a clinical study, curcumin was found to be equally effective at treating arthritis. To relieve chronic pain and inflammation, encourage your relative to take one or two 400- to 500-milligram capsules of extract three times a day. It's okay to take curcumin for arthritis indefinitely.

Stock up on another curative condiment. Unlike many arthritis medications that may wreak havoc on your digestive system, ginger is a stomach soother. Long used as a treatment for nausea, research now suggests that it may help ease the aches and pains of arthritis, says Dr. Broadhurst.

In a study from Denmark, three-quarters of the people with arthritis who took a daily dose of ginger reported some relief from pain and swelling without any side effects.

For the best medicinal benefits, look for fresh, organically grown rhizome, sometimes mistakenly referred to as a root. If it is old, shriveled, moldy, or chemically treated, it will not yield the same amount of active substances. To keep a steady supply on hand, peel the ginger and cut it into thick slices. Place them in a clean jar, pour in enough vodka (as a preservative) to cover, and put a lid on the jar. You can store it in the refrigerator indefinitely. Your relative should eat about 1 teaspoon of grated ginger every day.

Give him guaiacum. This is an herb specifically for the pain and swelling caused by rheumatoid arthritis, says Keith Robertson, a medical herbalist from Glasgow, Scotland. It stimulates bloodflow to the affected area and flushes away the dead and damaged cells caused by inflammation.

To make the decoction, put 1 teaspoon of guaiacum wood chips in 1 cup of water and bring to a boil. Simmer for 15 to 20 minutes, then strain. When your relative has a lot of pain and inflammation, have him drink three cups of the decoction daily.

Ice down the area. If your relative has swelling, especially after any physical activity, wrap some ice in a thin towel and place it on the area around the affected joint, says Keith Jones, head trainer for the Houston Rockets basketball team. "Ice the area for 15 to 20 minutes after exercise to reduce the discomfort and minimize the amount of swelling."

Or as an alternative to ice packs, Pesanelli recommends applying a bag of frozen peas to the affected area because it can contort to the shape of the hurting joint. After you've used the peas once, you can just toss them back into the freezer compartment, get them iced, and use the same bag again. But since bacteria can quickly multiply in food that has been thawed and refrozen, make sure to clearly label the bag so that you don't accidentally try to serve those peas for dinner.

Dementia

Spend more than a few minutes with your parents or grandparents, and you'll probably start hearing jokes about getting senile—usually because someone lost the car keys or forgot to show up for a doctor's appointment.

Despite the occasional humorous comments about memory loss, one of the main fears that people have is of losing their mental abilities as they get older. Everyone needs to understand that there is a difference between occasional lapses in memory, which are a normal part of aging, and dementia, which represents serious declines in memory and thinking.

Problems with memory and judgment that interfere with the conduct of daily life, such as getting lost in familiar places, forgetting important dates and appointments, or writing the same check twice, are signs of dementia, not normal aging. In the past, doctors considered these early changes associated with dementia to be normal aging and used the term *senility*. They now recognize that dementia is the result of specific conditions due to the progressive loss of brain cells.

The most common cause of dementia is Alzheimer's disease, which damages nerve cells in the brain and has no cure. Dementia can also be caused by stroke and other circulatory problems or nutritional deficiencies. It can even be a side effect of medications. The good news, however, is that some types of dementia can be reversed when they're treated quickly, so it's essential to have your loved one see a doctor at the first sign of problems, says Patricio Reyes, M.D., professor of neurology and director of the Alzheimer's Disease and Dementia Center at Thomas Jefferson Medical College of Thomas Jefferson University in Philadelphia. Even when the physical damage can't be reversed, it may be possible to slow or even stop the progression of symptoms, he explains.

WHEN TO SEE THE DOCTOR

Dementia often comes on very slowly, so family members can miss the early warning signs. Yet prompt medical attention is essential. For example, taking the appropriate medicines early on can help delay the progression of Alzheimer's. Make an appointment with your doctor if you notice any of the following symptoms in a loved one.

- Recent memory loss that affects job skills

- Difficulty performing familiar tasks—for instance, preparing a meal and forgetting to serve it, as well as not recalling who made it

- Problems with language, such as forgetting simple words or substituting inappropriate words

- Disorientation of time and place—becoming lost on his own street, not knowing where he is, how he got there, or how to get home

- Poor or decreased judgment, such as entirely forgetting a child under his care or wearing several shirts or blouses

- Problems with abstract thinking—not remembering completely what the numbers are in a checkbook and what needs to be done with them

- Misplacing things—for example, putting an iron in the freezer or a watch in the sugar bowl

- Changes in mood or behavior or unexplained mood swings

- Changes in personality, which can be drastic—for instance, becoming extremely confused, suspicious, or fearful

- Loss of initiative or becoming very passive

Protecting the Mind

People are living longer than ever before, thanks to improvements in medical care as well as lifestyle factors, such as giving up smoking and eating healthier diets. But along with the increase in longevity has come an increase in dementia, says Dr. Reyes. The brain, some experts believe, simply isn't designed to stay healthy for so many years. Research has shown, however, that there are ways to protect the brain from long-term damage. They are worth trying because dementia is very common. In the United States, 10 percent of those over age 65 suffer from Alzheimer's disease. The percentage increases to nearly 50 percent in those 85 and older.

Doctors don't know for sure what causes many cases of dementia, and medical treatments so far have had limited success. But there are ways to help keep blood vessels and nerves in the brain healthy. Here's what doctors advise.

Stock up on antioxidants. Oxygen is essential for life, but the body naturally transforms some of this life-giving substance into dangerous molecules called free radicals. Free radicals damage tissues throughout the body, including blood vessels in the brain. Researchers believe that these molecules play a pivotal role in the development of Alzheimer's disease and other forms of dementia.

Studies have shown that nutritional supplements containing antioxidants can help prevent this damage from getting started. Antioxidants are found in fruits, vegetables, and other foods, but in amounts that may be too small to fully protect the brain. With supplements, however, it's easy to get the recommended amounts. Important antioxidants include:

- Vitamin E. "Physicians are recommending that people at risk for Alzheimer's disease take 800 IU of vitamin E a day," says Stanley Birge, M.D., director of the Older Adult Health Center at Washington University School of Medicine in St. Louis. (People who are most at risk for Alzheimer's are those who have had a loss of height greater than 2 inches, didn't use estrogen after menopause, have symptoms of depression, and don't exercise regularly.) If you are considering giving your loved one amounts above 400 IU, discuss it with your doctor first. One study using low-dose supplements showed an increased risk of hemorrhagic stroke.

Herbal Medicine for the Mind

Many scientific studies have found that the herb ginkgo may be helpful for treating conditions associated with aging, such as memory loss and reduced blood circulation in the brain. Ginkgo helps with circulation in the brain by interfering with a substance in the blood called platelet activation factor. This is important because impaired circulation is thought to play a role in the development of Alzheimer's disease. While it's not proven to help with Alzheimer's, at least one study suggests that ginkgo may be helpful. In this study, German researchers found that people taking a standardized ginkgo extract had significantly improved memory and reaction times compared to those taking placebos.

"Ginkgo is believed to have antioxidant properties as well," says Patricio Reyes, M.D., professor of neurology and director of the Alzheimer's Disease and Dementia Center at Thomas Jefferson Medical College of Thomas Jefferson University in Philadelphia. "There's no solid scientific evidence that it's effective, but I think it has potential."

Researchers haven't determined what the ideal dose of ginkgo might be, Dr. Reyes adds. For now, the best advice is to give your loved one ginkgo capsules that have a standardized dose, following the directions on the package label.

- Vitamin C. "We recommend taking 500 milligrams of vitamin C a day," says Dr. Birge. "It potentiates the action of vitamin E, and it also has antioxidant effects of its own."

See that he gets enough vitamin D. The body uses this nutrient to produce a chemical called acetylcholine, which is essential for keeping brain cells healthy. "Vitamin D also plays a role in preventing depression and seasonal affective disorder, both of which can lead to symptoms of dementia," Dr. Birge adds.

The recommended daily amount for vitamin D in older adults is 600 IU—about the amount in five glasses of milk. Older people frequently need more than this because they may be resistant to its effects, says Dr. Birge. "The best way to get more vitamin D is to drink a couple glasses of milk a day and supplement that with a multivitamin that provides another 400 IU," he adds.

One way to tell if someone in your family isn't getting enough vitamin D is to feel the fingernails. Unusually soft and thin nails that tear easily are a common symptom of vitamin D deficiency or resistance to vitamin D, Dr. Birge says.

Think zinc. The central nervous system needs zinc in order to function properly. Paradoxically, many people are deficient in zinc because they're trying to keep their hearts healthy by cutting back on red meat. "Meats are our major source of zinc," says Dr. Birge. Eating meat a few times a week and taking a multivitamin that contains zinc will usually provide all that the body needs, he says.

Consider estrogen supplements. For women past menopause, estrogen replacement therapy appears to provide powerful protection against dementia. This hormone has been shown to improve circulation in the brain and stimulate the growth of nerve cells.

Studies have shown, in fact, that women have about the same risk as men of developing Alzheimer's disease *unless* they're taking estrogen. Those taking estrogen supplements after menopause can reduce their risk of Alzheimer's by 50 to 70 percent, says Dr. Birge. Unfortunately, among women who already have Alzheimer's, taking estrogen cannot slow the progression of the disease.

One problem with estrogen is that it may increase the risk of breast cancer in some women. You'll need to ask your loved one's doctor if the benefits of taking estrogen will clearly outweigh the possible risks.

Keep an eye on blood pressure. High blood pressure is a leading cause of stroke and other types of vascular changes that can lead to dementia, says Dr. Reyes. Make sure that the elderly people in your life get their blood pressure checked at least once a year—more often if they've already been diagnosed with hypertension, he advises.

Make a list of medications and review it with the doctor. It's not uncommon for people 65 and older to be taking five or more medications at any one time. The medications can interact with each other and cause side effects. Doctors refer to this as "polypharmacy," and it's a common cause of dementia, says Dr. Reyes.

Drugs that have been linked to dementia include heart medications and drugs used for controlling incontinence. "In some cases, once the medications have been changed or adjusted, the dementia will start to clear up," says Dr. Reyes.

Dealing with Dementia

Living with someone who suffers from dementia can make every day seem like a roller coaster of emotions. Even when dementia is in its earliest stages, it's common for people to feel confused and frightened by the changes they're experiencing. As the disease progresses, their behavior may get increasingly erratic and emotional.

"We can only guess what they must be feeling," says Mary B. Moorhead, an elder-care specialist and licensed family therapist in Berkeley, California. "We've learned that some people with dementia know that something's wrong with their minds, and they must have this horrid sensation of not knowing what's going on around them."

Caring for someone with dementia invariably turns into a full-time job, Moorhead adds. Not only will you be dealing with their physical and emotional difficulties, but you'll have to cope with your own emotions (and exhaustion) as well. Here are some ways to make every day a little bit easier.

Write things down. People in the early stages of dementia can usually manage most of life's little details, but not all of them. In early dementia, it's common for people to forget to eat meals or take medications.

Since you can't be available to help 24 hours a day, Moorhead recommends giving lots of reminders. With early dementia, for example, you could put a big note on the refrigerator reminding your loved one to eat lunch. You may even find yourself papering the walls with signs such as "Watch out for the last step" or "Bathroom, this way."

Make every day predictable. The brain is only capable of processing a certain amount of information. For those with mid-to-late dementia, having too many choices or getting too much information at once can make them even more frustrated and confused. It's essential to create routines and then stick with them, Moorhead says. For example, serve meals at the same times every day. Establish regular bed and wake-up times. These and other routines will help your loved one relax and feel more comfortable.

Find outlets for energy. Unlike most physical illnesses, dementia often damages the mind while leaving the body unaffected. People with mid-to-late dementia need just as much exercise as they always did, Moorhead says. If they don't get it, they often get agitated and restless. In some cases, a lack of exercise may contribute to a condition called wandering, in which people pace aimlessly for hours, often in the middle of the night. "Just taking them for walks at the same times every day may be enough to control the wandering," Moorhead says.

Pick up an identification bracelet. Because people with mid-to-late dementia often forget where they are or where they're going, it's not uncommon for them to wander out the door, through the neighborhood, or even out of town. "We always recommend fitting them with a wristband that has their name and phone number, just in case they get lost," Moorhead says. You can buy or order identification bracelets and necklaces at drugstores. The Alzheimer's Association also has a program called Safe Return, which involves sewing information labels in clothing of those with mid-to-late dementia.

Learn to recognize common triggers. Agitation and even violence are common in those with mid-to-late dementia. Even though family members often say that the agitation "just happens," in most cases it's caused by something very specific.

"For some people, having others touch them will set them off," Moorhead says. "For others, it might be certain words or activities. You just have to be sensitive to how they're going to react. Avoiding their triggers will make life a lot easier for everyone."

Use distraction, not confrontation. You can't have logical discussions with people who have mid-to-late dementia. They get upset by all sorts of things, real or imagined. It won't do any good to explain to them that their sandwich isn't burned or that there isn't something scary hiding in the closet. If anything, they'll just get more frustrated when you argue.

"Rather than having an argument, try to redirect their attention to something else," Moorhead suggests. "Ask if they'd like to go for a walk or fold some laundry. That's often enough to get their minds off whatever's bothering them."

Try to anticipate needs. It's impossible to truly get into the mind of someone with mid-to-late dementia, but you can learn to predict behavior. This makes it easier to prevent some of the most common causes of conflict.

For many caregivers, for example, one of the hardest tasks is dealing with the loss of bowel or bladder control. "Having to wash people and change their clothes every day can be incredibly draining," Moorhead says. "But you can often figure out how to circumvent this—maybe by taking someone to the bathroom every few hours, or by figuring out when they're most likely to have accidents."

Remove confusing objects. One of the curious symptoms of mid-to-late dementia is that people often forget what certain objects are for, but they still remember the shapes—and then they associate those shapes with other things. What this means, for example, is that someone may see a circular trash can and confuse it with a toilet.

"You have to spend some time trying to figure out what's most confusing for them. It's different with everyone," Moorhead says. Once you identify objects that are causing confusion, you can simply remove them or put them out of sight by taking trash cans out of the bedroom, for example.

Keep life calm and quiet. "If you have 10 grandkids coming over, the dog's barking, and everyone's running around, it's going to be overwhelming," Moorhead says. You'll want to keep the environment as calm and peaceful as you can.

Do some home improvements. Few things are more frightening than coming home after work and finding every burner on the stove going full blast, or discovering that the bathtub is overflowing. Since people with mid-to-late dementia are often physically active, they may spend their days picking things up, turning things on, or opening things. Sooner or later they're going to get hurt if you don't take precautions. For example:

- Take the knobs off the stove when it's not in use.

- Install childproof latches on cabinet doors.

- Pick up toys or other objects from the floor.

- Lower the temperature of the water heater so it's not scalding—somewhere under 120°F. You can adjust the temperature by turning a screw (or screws) located behind the removable panels on the front.

- Secure carpets with rubber underpadding.

- Put poisonous houseplants out of reach.

Communicate simply—and often. Research has shown that people with Alzheimer's who spend the most time reminiscing or simply talking with their loved ones tend to have less declines in mental ability. Even though they may not be able to talk as clearly or logically as they used to, they still crave human contact, Moorhead says.

Try to keep conversations at a level your loved one is comfortable with. Speak slowly. Use short words and sentences. Or ask simple questions that require only yes or no answers.

Take care of yourself, too. "It's extremely helpful for people caring for those with mid-to-late dementia to talk to other people who are going through the same thing," says Dr. Birge. "Contact your local Alzheimer's Association. They have outstanding support groups. The sooner you get involved, the better."

These groups aren't limited to family members of those with Alzheimer's, he adds. Regardless of the form of dementia you're dealing with, you'll find other people who will be eager to share their experiences. The Alzheimer's Association in your area will be able to tell you whom to call.

Heart Palpitations

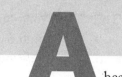

A heart palpitation is really a mild electrical malfunction. The heart has its own electrical system. Each electrical impulse triggers a heartbeat. If something interferes with the transmission of these electrical impulses, an irregular heartbeat may occur. A person will feel a thumping, pounding, racing, or fluttering sensation in the chest or will feel as if her heart skipped a beat. But just as quickly as the heart gets off track, it usually goes back to normal.

Other than the knowledge that the heart is beating to a different drum, heart palpitations are typically nothing to worry about. "Often, there's no treatment necessary. Rarely is it very serious," says Gary Francis, M.D., director of the coronary intensive care unit at the Cleveland Clinic Foundation in Ohio.

If your loved one has the rare and occasional heart palpitation, assume that she is fine, he adds. If her heartbeat does skip off tempo, here are a few measures to make it return to its normal rhythm. You can also help your loved one take a few steps to keep her drum on a steady beat in the first place.

Tell her to cough. Your loved one should cough during the next heart palpitation episode. The force of the cough will sometimes get a heart back on its regular track, says Robert March, M.D., professor of cardiovascular surgery at Rush–Presbyterian–St. Luke's Medical Center in Chicago. "A good cough can break the pattern of the palpitation."

Suggest getting comfortable. When your loved one's heart thumps a little off beat, advise her to sit down, says Michael A. Brodsky, M.D., professor of medicine in cardiology at the University of California, Irvine, Medical Center. If she can, she should elevate her feet, he adds. Your relative should take a few moments to relax and let the heartbeat get back to normal.

Try water to get the beat back to normal. Recommend that she splash her face with cold water (not ice water) during her next heart palpitation. The cold water may activate a part of the nervous system that could return the heart rate to normal, Dr. Brodsky says. Your relative can also sip cool water slowly. That may also help stop the palpitations.

Slow down the breathing. Many heart palpitations are brought on by stress or anxiety, warns Dr. March. Your loved one should take a deep breath and then slowly exhale. She should repeat this breathing slowly until she calms down. Just the act of relieving tension may bring her heart back in step.

Blow to get the rhythm right. A move called Valsalva's maneuver will derail heart palpitations, explains Dr. Francis. To do it, your loved one should pinch her nose and close her mouth, then blow out while keeping the nose and mouth shut. The built-up pressure in the nose and mouth can force the heart back into its normal rhythm, he says.

Talk to her. Although many of these tips are things your loved one

WHEN TO SEE THE DOCTOR

For occasional heart palpitations, your loved one doesn't need to see the doctor, says Gary Francis, M.D., director of the coronary intensive care unit at the Cleveland Clinic Foundation in Ohio. Her heartbeat usually will go back to normal rather quickly. But sometimes, palpitations may be a sign of another, more serious kind of heart problem. At the onset of palpitations, advise your loved one to talk to her doctor at once if she has a previous history of heart disease. And even if your relative doesn't have heart disease, she should get in touch with the doctor if:

- She also has chest discomfort or chest pains

- She feels breathless or dizzy

- The palpitations become more frequent than usual

has to do for herself, you can help more directly. How? Just sit and talk to her when she's having an episode, calming her down while waiting for something to happen, suggests Dr. Brodsky. Of course, you can also get emergency help if it turns out that your loved one needs it, he says. And if your relative doesn't need medical attention, you'll at least be able to calm her down, which could help offset the palpitations.

Advise alcohol avoidance. For some people, a cocktail sends their hearts aflutter. If your loved one has heart palpitations after drinking alcohol, she should put the drinks away, Dr. Brodsky advises.

Some people may experience heart palpitations after one drink, others after a few more, and some people may not have a problem at all. "Everyone has his own threshold," Dr. Brodsky adds. So it's important for you and your loved one to remember what her threshold is and make sure she doesn't go over it.

Suggest chilling with the coffee. This doesn't mean drink iced coffee. Your loved one should keep her coffee-cup count to a minimum, Dr. Brodsky says. For some people, coffee or caffeinated products such as soda or chocolate cause heart palpitations, and it may take no more than a smidgen of caffeine to start the arrhythmia. But that's not true for everyone. "Some people just smell the coffee and experience heart palpitations," notes Dr. Brodsky. "Others can drink 15 cups a day and have no problems."

Ask her to consider quitting for good. Nicotine can sometimes cause an irregular heartbeat, Dr. March says. For the overall health of the heart as well as for control of heart palpitations, your loved one should stop smoking. (For more information about quitting smoking, see the Smoking chapter on page 236.)

Hip Pain

The 20th century wasn't kind to the hip. Between swing, the twist, and inventions like the Hula Hoop, our hips have had a lot of work to do. Yet these gyrations and dance sensations were hardly the hip's worst enemies. It's what people *didn't* do in these sedentary times that have helped cause so many people to have hip problems. And what they didn't do was exercise.

"If anything, swinging our hips on the dance floor, walking to the post office, or just doing a few stretching exercises every day helps keep the muscles and bones of the joint strong. But we've gotten away from doing those things. The vast majority of Americans have become couch potatoes, and they're paying the price for it later in life in the form of thinner, weaker bones and an increased potential for hip fracture," says Jan I. Maby, D.O., director of the Geriatric Medical Home Care program at Mount Sinai Medical Center in New York City.

But it's never too late to make lifestyle changes, including regular exercise, to ease mild hip pain, strengthen weak bones, and reduce your loved one's (and your) susceptibility to hip fractures, Dr. Maby says. In fact, many of the underlying causes of hip pain in older Americans, such as arthritis, bursitis, and tendinitis, can easily be treated with these home remedies.

Have him heat up. Heat is one of your relative's most potent allies against occasional hip pain, says Scott Marwin, M.D., vice chairman of the department of orthopedics at Long Island Jewish Medical Center in New Hyde Park, New York. Try placing an electric heating pad over his hip for 20 minutes, three or four times a day, he suggests. If you don't have a heating pad, soak a towel in hot water, wring it out, and apply that.

Chill it out. If heat isn't helping, apply ice where your relative feels hip pain to help reduce pain and swelling, says Craig Cisar, Ph.D., professor of exercise physiology at San Jose State University in California. To protect his skin, put a towel between the skin and the ice. Ice may be used for 15 to 20 minutes every 1 to 2 waking hours.

Try an anti-inflammatory. Over-the-counter extra-strength anti-inflammatory medications such as ibuprofen can reduce swelling and ease hip pain caused by arthritis, bursitis, and other muscle or joint injuries, says Jacob Rozbruch, M.D., orthopedic surgeon and assistant professor of medicine at Albert Einstein College of Medicine of Yeshiva University in New York City. If the recommended dosage on the label doesn't help ease the pain, alert his doctor. Your loved one may have a

WHEN TO SEE THE DOCTOR

In general, any pain in the hip region, particularly if it radiates down into the groin, should be evaluated by a doctor to rule out any serious problem like hip fracture or joint degeneration, says Jacob Rozbruch, M.D., orthopedic surgeon and assistant professor of medicine at Albert Einstein College of Medicine of Yeshiva University in New York City. In addition, be wary if your relative has the following symptoms.

- The hip pain was caused by a fall or injury, even a minor one.

- The pain persists after a couple of weeks, despite self-care and home remedies.

- Your relative can't bear weight on the hip.

- The pain occurs while he lies in bed at night, or it disrupts sleep.

- He has difficulty walking or moving.

- Your relative also has open sores on his feet or leg pain.

hip fracture or another serious underlying problem that should be evaluated, he says.

Size up some assistance. A cane or walker can be your loved one's best friend if it eases his hip pain and helps him stay independent, Dr. Maby says.

If your relative needs a cane or walker for stability, be sure it is the right size, Dr. Marwin says. An ill-fitting assistive device will increase hip pain, not relieve it. Ask his doctor to refer you to a medical supply store where your loved one can be properly measured and outfitted with an appropriate cane or walker.

When your relative uses a cane, have him follow these directions from Dr. Marwin: Hold the cane in the hand opposite the injured hip. Move it forward at the same time that you step out with your injured hip, so you're distributing weight away from your bad hip and onto the cane. Then move your good hip forward as you take another stride.

Talk to him about losing weight. Getting rid of excess body weight can help relieve the strain on his hips, Dr. Marwin says. In fact, each pound lost will take 2 to 3 pounds of pressure off his hips.

"As we get older, it becomes more difficult for the muscles to offset the increased weight. As a result, the joints bear more and more of the brunt of the load, and they degenerate," Dr. Marwin says. "So staying at a good weight and staying physically fit are two of the best things we can do to preserve the hips."

Recommend some stretches. Stretching exercises often can relieve both hip and back pain by strengthening common muscles and increasing flexibility, Dr. Rozbruch says.

Over time, Dr. Rozbruch says, loosening the hips will translate into more fluid, graceful, and pain-free movement. If your loved one wants to try this therapy, have him follow these instructions. He can do these stretches once a day to coax hip muscles into lengthening gently and slowly. But if he starts to feel pain, he should stop. (And if your relative has a herniated disk, you should consult his doctor or a physical therapist before trying any of these stretches.)

1. Lie down on a bed or on the floor on a mat, with your knees bent and your feet braced about 24 inches high on a wall, letting your head, upper body, and arms relax completely on the floor. (Hint: The farther from the wall you are, the easier this stretch will be.)

You can support your head with a pillow or towel. Keep your buttocks on the floor. Keeping your right foot on the wall, cross your left foot over your right thigh, bringing the outer edge of your foot just below your right knee. If you are too stiff to reach that point, let your left leg cross farther over your right leg as much as needed.

Then, lift your right thigh toward your chest and reach your hands through to interlace around the back of the thigh. Create just the amount of stretch that is good for you by slowly drawing your right leg toward your chest. Hold for up to 1 minute. (If the reach is too difficult, use a towel to raise your thigh to your chest without lifting your head and shoulders off the floor.) Release and repeat on the other side.

Note: You should feel this in the back of your left thigh, hip, or outer buttock, not in your lower back.

2. Lie down on your back on a bed or on the floor on a mat, with your legs extended and your feet wedged snugly and pressing against a wall. You can support your head with a pillow or towel. Make sure that your toes point up toward the ceiling. On an exhalation, slowly draw your left knee toward your chest, interlacing your hands behind your knee/upper thigh. Hold this position for up to a minute, breathing evenly, then release. Repeat with your right leg. Avoid letting your straight leg bend and rise up. The most important part of this stretch is keeping one thigh pressed down onto the floor while you're flexing the other. Getting your knees to your chest is secondary.

Incontinence

If your loved one has a problem with incontinence, it might be a little reassuring to hear that it's a common concern among older people. But is that the kind of reassurance she really wants? More likely, both of you would like to know that there are things you can do about it.

Well, there are.

"Incontinence is never normal at any age," says Neil Resnick, M.D., professor of medicine at Harvard Medical School. "It's not a function of age nor of gender. Incontinence is almost always treatable and very often curable."

At least 13 million Americans experience urinary incontinence, the involuntary release of urine. And it's not at all fair to both sexes. About 11 million of those 13 million are women. In fact, one out of every three women experiences some degree of urinary incontinence during her lifetime.

In most cases, the doctor can suggest not only solutions but also some methods you can try to help your loved one.

Suggest learning Kegel exercises. Pelvic muscle exercises, also known as Kegel exercises, help many women with the most common kinds of incontinence, says Dr. Resnick.

Kegels strengthen the pelvic floor muscles that support the bladder. When those muscles are stronger, it is easier to tighten up in the area that controls the release of urine.

To do Kegels, your relative will need to quickly contract her pelvic floor muscles as if she were stopping a stream of urine. She should hold the contraction for about 3 seconds, then relax her muscles for an equal length of time. This pair of movements should be counted as one exercise. Doing these exercises 45 times each day, divided into three sessions of 15 exercises each, for at least 6 weeks can help control incontinence, says Dr. Resnick. Just like strengthening the biceps or doing any other muscle-building exercise, it takes time.

The great thing about Kegels is that she can do them anywhere—in the car while driving, during a card game, while washing dishes—and no one has to know. And they really do work if they're done right, notes Dr. Resnick.

Remind your loved one that when it comes to Kegel exercises, as with any exercise program, the beneficial effects last only as long as the exercise continues, says Dr. Resnick. One study found that women who practiced Kegels three times a week had the most success, even after 5 years.

Recommend trying an herbal toner. Horsetail is an abrasive plant that was once used to polish metal and wood. The primitive perennial contains large amounts of silica, which helps support the regeneration of connective tissue. If your relative has stress incontinence due to weak muscle tone, a daily dose of silica-rich horsetail tea combined with a regimen of Kegel exercises can help restore muscle tone in her urinary tract, says Lynn Newman, a medical herbalist in Glen Head, New York.

Since a large proportion of its silica content is water soluble, take horsetail as a tea. Bring 1 cup of water to a boil, remove it from the heat, and add ½ teaspoon of dried herb. Steep for 15 to 20 minutes, then

WHEN TO SEE THE DOCTOR

Occasionally, incontinence is a symptom of a serious underlying problem, like a brain tumor, urethral blockage, ruptured disc, or multiple sclerosis, according to Neil Resnick, M.D., professor of medicine at Harvard Medical School. In most cases, these conditions are treatable if found early, so you shouldn't delay diagnosis.

If your loved one's doctor says that nothing can be done about incontinence, don't necessarily accept that as the final word, says Dr. Resnick. Since research into new solutions is being done all the time, you may want to find a doctor who's up-to-date on the subject.

strain. Encourage your relative to drink one cup of tea daily or to take 10 to 12 drops of alcohol-free extract twice a day for a month.

Since horsetail can irritate the digestive tract if used daily for more than 6 weeks, Newman recommends the following monthly routine: She should drink a cup of tea every day for a month, take a week off, then resume taking the tea for another month. If your loved one takes horse-tail as an extract, says Newman, add each dose to 1 cup of water and advise her to adhere to the same monthly pattern as with the tea. To get the maximum benefit from the herb, however, she should also include three sets of Kegel exercises in her daily routine.

Try "bladder drills." For people with urge incontinence, the so-called bladder drills can help them reassert control, says Phillip Barksdale, M.D., a urogynecologist with Woman's Hospital in Baton Rouge, Louisiana.

To do them, your loved one needs to urinate at set intervals, every hour or two, to keep the bladder from getting too full. After she achieves dryness for a few days, she should increase the intervals, says Dr. Barksdale. If she takes her time, your loved one should be able to control urination for several hours.

Ease the irritation. An overactive, irritated bladder can send your loved one running to the bathroom. Corn silk and agrimony work together to soothe the irritation, says Claudia Wingo, R.N., a medical herbalist in College Park, Maryland.

As a treatment for incontinence when bladder irritation is the cause, agrimony works best in combination with corn silk. Known for its diuretic properties, corn silk may seem like an herb to avoid for bladder control. Actually, the nourishing tea made from the stamens of this everyday vegetable contains mucilage that helps soothe the walls of the urinary tract, explains Silena Heron, N.D., a naturopathic physician and professor at Southwest College of Naturopathic Medicine and Health Sciences in Tempe, Arizona.

Finding good-quality corn silk can be a challenge. It's often simpler just to use your own, says Dr. Heron. Buy organic corn on the cob and save the silk as you husk the corn. Trim away any brown or dried-up areas. Chop it and use it in salads or dry it in a food dehydrator or on a ventilated rack. The silk tastes like fresh corn.

To make sure that your loved one always has a supply of ready-to-drink tea on hand, make it at night before you go to bed, says Wingo. Place 1 heaping tablespoon of a blend of equal parts dried corn silk and agrimony in a 1-quart jar. Cover the herbs with boiling water and steep overnight. "You'll have a nice, strong tea the next day," she says. She should drink three cups of tea every day. You can use this remedy daily for up to a year.

Try hawthorn to spur healing. Used primarily for heart and circulatory disorders, a daily dose of hawthorn can also promote healing of the muscles, ligaments, and nerve tissue of the urinary tract, says Erik Von Kiel, M.D., D.O., a holistic physician in Allentown, Pennsylvania. Known as a symbol of hope in the Middle Ages, hawthorn is a powerful antioxidant whose main medicinal benefit comes from its high bioflavonoid content.

Dr. Von Kiel recommends taking the concentrated extract of the herb—which is a tarlike syrup—for this problem. Your relative can lick it off a spoon, or you can make her a tea by adding ¼ teaspoon of the extract to 1 cup of warm water. Let the mixture stand for 10 minutes before serving. Give your loved one ¼ teaspoon of solid extract three times a day. You can also use a tea bag instead of the extract. Although you may see some improvement after giving it to her regularly for a week, typically it may be 1 to 3 months before you notice more bladder con-

Medication Alert

Some muscle relaxants such as the product dantrolene (Dantrium) can cause incontinence by relaxing the muscles that support the bladder, says W. Steven Pray, Ph.D., R.Ph., professor of nonprescription drug products at Southwestern Oklahoma State University in Weatherford. Caffeine can be a culprit as well, he says. This includes caffeine in aspirin-based analgesics such as Excedrin.

trol. You can use the same dose daily or every other day for a year or longer, says Dr. Von Kiel.

Have her keep track. Before your relative sees her physician, it's a good idea for her to keep a diary of her urinary habits for 2 days, advises Dr. Resnick. She should write down when she urinates and when she experiences leaking, and note activities that may have triggered leaks, such as sneezing, coughing, or exercising. It may also be helpful to estimate the amount of leakage experienced. Also tell your loved one to note whether she leaked just a few drops of urine, a few teaspoons or tablespoons, or enough to soak a pad or her clothes. These notes may be able to help the doctor determine what type of incontinence she has and the proper course of treatment.

Soothe the bladder. While it may be better known for its power to induce a calm, euphoric state of mind, kava is a valuable herb to help settle an irritable bladder, says Wingo. As people age, the bladder can become overactive, causing contractions that are too strong to control; this is called urge incontinence. People feel an overwhelming urge to urinate but can't get to the bathroom before the bladder releases the urine. Taking kava can help quiet and soothe the bladder and the pressing urge to urinate. But don't give it to your loved one before going to bed, she advises, as it can increase urination through the night. Give your loved one 30 drops of tincture with water three times a day.

Note: A tincture is a highly concentrated herbal liquid. It's made by soaking leaves in alcohol or glycerin—which extracts the herb's medicinal properties—for at least 6 weeks. Tinctures are sold in health food stores in small bottles with eyedroppers to give doses. Be sure to always store them out of the reach of children.

Recommend that she watch what she drinks and when. Alcohol and caffeinated beverages like coffee and tea stimulate urine production. Advise her to limit her consumption to no more than one or two servings a day or, better yet, to eliminate these drinks, suggests Dr. Barksdale. These measures will help your relative with her bladder drills, reducing the urge to go more often. Also, she should reduce the fluids she drinks in the evening. Less stress on the bladder will help her be more comfortable between nighttime bladder drills.

Keep an eye on "drought" conditions. Your relative may be tempted to drink less throughout the day so she won't have to go as often. But it's important to continue drinking normal amounts of fluids for health reasons, says Dr. Barksdale. If your loved one consciously resists drinking when thirsty, the deprivation can quickly lead to dehydration, especially for an older person.

Suggest being precise. Many people with incontinence can be taught by a therapist to contract their pelvic muscles at the moment of physical strain, says Dr. Resnick.

"Usually, you have advance warning that a cough or a sneeze is coming," he says. If your relative practices doing a Kegel exercise at that exact moment, she can prevent incontinence.

Try treating the triggers. Sometimes, treatment of an allergy or cough can "cure" incontinence, says Dr. Barksdale. Once the physical trigger is removed, incontinence often goes away.

Suggest using absorbents wisely. Traditionally, people with incontinence have turned to various absorbent products, like maxipads or disposable adult undergarments.

While absorbent products are still the most widely used means of dealing with incontinence, your loved one should not rely on them exclusively. Dr. Resnick and Dr. Barksdale stress that they should be used only in addition to a doctor's treatments and your relative's own restraining measures.

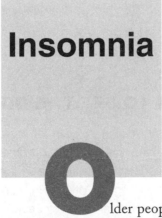

Insomnia

Older people need just as much sleep as other adults, about 8 hours a night on average. Their ability to sleep, however, can be compromised for a variety of reasons.

As a natural part of aging, older people tend to be more easily roused from slumber. Over time, their sleep cycles can change, too, so suddenly they feel more tired earlier in the evening. Insomnia enters the picture when they fight the urge to sleep and stay up later in the evening but then cannot remain asleep in the earlier hours of the morning.

Then there are the times when your loved one (and you, too) will experience an occasional bout of sleeplessness because of stressful and worrisome events in his waking life. The changing nature of life, adjusting to retirement, or bereavement may cause situational, or transient, insomnia. The important thing is to keep these periods in perspective, says Michael Vitiello, Ph.D., professor of psychiatry at the University of Washington in Seattle.

Insomnia is wearisome, but it's usually not considered a serious hazard to health. If insomnia lasts for more than 2 weeks, have your loved one see the doctor. In the meantime, here are some suggestions to help him get to sleep.

Recommend resetting the clock. The circadian rhythm, the body's internal clock that tells it when to sleep and when to be awake, can be influenced by the body's exposure to the sun. This knowledge can be very useful if your relative starts wanting to sleep at 7:00 P.M. and starts waking up at 3:00 A.M. That's a sign that his internal clock may be out of whack and needs some resetting.

To get your relative's body clock adjusted, he should get as much light exposure as possible toward the end of the day, recommends Sonia An-

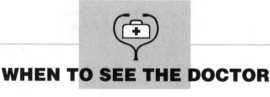

WHEN TO SEE THE DOCTOR

If your loved one's insomnia persists for more than 2 weeks or makes him feel so drowsy during the daytime that it impairs his ability to perform important tasks such as driving a car, consult with a sleep specialist, says Michael Vitiello, Ph.D., professor of psychiatry at the University of Washington in Seattle. Your relative may have a more serious underlying sleep disorder that needs to be treated by a professional.

coli-Israel, Ph.D., director of the sleep disorders clinic at the Veterans Affairs Health Care System in San Diego. This has the effect of moving the body's clock ahead a few hours so that he feels like going to bed at his more usual time. Your loved one should eat lunch outside, go for a walk in the afternoon, and when he has to spend time outside in the morning, he should wear sunglasses so that his eyes are exposed to a little less light. All of these strategies will move his daylight exposure to later in the day, rather than earlier. Your relative should see results in about 2 weeks, says Dr. Ancoli-Israel.

Tell him to get into a routine. If your loved one goes to bed and gets up at the same time 7 days a week, his body will thank him by becoming accustomed to that rhythm and sleeping during those hours, Dr. Ancoli-Israel explains.

Try giving valerian. Valerian root may help him sleep, suggests Varro E. Tyler, Ph.D., Sc.D., distinguished professor emeritus of pharmacognosy at Purdue University in West Lafayette, Indiana. Valerian is an ancient herb that is helpful in adjusting sleep over a period of time, but you don't need to grow it fresh or grind up the root.

Dr. Tyler recommends buying concentrated valerian and using an amount equivalent to 2 to 3 grams of root a day. Valerian is also available in capsule form. Look for a standardized extract (0.8 percent valeric acid) and follow the directions on the label. Don't give valerian to your loved one if he takes sleep-enhancing or mood-regulating medications such as diazepam (Valium) or amitriptyline (Elavil). If stimulant action occurs, discontinue use. In infrequent cases, this herb may cause heart palpitations and nervousness in sensitive individuals.

Calm him with passionflower. Passionflower, with its exotic-looking blooms, makes a strikingly beautiful houseplant. When dried and crushed and included in an herbal sleep formula, it also does an excellent job of alleviating nervous restlessness.

"Passionflower is often found in combination with valerian root," says Connie Catellani, M.D., medical director of the Miro Center for Integrative Medicine in Evanston, Illinois. It's a safe combination that may work better than either herb alone. "They seem to enhance each other's effects, making the remedy more likely to work." One hour before bedtime, give your relative 4,000 to 8,000 milligrams of dried passionflower in single-herb capsules, or give him a combination formula according to package directions. It's okay for your relative to take these herbs on an

AN HERBAL PILLOW THAT HELPS SLEEP

This may seem like an unusual remedy, but using tiny, hand-made pillows stuffed with sleep-inducing herbs is a time-honored path to dreamland. And they work well for everyone, including children and the elderly, says Phoebe Reeve, an herbalist in Winchester, Virginia.

"It's something that's beautiful and natural, and that in itself is soothing," she says. "Plus, the scent is physiologically and psychologically soporific." That means that the fragrance is re-laxing for body and soul.

If you can't find all of these dried herbs, any combination or even just one can help your relative sleep better. The pillow is not meant to cradle the whole head when he's sleeping; instead, he just places it near his nose when he lies down. "It's also something nice to hold on to while sleeping," says Reeve.

	Cotton fabric such as muslin
1	tablespoon lavender
1	tablespoon chamomile
1	tablespoon hops
1	tablespoon mugwort
1	tablespoon rose

Cut two small rectangles of the same size from the piece of fabric. (Reeve recommends 4" by 4", but you can make the pillow a bit bigger if you prefer.) Sew the right sides of the fabric together on three sides, then turn the pieces inside out.

Mix the lavender, chamomile, hops, mugwort, and rose to-gether. Use the mixture to stuff the pillow, then sew it shut.

To reactivate the scent of the herbs, sprinkle vodka or any odorless grain alcohol on the pillow and let it dry. This pillow should remain effective for about a year, when you can refill it with a new batch of herbs.

ongoing basis. Since you'll probably find capsules of passionflower in doses of less than 1,000 milligrams, you can expect to give him quite a few capsules to get the effective amount.

Catch some kava. For acute insomnia, such as that brought on by jet lag, you may want to try the herbal remedy kava, says Dr. Tyler. This herb is also prepackaged, but you want to check the label to make sure it has the active constituents kavapyrones or kavalactones.

Encourage your relative to take between 60 and 120 milligrams before bedtime to help induce sleep. But because kava has a sedating effect, he shouldn't take it if he's already taking a sedative before bedtime, Dr. Tyler warns. Make sure that your loved one *never* takes kava with alcohol or barbiturates. Also, he shouldn't take more than the recommended dose. Finally, he should use caution when driving or operating equipment, as this herb is a muscle relaxant.

Soothe the stomach for better sleep. A rarely mentioned cause of insomnia is indigestion. If your relative is having trouble sleeping because of something he ate, or if his stomach hurts because something is bothering it, chamomile's antispasmodic action makes it a worthy cure.

Tea is probably the most pleasant way to have chamomile. You can buy it in single-cup tea bags at just about any grocery store or buy the dried flowers in bulk and brew your own. Use 1 rounded tablespoon of herb and cover with 1 cup of boiling water to make one serving. Steep for 10 minutes, then pour through a tea strainer or mesh sieve into a mug. Give your relative one cup of tea before bed.

Chamomile is so safe and mild that you can feel free to use it to wash down any other sleep-inducing herbs that you might choose to give him, and he can take it indefinitely without a break, says Dr. Catellani.

Suggest eating light late at night. A big meal late at night may make your relative sleepy, but then again, it might not. If he is prone to heartburn or gastroesophageal reflux, problems that tend to increase with age, having a huge dinner late will keep him up, says Phyllis Zee, M.D., Ph.D., professor of neurology at Northwestern University Medical School in Chicago. He should try to eat earlier in the evening.

Give him some warm tryptophan and cookies. Of course, if your loved one eats an early dinner, it may not be enough to tide him over until bedtime. And hunger pangs can certainly keep him awake. So tell him to get a snack to alleviate hunger before bedtime, suggests Dr. Vi-

Medication Alert

Certain medications that older people may be taking can interfere with their ability to fall asleep, explains Phyllis Zee, M.D., Ph.D., professor of neurology at Northwestern University Medical School in Chicago. Check with the doctor if you think your relative's medications may be causing insomnia. Still, he should never stop taking them without the doctor's consent. Here are some of the usual insomnia-causing suspects.

- Antidepressants such as fluoxetine (Prozac)

- Medications for chronic pulmonary disease and emphysema, such as prednisone (Deltasone), theophylline (Respbid), and beta-blockers like propranolol (Inderal), which can aid breathing but be so stimulating that they interfere with sleep

- Diuretics for high blood pressure, which can interfere with sleep indirectly because your loved one will have to get up in the night to go to the bathroom

tiello. He recommends that your loved one include some warm milk in that snack because milk contains tryptophan (a food substance that helps people feel sleepy). Other foods such as turkey, fish, and bananas are also rich in tryptophan.

Advise exercise. Exercise has been shown to help sleep, says Dr. Zee. And it doesn't have to be strenuous aerobic exercise either. In fact, the timing of the exercise is more important than how strenuous it is. Exercise will initially make your loved one more alert, but 4 to 6 hours later, his body temperature and metabolism drop, which prepares his body for sleep, explains Peter Hauri, M.D., codirector of the Mayo Clinic Sleep Disorders Center in Rochester, Minnesota.

Your loved one should schedule his workouts for 4 to 6 hours before bed, so his body temperature and energy will be declining just about the time he needs to get to sleep. Any closer to bedtime, and he'll be too stimulated to sleep.

Watch what he drinks. Caffeinated beverages interrupt sleep, so your loved one shouldn't drink them after noon. And he'll want to avoid alcoholic drinks before bedtime, too. Alcohol initially has a sedating effect, but as the body turns it into energy, it becomes stimulating, causing wakefulness in the night, says Margaret Moline, Ph.D., director of the Sleep-Wake Disorders Center at the New York Presbyterian Hospital–Cornell Medical Center in White Plains, New York.

Intermittent Claudication

Even in bygone days when doctors were scarce and do-it-yourself medicine was all the rage, some ideas were really weird. Take, for instance, this oddball cure for leg pain: "Rub leg with turpentine and sit before the fire until leg begins to tingle." Fortunately, this dubious remedy was just a flash in the pan that never really caught fire, so to speak.

Nowadays, there are vastly safer natural remedies for intermittent claudication, a type of persistent leg pain that affects 1 in 10 Americans over age 70. The condition is named for Roman emperor Claudius, who, like many people who have this condition, had a noticeable limp. It is caused by hardening of the arteries supplying blood and oxygen to the lower limbs. High blood pressure, diabetes, smoking, high cholesterol—

the very same lifestyle factors that promote heart disease—all contribute to this condition, which can cause a burning, cramplike pain in the legs, feet, hips, thighs, or even the buttocks.

The pain typically strikes after a person has walked a short distance, often as little as a block. After he's stopped and rested a few minutes, the pain usually disappears. When your loved one has intermittent claudication, the pain recurs once he begins exerting himself again. As the arteries become more clogged, the distance he can walk before experiencing pain gradually decreases.

"Intermittent claudication definitely interferes with living well. But up to 90 percent of people who have it never report it to their doctors. Most people consider it just a part of getting old. They think, 'Oh well, I just can't do what I used to do,'" says Steven Santilli, M.D., associate professor of surgery at the University of Minnesota and a vascular surgeon at the Veterans Administration Medical Center, both in Minneapolis.

That fatalistic attitude is unjustified, Dr. Santilli says. "Lifestyle changes like quitting smoking and getting regular exercise can have a

WHEN TO SEE A DOCTOR

Ignoring persistent leg pain can be dangerous, says Jay D. Coffman, M.D., chief of peripheral vascular medicine at Boston University Medical Center. "Many people who have intermittent claudication also have hardening of their coronary arteries and are more susceptible to heart attacks and strokes."

Your loved one should tell the doctor about any leg pain that happens even when he's not exercising, says Steven Santilli, M.D., associate professor of surgery at the University of Minnesota in Minneapolis. Also inform your physician if your loved one is suddenly unable to walk as far as before, or if his legs start to hurt consistently after walking a short distance, he adds.

huge impact on this condition. There is really no reason your loved one should have to live with intermittent claudication," he says. Here are a few effective ways to put the zing back into his step.

Advise him to walk it off. Walking—the very activity that usually induces the pain associated with claudication—also is one of the surest ways to stop it, doctors say.

"Some people look at me like I'm crazy when I tell them that they need to get out there and walk more, not less. They want pills. But the truth is, we really don't have a drug that will treat claudication as effectively as walking," says Jay D. Coffman, M.D., chief of peripheral vascular medicine at Boston University Medical Center.

Walking enhances the ability of the leg muscles to extract oxygen from blood, Dr. Santilli says. So if your loved one walks more, not less, his leg muscles will learn to use oxygen more efficiently and will be less likely to develop cramps and leg pain.

Your relative should set aside about an hour a day 5 days a week for walking, he suggests. While walking, he should avoid stopping when the first twinges of pain hit. Instead, he should let the pain intensify a bit, then pick out a nearby goal, like the next telephone pole, and vow to reach it before resting. Once the pain subsides, he should get moving again. When he feels the next surge of pain, he should again focus on another goal—say, the length between two telephone poles—that's just a bit more ambitious than the first goal. He should keep going on like this for the full hour.

Your loved one shouldn't worry about the amount of times he has to stop or the speed at which he walks, Dr. Santilli says. In the beginning, some people who try this approach have to stop and rest every 2 to 3 minutes. That's okay. If your loved one sustains this effort for several weeks, his pain should subside, and the distance between rest stops should increase, he says. In fact, researchers have found that many people with intermittent claudication who use this technique are able to double their walking distance in just 2 to 3 months.

Tag along. A companion can encourage your relative to keep moving and reinforce his determination to beat intermittent claudication. And who better than you? But if you can't because of time concerns, ask your loved one's spouse, your husband, or one of your kids to be a walking partner. Walking with your relative provides not only healthy benefits for both of you but also more one-on-one time with your relative.

Recommend walking inside. Rather than ditching the walk on unseasonably hot or cold days, your loved one can go to an indoor shopping mall where he can do his routine in temperature-controlled comfort, recommends Dr. Coffman.

Enlist this circulatory commando. "We usually think of ginkgo for the brain, but it's really excellent for overall circulation," says Mindy Green, an herbalist in Boulder, Colorado. Indeed, at least 13 studies have been done on ginkgo's ability to help people with intermittent claudication. Germany's Commission E, which evaluates herbs for safety and effectiveness, concluded that in 4 of these studies, the increase in pain-free walking distance was statistically significant and clinically relevant. Encourage him to take standardized tablets or capsules according to the manufacturer's directions.

Go with a kitchen cure. No one knows why, but garlic does seem to help increase circulation throughout the body, according to Terry Willard, Ph.D., a clinical herbalist from Calgary in Alberta, Canada. Capsules are the easiest—and least smelly—way to get garlic. Suggest that he take two capsules two or three times a day for 2 to 6 months until he no longer has symptoms.

Try a curing combo. The amino acid arginine is involved in the production of nitric oxide, a chemical released by the cells lining the artery walls. Nitric oxide allows blood vessels to relax and open up, thus helping with circulation, explains Decker Weiss, N.M.D., a naturopathic physician at the Arizona Heart Institute in Phoenix. A standard dose is a 500-milligram capsule up to three times a day.

Along with arginine, Dr. Weiss recommends magnesium, an essential mineral. Magnesium is known for its ability to relax the muscles that wrap around blood vessels, so it can help dilate arteries that have been clogged by cholesterol deposits.

Your loved one might have a deficiency of magnesium if he is taking drugs meant to help heart problems, such as diuretics. Some people have deficiencies if they're taking commonly prescribed digitalis heart medications such as digitoxin (Crystodigin) or digoxin (Lanoxin). Signs of magnesium deficiency include muscle weakness, nausea, and irritability.

Most people can safely take up to 350 milligrams of supplemental magnesium a day, Dr. Weiss says. He recommends it in the form of magnesium orotate or glycinate.

Administer antioxidants. People with intermittent claudication usually do better in general if they are taking antioxidant nutrients such as vitamins E and C, which may help prevent the early stages of atherosclerosis (hardening of the arteries), Dr. Weiss says.

Vitamin E has a long history of use for intermittent claudication. In one study conducted in Sweden, researchers found that they could reduce symptoms if they gave people supplements of 300 IU a day.

For smokers, however, supplementation with vitamin E doesn't seem to reduce the symptoms of intermittent claudication. It's quite possible that the vitamin can't entirely overcome the harmful effects that smoking has on the circulatory system, Dr. Weiss says. Breaking the habit comes first: Often, when people stop smoking, intermittent claudication disappears with time.

Dr. Weiss gives many of his patients with atherosclerosis 400 to 800 IU of vitamin E and 1,000 to 3,000 milligrams of vitamin C a day. Vitamin E helps prevent the oxidation of harmful LDL cholesterol, an important factor in cholesterol blockage. Vitamin C regenerates vitamin E and helps the cells lining the blood vessel walls produce nitric oxide, which keeps blood vessels open and dilated. For vitamin E, you should use natural d-alpha-tocopherol and mixed tocopherols, says Dr. Weiss.

Offer food fixes. "Ginger can be a wonderful addition to a treatment program for intermittent claudication, especially if the person also has arthralgia, or pain in the joints," Dr. Weiss says. Like ginkgo, ginger helps keep platelets from getting too sticky, so it keeps the blood flowing smoothly. Most research studies use about 1,000 milligrams a day of powdered gingerroot, which is about what you'd get from a ¼-inch slice of fresh root. Ginger is safe to take long-term, he says.

Another common food, pineapple, also offers some relief in supplement form. An enzyme in pineapple called bromelain helps keep blood from clotting too readily and may also help existing clots dissolve. "I might use this if someone with circulatory problems also has had clotting problems in the legs, such as thrombophlebitis," Dr. Weiss says. Give your relative bromelain between meals; otherwise, it will be used up digesting meals. A common daily dose used in studies ranges from 60 to 160 milligrams. Dr. Weiss usually recommends much more to his patients—500 milligrams—twice a day, as long as needed. With the doctor's supervision, take note of how your loved one's body reacts.

Talk to him about quitting. People who smoke are twice as likely to develop intermittent claudication as nonsmokers, Dr. Santilli says.

Smoking constricts blood vessels and makes it harder for the leg muscles to work properly. But even if he has smoked for years, quitting now will improve circulation in his legs and help relieve the pain, he says. (For more information on how you can help your loved one quit smoking, see the Smoking chapter on page 236.)

Be firm about fat. Eating too much artery-clogging fat will only worsen intermittent claudication, Dr. Santilli explains. That's because a fatty diet can cause hardening of the arteries, which in turn causes intermittent claudication. For every bite of meat, give him four bites of fruits, vegetables, beans, and grains. It will help keep your relative on track for a low-fat lifestyle. If your loved one just can't live without at least some fatty foods, make foods like gravy, bacon, or fried chicken a once-a-month treat.

Macular Degeneration

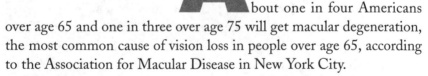

About one in four Americans over age 65 and one in three over age 75 will get macular degeneration, the most common cause of vision loss in people over age 65, according to the Association for Macular Disease in New York City.

The disease is caused by a breakdown of the macula, a dot-size part of the retina that allows a person to read, thread a needle, and see other fine details clearly, says Anne Sumers, M.D., an ophthalmologist in Ridgewood, New Jersey, and a spokesperson for the American Academy of Ophthalmology. When the macula doesn't work properly, it causes blurriness or darkness in the center of vision.

Macular degeneration may be linked to aging, since it most often strikes in later life. But what really triggers this malfunction is still a mystery, Dr. Sumers says. Some of the suspects include diabetes, family history, atherosclerosis (hardening of the arteries), and ultraviolet (UV) light.

There is no cure for macular degeneration. In a few instances, laser surgery can prevent progression of the disease, but it can't restore vision that has already been lost, Dr. Sumers says. Because side vision is usually not affected, people often can continue many of their favorite activities by using low-vision aids such as magnifying glasses.

"Many people with macular degeneration have functional vision for many years, which enables them to see well enough to complete household tasks such as cooking and laundry but may not allow them to read regular print in a newspaper. They might even continue to drive with their doctor's approval," Dr. Sumers says. "It is not necessarily a sentence of blindness. People should not get depressed when they get the diagnosis. There are lots of things they can do to continue living a full and active life despite this disease."

Here are some ways you can help your older loved one with this disease.

Advise him to avoid direct sunlight exposure. This places an additional strain on the retina and damages the light receptors in the eye, says James G. Ravin, M.D., clinical associate professor of ophthal-

WHEN TO SEE THE DOCTOR

Take your relative to the doctor immediately if:

- He notices irregular patches of dimness in his vision

- He has or experiences a sudden loss of vision, even if fleeting

- It's hard for him to read or words appear blurred on a page

- He notices a dark or empty area in the center of his vision

All are possible symptoms of macular degeneration and need to be checked out right away.

mology at the Medical College of Ohio in Toledo. When outside, he should wear a pair of sunglasses that filters out UV rays. "People should try to avoid exposure between 10:00 A.M. and 2:00 P.M., when the UV rays are most intense. The closer one lives to the equator, the more he needs to protect his eyes," he says.

Suggest fighting it to the "finich" with spinach. Dr. Sumers recommends eating five to nine servings of fruits and vegetables daily, including at least one serving of dark green leafy vegetables. Dark green vegetables, particularly spinach, are the ideal food for the eyes, she says, because they contain an array of nutrients, including zinc, beta-carotene, and magnesium, that may improve bloodflow to the eye and protect the retina from the worst effects of macular degeneration.

Normal chemical reactions caused by the effect of light on the macula may activate oxygen and cause macular damage over time. Some vitamins and minerals like beta-carotene function as antioxidants, chemicals that work against this activated oxygen, and perhaps protect the macula from damage. In addition, zinc, one of the most common minerals in the body, is highly concentrated in the eye, particularly in the retina and tissues surrounding the macula.

"There's a reason why Popeye always says, 'I'm strong to the finich 'cause I eats me spinach,' " says Stuart P. Richer, O.D., Ph.D., chief optometrist at the Department of Veterans Affairs Medical Center in North Chicago. "Dark green leafy vegetables are very important to the overall health of the eyes. I tell my patients to eat the equivalent of 2½ to 5 ounces (½ to 1 cup) of frozen spinach a day." That's the same as one-quarter to one-half of a 10-ounce box. For variety, he suggests that your loved one try collard greens, kale, or romaine lettuce.

Give him ginkgo for his vessels. One of the best ways your loved one can avoid deterioration of the tissues in his eyes is to maintain the health of the blood vessels and capillaries that supply them, says Alice Laule, M.D., who practices holistic medicine and ophthalmology in Harrison, Arkansas. Several studies have shown that ginkgo does exactly that. It also helps thin out the platelets in the blood that can sludge up circulation. Give him 60 to 80 milligrams in capsule form or 15 drops of tincture in 1 cup of cold water twice a day.

If you decide to give the tincture to your relative, Dr. Laule warns that the taste isn't great, so you may want to dilute it. Instead of putting 15 drops in 1 cup of water, you can add them to a glass or two. "Some people would rather drink a little bit of really bad-tasting stuff, and others would rather drink a lot of moderately bad-tasting stuff," she says. "It doesn't matter, just so they can get it down."

Morning and evening doses, before or after meals, are fine for both capsules and tincture. Your loved one can take this herb on an ongoing basis, she says.

Note: A tincture is a highly concentrated herbal liquid. It's made by soaking leaves in alcohol or glycerin—which extracts the herb's medicinal properties—for at least 6 weeks. Tinctures are sold in health food stores in small bottles with eyedroppers to give doses. Be sure to always store them out of the reach of children.

Look for grape seed extract. The pip, or seed, of the grape, is an especially rich source of flavonoids, according to Dr. Laule. Health food stores often sell this in an antioxidant mixture containing vitamin C. Since antioxidant vitamins are considered vital for maintaining vision, that makes a potent eye-saving combination. Give him a 50-milligram capsule of extract twice a day. He can take this on an ongoing basis.

Brew some clove tea. To make a vision-protecting tea for your loved one, pour 8 ounces of boiling water over 2 teaspoons of whole cloves and a piece of cinnamon stick, if desired, for extra flavor. Steep for a few minutes, then strain the tea and serve it while it's hot. He can drink one to three cups of tea a day.

"I would recommend three cups a day for the short term, but if you intend to use it for more than 4 to 6 months, it's better to stick to one or two cups a day," says C. Leigh Broadhurst, Ph.D., a nutrition consultant and herbal researcher based in Clovery, Maryland.

The oil in cloves is a powerful antioxidant, according to James A. Duke, Ph.D., an herbalist and ethnobotanist in Fulton, Maryland, and author of *The Green Pharmacy*. Studies have shown that it helps prevent the breakdown of important chemicals that help keep the retina healthy.

Remember that bigger is better. Large-print books and playing cards, television remote controls with large readable buttons, and other oversize products can help your relative continue doing activities that he enjoys, Dr. Sumers says. Some companies even sell telephones with large numbers and extra-large wall clocks and calculators. Ask your ophthalmologist if these products are available in your area. Or for a catalog of items designed to make life a little easier for people of low vision, write to Lighthouse International, a nonprofit agency for

Medication Alert

A ntimalarial drugs such as chloroquine (Plaquenil), which are also used to treat lupus and rheumatoid arthritis, can spark chloroquine retinopathy, a condition that has many of the same symptoms as macular degeneration, says Samuel L. Pallin, M.D., an ophthalmologist and medical director of the Lear Eye Clinic in Sun City, Arizona. The difference is that chloroquine retinopathy is reversible, while macular degeneration is not. If your loved one is on one of these drugs and develops signs of macular degeneration, consult the doctor. In most cases, once he stops taking the offending medication, the symptoms will disappear and vision will return to normal.

people who have partial sight or are blind, at 111 East 59th Street, New York, NY 10022. The catalog is available in large-print, braille, and audiotape versions.

Buy a magnifying glass. A high-quality magnifying glass is a must if your loved one with macular degeneration wants to read, says Charles R. Fox, O.D., director of vision rehabilitation at the University of Maryland School of Medicine in Baltimore. You don't have to buy it from a vision rehabilitation center or mail-order service; buy it at Brookstone, the Nature Store, or another gizmo and gadget store. It can be just as good as one you'd get from a low-vision center and often will be cheaper, he notes. To make sure that you get a high-quality magnifier, have your loved one put the magnifier flat on a piece of lined paper and raise it up until the lines look bigger. It helps to use just one eye for this. The lines should look bigger, but just as sharp. Make sure that there are no distortions, no waves, and no breaks.

Get him close to the TV. If your relative has trouble watching television because of macular degeneration, tell him to try sitting as close as possible to the set, Dr. Fox suggests. "If the television is far away from your loved one, the black hole in the center of his vision may cover the whole screen. Bring the television closer and closer, and the black hole covers less and less of the screen. So if it helps to sit 3 feet away from the television, he should do it."

Buy 100-watt soft bulbs. They will brighten your living space and cut down on glare, Dr. Fox says. Make sure that your lamps or light fixtures can handle the additional wattage. Many have a maximum safe rating of 60 watts, which is usually labeled on the lamp, near the socket that holds the bulb. Get a gooseneck or swing-arm adjustable lamp from a home center or office supply store so your loved one can shine the light directly onto the material he is reading.

See if he'll consider quitting. Your loved one should quit smoking, urges Dr. Sumers. People with macular degeneration who continue to smoke are three times more likely to go blind than those who quit, she says. Over-the-counter nicotine patches and gums can help your loved one kick the habit and retain his usable sight. (For more information about quitting smoking, see the Smoking chapter on page 236.)

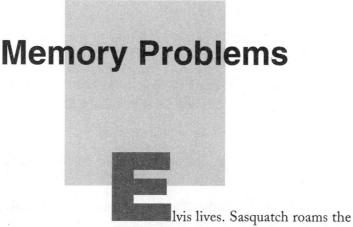

Memory Problems

Elvis lives. Sasquatch roams the forest. Aliens have landed. Yes, modern myths abound. But few are as pervasive or damaging as the misconceptions about aging and memory. Just take a gander at these tall tales.

- We lose 10,000 brain cells a day, and one day we'll run out.

- Our memory gets worse as we get older, and we can't do anything about it.

- Forgetfulness is a sign that something is wrong with our brains.

Not one of these statements is true, yet thousands of people over and under 60 continue to believe them, says Barry Gordon, M.D., Ph.D., behavioral neurologist at Johns Hopkins University School of Medicine in Baltimore.

"These myths about memory give people over 60 a fatalistic attitude

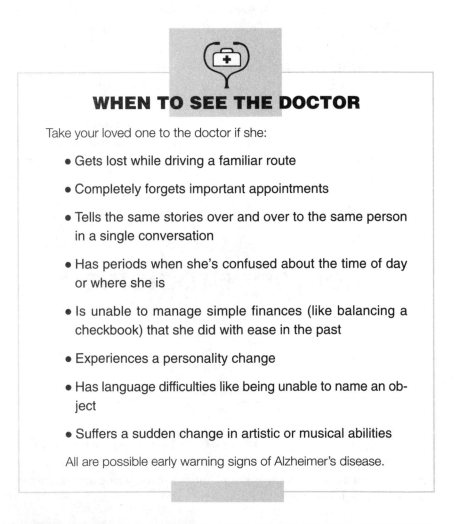

WHEN TO SEE THE DOCTOR

Take your loved one to the doctor if she:

- Gets lost while driving a familiar route

- Completely forgets important appointments

- Tells the same stories over and over to the same person in a single conversation

- Has periods when she's confused about the time of day or where she is

- Is unable to manage simple finances (like balancing a checkbook) that she did with ease in the past

- Experiences a personality change

- Has language difficulties like being unable to name an object

- Suffers a sudden change in artistic or musical abilities

All are possible early warning signs of Alzheimer's disease.

about these problems that is often quite harmful to self-esteem," Dr. Gordon says. "While it is true that many people will have a worsening of memory with age, it is also true that some of these problems are reversible. They can be helped with a few simple coping strategies."

If a person has a mild memory loss, it doesn't necessarily mean her brain is rotting, says Dr. Gordon. It could be a simple problem that is easy to remedy. Here's a look at a few simple ways to help your loved one sharpen her memory.

Encourage her to work out her mind. Regular mental exercise like memorizing names, shopping lists, and other important information is vital to keep the memory sharp, says Alan S. Brown, Ph.D., professor of psychology at Southern Methodist University in Dallas.

"People in their sixties, seventies, and eighties tend not to practice using their memories as much as they did when they were younger," he says. "Many people in this age group, for instance, rely on lists, and that's a fine technique if it isn't overused. But if a person becomes overly dependent on lists, that can actually diminish the ability to concentrate and recall."

So at least once a week, encourage your older loved one to try making a mental rather than written list to shop, clean the house, or run daily errands. Memorizing these tasks is one of the best and simplest brain-stretching exercises she can do, according to Dr. Brown.

Suggest aerobics to work the body—and the mind. Aerobic exercises like brisk walking or swimming can improve memory 20 to 30 percent, Dr. Gordon says, although he recommends that your loved one check with the physician before beginning any exercise program.

Make sure she gets her rest. When your loved one is tired, it will be harder for her to focus her attention and recall will suffer, says Janet Fogler, a clinical social worker at Turner Geriatric Services at the University of Michigan Health System in Ann Arbor.

A good night's sleep also will help your loved one's brain process and store new information, Dr. Gordon says. Although most people get 6 to 8 hours of sleep a night, the amount an individual needs will vary. She should try to get enough sleep so that she feels well-rested when she wakes up, he suggests.

Supplement her memory. A high-potency multivitamin/mineral supplement will supply many of the antioxidant, anti-inflammatory nutrients needed to help control memory loss, according to Steven J. Bock,

M.D., a family practitioner, acupuncturist, and director of the Center for Progressive Medicine in Rhinebeck, New York. Look for a supplement that delivers a daily intake of at least 10,000 IU of vitamin A, 15,000 IU or more of beta-carotene and other carotenoids, 50 to 100 milligrams of many of the B vitamins, 1,000 milligrams of vitamin C, 200 IU of vitamin E, 20 milligrams of zinc, 2 milligrams of copper, 2 to 3 milligrams of manganese, 200 micrograms of selenium, and 200 micrograms of chromium.

Consider these compounds. Phospholipids are compounds that help form the neurons' outer covering, or membrane, and aid communication between brain cells. But they decline with age, possibly hurting memory. Since phospholipids aren't prevalent in the diet, the best way to replace them is with a daily supplement, says James Hughes, M.D., medical director of the Hilton Head Longevity Center in Bluffton, South Carolina. Look for a 200- to 300-milligram capsule that contains the following phospholipids: phosphatidylserine, choline, and inositol.

Fatten her up. But not with butter or greasy foods. Essential fatty acids, or EFAs, are a major component of neuron membranes and can help protect memory, explains Dr. Bock. He recommends 2 tablespoons a day of flaxseed oil, which is rich in EFA.

Try another brain feeder. The nutrient acetyl-carnitine can help improve memory, says Alan Brauer, M.D., founder and director of the TotalCare Medical Center in Palo Alto, California. Scientists theorize that it boosts energy production in the brain; improves function in the brain's "glutamate receptors," which are responsible for learning; and may stop the formation of lipofuscin, a kind of "age spot" of the neurons that can interfere with memory. He recommends 250 to 2,000 milligrams of acetyl-carnitine a day.

Consider buying this mental messenger-maker. Neurotransmitters are the chemicals that relay messages between neurons. So when levels of neurotransmitters are low, memory suffers.

The supplement DMAE (short for dimethylaminoethanol) supplies a compound called methyl that the body needs to manufacture neurotransmitters, says Ross Hauser, M.D., director of physical medicine and rehabilitation at the Caring Medical Rehabilitation Service in Oak Park, Illinois. Your loved one should follow the dosage recommendation on the label. According to Dr. Hauser, DMAE may also help elevate mood and increase physical energy.

What You Should Ask the Doctor

Most conventional physicians have no treatments for non-Alzheimer's, age-related memory loss, says Alan Brauer, M.D., founder and director of the TotalCare Medical Center in Palo Alto, California. Still, here are some important things you should ask the doctor about if your relative is suffering from memory loss.

Evaluation for illness and chronic pain. "In treating memory, the doctor should first look for physical disorders and attempt to correct them," he says.

Hormonal tests. Testosterone, estrogen, progesterone, cortisol, DHEA, and many other hormones affect memory, and unless those levels are healthy, your loved one is not going to make any significant improvements in memory.

Evaluation for clinical depression. The most common medical cause for memory loss is clinical depression.

Evaluation of memory. Look for a doctor with an in-office test that can evaluate your loved one's memory. The doctor can repeat the test during your loved one's treatment to track her progress.

Prescription medications. Some are memory-enhancing in the proper (usually small) dosages, including ergoloid mesylates (Hydergine), selegiline HCl (Eldepryl), vasopressin (Pitressin or Pressyn), and piracetam (Nootropyl).

Evaluation of nutritional supplements. Dr. Brauer reviews his patient's supplement intake, revising it if necessary.

Lifestyle factors. A good memory evaluation should include questions about exercise, diet, and levels of stress, and include advice to help establish a memory-enhancing lifestyle.

Don't forget this plant. The herb periwinkle can speed up brain activity. One of the extracts of periwinkle seeds works as a powerful enhancer of memory function by improving bloodflow to the brain. In one scientific study, secretaries who took *Vinca major* (a particular species of the plant) improved their ability to remember sequences of words by 40 percent. Your loved one should take 20 to 40 milligrams a day, says Dr. Hauser.

Suggest another herbal memory booster. A supplement of ginkgo biloba can help protect memory in two ways, Dr. Brauer says. It improves circulation to the brain and is a potent antioxidant. He recommends 120 to 240 milligrams a day.

Help her get organized. If your loved one randomly scatters bills, car keys, and glasses around the home or office, she'll have trouble finding them simply because she probably wasn't paying attention when she set them aside, Fogler says. Your relative should designate a hook for keys and always hang them there. She should toss old magazines and newspapers at least once a week. Finally, Fogler suggests, it would be a good idea to keep a wastebasket near where she checks her mail so she can throw away unwanted mail immediately.

She should stop for a second. Most of us—whether older or younger—have experienced at least one anxious instant when we couldn't remember if we fed the cat or turned off the iron. Usually, that's a sign that we were distracted. So if this happens to your loved one, advise her to always pause, take a deep breath, and relax before dashing out the door, says Danielle Lapp, a memory training researcher at Stanford University. Also, she should take a moment to ask herself some questions, like: Where am I going? What am I doing? What do I need? Have I forgotten anything important?

Encourage her to talk to herself. Talking to themselves as they do a task can help older folks focus their attention and make things easier to remember, Fogler says. As your loved one straightens up her house, for instance, she can literally talk her way through the process. She could say: "I'm putting these old clothes in a white cardboard box marked with a red X. Now I'm carrying the box down to the basement. I'm placing the box on the floor behind the blue lounge chairs that we use on the patio during the summer." When she wants to find the box, she can talk her way back through what she did, and it probably won't be hard for her to find it, she says.

Suggest making the ordinary extraordinary. A good reminder can be unconventional or even weird, Fogler says. The next time your relative needs to remember an errand, maybe she can try placing a sock in the refrigerator. The sight of that sock will probably jog her memory the next time she opens the fridge.

Tell her to make the connection. It may take more effort to retrieve information as your relative gets older, but she shouldn't give up, Lapp says. Recommend that she try to organize her thinking, in other words, to keep her memory scanner in the area of the subject. If a movie title escapes her, for example, she should keep talking about the movie. She could name as many actors and actresses in the movie as possible. That may trigger the recollection, she says.

Recommend relaxation. Relaxation techniques like deep breathing can reduce stress and boost the ability to recall, Lapp says. Here's some instructions for your loved one in case she wants to try this:

Sit comfortably, without tensing your muscles, and close your eyes. Let your arms and legs rest limply. Keep your mouth closed and inhale deeply and gradually through your nose until your lungs are full. Now exhale slowly, again through your nose, until all of the air is out.

As you continue breathing deeply, listen to the rhythm of air rushing in and then slowly seeping out. Notice how it sounds like waves crashing gently against the shore. Visualize the motion of the waves, their sound, and the smell of the sea breeze. Enjoy the sensations. Use this visualization technique as often as you can, particularly when you feel tense and are having difficulty remembering things, Lapp says. Try it while at work or while waiting in line. The visualization part of the exercise is enough to lessen anxiety when you have trouble remembering a piece of information.

Mobility Problems

Mobility is freedom. Each step is a declaration of independence. Each time your loved one stands, he becomes a statue of liberty.

"Without mobility, the quality of life is greatly diminished," says Sandy O'Brien-Cousins, Ed.D., professor of exercise gerontology at the University of Alberta in Edmonton, Canada. Stiffness in the joints doesn't necessarily stop older people in their tracks. But it definitely takes more energy to do things; eventually, your loved one will have trouble getting around and may lose her independence.

"We're taught that it is okay to take it easy when we get older," says Wayne Phillips, Ph.D., professor of exercise science at Arizona State University in Tempe. "It's considered the reward for working hard throughout your life. But taking it easy after age 60 isn't a reward. It turns out to be a penalty. It causes much of the loss of mobility that we attribute to aging. We can reduce our risk of these problems if we just stay active." In other words, we really have to move it or lose it. Staying active helps your loved one maintain all of the components—muscles, bones, flexibility, and balance—that she needs to remain mobile, he says.

"Studies have shown that people well into their nineties can improve their mobility. Some of these people were using walkers, canes, and wheelchairs. But when they added strength training and other activities to their daily lives, they were able to rehabilitate themselves and set these assistive devices aside," says Bryant Stamford, Ph.D., director of the health promotion and wellness center at the University of Louisville in Kentucky.

Here are some hints for helping your loved one stay active.

Keep her active. You and your loved one should look for ways to help her use more energy and become more active, either by doing things a little faster or a little longer than normal, Dr. Phillips says.

For example, if your loved one wants to do things faster than normal and it usually takes her 20 minutes to vacuum the house or rake up leaves in the yard, she can try doing it in 15 minutes, he says.

If your relative wants to use more energy by taking longer than normal to do things, she should think about ways to break a single task into many. Instead of piling folded clothing on the stairs and letting it sit there until she can carry it up in one trip, she can take each piece up the stairs as she finishes folding it. When putting away groceries, she can put each item on the table, then move each one to a counter, and finally put it where it belongs. If your loved one gardens, she can kneel down and stand up each time she digs up a weed. Painting the house? She can go up and down the ladder more times than necessary.

Talk to her about being more self-reliant. "Too many people want to rescue older people from difficult situations," says Dr. Stamford. If you both agree that it would be good for your loved one to be more self-

WHEN TO SEE THE DOCTOR

Any mobility problem, including walking difficulties, should be evaluated by a physician because it could be a sign of a more serious, underlying condition, says Helen Schilling, M.D., medical director of HealthSouth-Houston Rehabilitation Institute in Texas. It is particularly important to take your loved one to the doctor as soon as possible if she:

- Has fallen

- Has difficulty getting into and out of chairs

- Holds on to chairs and other furniture to balance and avoid falling

- Is reluctant to go outside without someone to hold on to for balance

reliant, talk about ways you can stop helping her so much. Perhaps you can let her carry the groceries or do other tasks without your help. Choosing appropriate tasks for this can be tricky to figure out. It depends on the physical condition of your relative and what she is capable of doing. Probably the best thing to do is to discuss what activities your relative will do on her own, then check with her doctor to make sure that they are okay. And of course, if your loved one really needs help with a task, she shouldn't be embarrassed to ask for help.

Medication Alert

A cornucopia of over-the-counter and prescription drugs can make it harder for your loved one to move about safely, says Helen Schilling, M.D., medical director of HealthSouth-Houston Rehabilitation Institute in Texas. So check with her doctor or pharmacist before your relative takes any drug or drug combinations, she suggests. Be particularly cautious when your loved one is using propoxyphene, acetaminophen, and other prescription pain relievers. These drugs can cause drowsiness and make your loved one less surefooted. In addition, be wary of:

- Alcohol

- Prescription antianxiety medications known as benzodiazepines (Valium, Xanax)

- Phenothiazines (Thorazine), which are used to treat nervous, mental, and emotional disorders

- Antihistamines, including diphenhydramine (Benadryl)

The advantage here is that your relative avoids getting weaker because of inactivity. You must resist the urge to help, however, unless she asks. After all, the only way your loved one is going to get better at lifting and carrying things is to do it. If she lets others do too many things for her, she'll get weaker. As she gets weaker, more things will be a challenge.

Go out for a stroll with her. Walking is moving at its finest, according to Dr. Stamford. It works out all of the muscles and strengthens bones. The more your loved one can do it, the better, he says. Even if your relative can walk only 2 to 3 minutes a day, she'll be on the path to a more active lifestyle. Be sure to talk with her doctor first and get his approval, and increase her activity level bit by bit.

Try the bookworm workout. Dr. Stamford recommends that your loved one get in the habit of carrying a box of books from room to room. It will help build the muscle strength she needs to stay mobile. She just has to put enough books in the box so that it weighs about as much as a sack of groceries. Every time she leaves a room, she should lift the box from the bottom with two hands, making sure to keep the back straight. She should hold the box close at chest level, with the elbows at a 90-degree angle.

Suggest doing a "chair-up." For your loved one to try the following mobility exercise, she will need a firm chair with sturdy armrests. Show or read her these instructions: Grasp the armrests and push off with your arms and legs, rising to a standing position. Then slowly lower yourself to a sitting position. Your loved one can try doing this exercise at least twice each time she sits down.

Get her to try another mobility maker. Show your loved one the following exercise: Lie with your back flat on the floor and try to get up any way you can. That way you'll exercise virtually every muscle in your body, says Dr. Stamford. He recommends doing this three or four times a day. Of course, before doing this or any other exercise, make sure your loved one has her doctor's approval. In fact, you may want to show these exercises to the doctor to make sure they'll be okay for your loved one to do.

Encourage her to lift everyday household objects. This will build the upper body and promote mobility, Dr. Stamford says. He recommends starting with an object that your loved one can comfortably lift 10 times, like an 18-ounce jar of peanut butter. Then she should add one lift each day until she reaches 25. Then she can try a slightly higher weight at 10 repetitions and repeat the cycle.

Help her with a stretching routine. Stretching can improve your loved one's flexibility and make getting around easier, Dr. O'Brien-Cousins says. Show her the instructions and illustrations and, if you have her doctor's approval, see if she is willing to try these twice a day. She should hold each stretch for 15 to 20 seconds.

Wrist Stretch ▶

Sitting on a sturdy chair with one arm straight out in front of you, pull the fingers of that hand toward you with your other hand until you can feel the stretch in your fingers and palm. Stretch your other hand the same way. Then repeat the exercise with each hand.

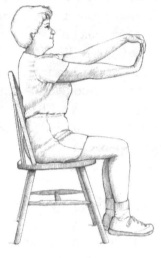

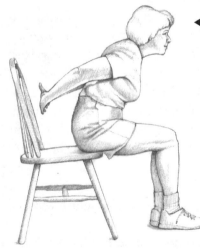

◀ Shoulder Stretch

Sit on the edge of a sturdy chair. Interlace your fingers behind your back with your palms facing away from your body. Bend forward at your waist, as far as you can, keeping your head above your hips with your eyes looking forward, not down at the ground. You'll feel the stretch in your shoulders.

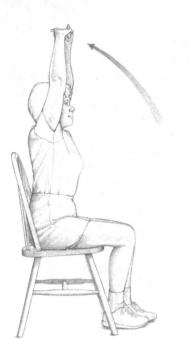

◀ Upper-Body Stretch

Sit on a sturdy chair. Intertwine your fingers in front of you, palms facing outward, and stretch your arms straight forward until you can feel pressure in the back of your hands, wrists, and arms. Keeping your fingers intertwined, raise your arms above your head briefly. You'll feel the stretch in your upper back and shoulders.

Calf Stretch ▶

Stand with your feet flat on the floor and your legs straight, a few feet away from a countertop or sturdy, immobile piece of furniture. Lean forward until your palms are resting against the edge of the furniture. Your toes should be facing directly forward, and your hips should also be pressing forward. Don't arch your back. You'll feel the stretch behind your lower legs at your calves.

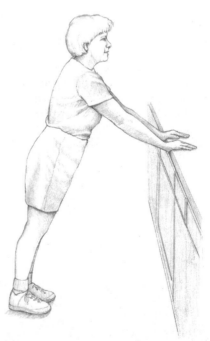

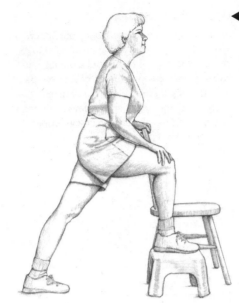

◀ Hip Stretch

Stand to the side of a sturdy chair with one hand resting on the back of it for balance. Place one foot on a sturdy stool or low step. Step back with your other foot so that your feet are a few feet apart but not so much that you find it hard to keep your balance. Keep both feet facing forward while you shift your weight forward onto your bent knee. Place your other hand on your bent knee. Feel the stretch above your flexed knee, and at the front of your hip and in the calf area of your rear leg. Switch your position and repeat with the opposite leg bent.

Swing Stretch ▶

Stand a few feet away from a sturdy piece of furniture such as a hip-high desk. Rest your hands on the desktop for balance. Shift your weight to one foot, then gently swing your other leg backward 10 to 12 times until you feel more limber. Switch your position and repeat with the opposite leg.

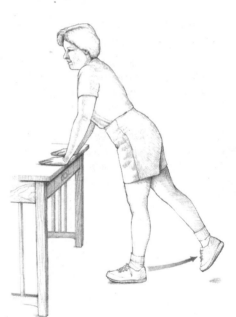

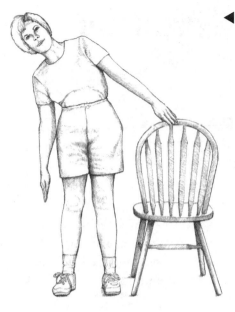

◀ Trunk Stretch

Stand tall with your feet shoulder-width apart, your feet flat on the floor, and your left hand resting on the back of a sturdy chair for balance. Slowly bend sideways to your right, sliding your right hand down your leg toward your knee. Try to keep your body aligned—don't lean forward or backward. Repeat with your other side. You should feel the stretch along the side of your trunk.

Cooldown Stretch ▶

Stand with your feet shoulder-width apart, with your feet flat on the floor behind a sturdy chair. With your hands on the back of the chair for balance, slowly bend your knees, keeping your back straight and your feet flat. Lower yourself a few inches while you breathe out and relax. Then return slowly to the upright position and relax again. Repeat about five times.

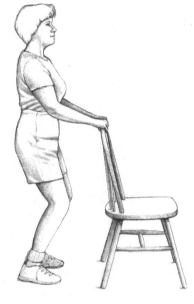

Muscle Soreness

Although it may not seem that way, sore muscles actually have a bright side. If people weren't active, they wouldn't get them. It's perfectly normal, says William J. Evans, Ph.D., director of the nutrition, metabolism, and exercise laboratory at the University of Arkansas for Medical Sciences in Little Rock. But, he adds, the symptoms will be much worse if a person has exercised too much too quickly.

Since there are so many health benefits to exercise, such as lowering cholesterol and helping to prevent bone and muscle loss, obviously your loved one won't want aches and pains to prevent him from keeping active. The trick is to make sure that exercise doesn't leave him groaning every time he moves the day after. And for that, there are plenty of things he can do before, during, and after a workout.

Most of these suggestions apply to dull aches and pains experienced during or after a workout. If your relative is experiencing acute pain, that's a signal from his body that something is not right. Encourage him to see the doctor if he has sharp pains, says Dr. Evans. He shouldn't try to exercise right through it.

Ice it down. Your loved one may be able to recover from muscle pain more quickly if you ice down the muscles that are complaining, says Dr. Evans. "Muscles swell somewhat when they get damaged from overuse. Ice can help to reduce the inflammation." Wrap a frozen ice pack in a thin towel and place it on the affected area for no more than 20 minutes each hour. You can repeat as often as necessary until the area is no longer sore. If an ice pack isn't handy, you can use a bag of frozen peas wrapped in a towel instead.

Alleviate with acetaminophen. Other over-the-counter medications will probably reduce pain, but acetaminophen is the best choice for muscle pain, says Dr. Evans. Why? Other possible painkillers on the pharmacy shelf—aspirin, ibuprofen, ketoprofen, and naproxen—all share a single drawback. These anti-inflammatory drugs block the body's production of chemicals that cause swelling and pain, but in so doing, they interfere with the body's muscle-repair process.

Acetaminophen, on the other hand, blocks pain impulses within the brain itself, allowing the muscle-repair process to proceed normally, says Dr. Evans. It's also the pain reliever that causes the fewest side effects when taken in normal amounts. Just make sure your loved one follows the directions on the label and never takes more than 12 of the 325-milligram pills in a single day.

Urge him to take a bath. When the aches and pains are particularly bad the day after your loved one has exercised hard, he should take a warm bath, says Priscilla Clarkson, Ph.D., professor of exercise science at the University of Massachusetts School of Public Health and Health Sciences in Amherst. He can soak for as long as he likes, she says. "The

WHEN TO SEE THE DOCTOR

Some muscle soreness is routine after a vigorous workout or overdoing it with a new activity, but you should be concerned if your loved one's pain doesn't go away relatively quickly, says William J. Evans, Ph.D., director of the nutrition, metabolism, and exercise laboratory at the University of Arkansas for Medical Sciences in Little Rock. "Report any pain that persists for more than a week to your doctor."

You should also be concerned if the pain is acute, he says. If the pain is sharp or stabbing, your relative might have a muscle tear or joint injury. This is the sort of thing that can be quite painful and lead to further injury, says Dr. Evans, so you'll want to get your relative checked out right away.

warm water helps the muscles relax and promotes circulation, which will have a soothing effect. The pain will come back 15 minutes or so after he gets out, but it still makes for a nice break."

Try a massage. Massage can significantly reduce muscle soreness, and it's a safe alternative if your relative doesn't want to take over-the-counter medication. In addition, it may decrease levels of cortisol (the stress hormone) and increase production of serotonin, a compound produced in the brain that has a calming, pain-killing effect, says Maria Hernandez-Reif, Ph.D., director of the massage therapy research program at the Touch Research Institute of the University of Miami School of Medicine. Here are some massage tips from Dr. Hernandez-Reif.

- Use a massage oil or lotion to make the experience a lot more pleasant. Put a little oil or lotion on the palm of your hand, then rub your hands together to warm it before beginning the massage. The heat helps loosen muscles more quickly.

- Don't skimp on the pressure. You'll know that you're not applying enough pressure if your loved one tells you the rubdown feels like light tickling. Ideally, you should cause some muscle stimulation but not so much that he feels pain.

- Rub the right way. Cup your hand and glide it along the skin's surface. This is most effective when you can massage a large surface all at once, like the side of the leg from the ankle to the knee. "It's taught in massage therapy classes to rub in one direction toward the heart," she says.

Note: Never apply pressure to any joint area, says Dr. Hernandez-Reif. You might injure that joint.

Take care of it before it kicks in. Even before your relative's muscles seize up, you can get a jump on the healing process with bromelain, an enzyme derived from pineapple, says Jacob Schor, N.D., a naturopathic physician in Denver. "If I know I'm going to be sore tomorrow—that I'm not going to want to get out of bed in the morning—I take bromelain."

When you overwork a muscle enough to cause pain, bits of muscle fiber actually break off. These tiny scraps of protein may clog the muscle and cause pain and inflammation. The body has to clean house. Bromelain helps by breaking down these proteins and digesting them. Once the waste products are eliminated, pain and stiffness go away, says Dr. Schor.

To speed up this muscle-repair work, encourage your loved one to take 500 milligrams of bromelain three times a day between meals until the pain goes away, says Dr. Schor. If he takes it with meals, bromelain's protein-digesting powers will work on the food, not on the muscle debris that's prompting the pain and the inflammation.

Be sure to check the product label to make sure that it specifies a strength of 1,800 to 2,400 milk-clotting units (mcu). "When it's not on the label, it makes me suspicious," cautions Dr. Schor. "The company may not know what it's doing, or it may have a very weak product and not want anyone to know." Bromelain is also sometimes measured in gelatin-dissolving units (gdu). Look for a range of 1,080 to 1,440 gdu.

Give your loved one a kitchen painkiller. For all-over muscle pain, try ginger, says Dr. Schor. "It's kind of like a home-style ibuprofen." Ginger is well-known for its anti-inflammatory properties. Like bromelain, it also contains an enzyme that can break down protein, he says. In ginger, this enzyme is zingibain. Ginger has more helpful components, including various antioxidants, which help neutralize the free-roaming, unstable molecules called free radicals that play a role in causing inflammation.

As a supplement, you can use it in tincture or capsule form. If your loved one is in a lot of pain, suggest that he take six 500-milligram capsules of the concentrated extract per day, says Dr. Schor.

Note: A tincture is a highly concentrated herbal liquid. It's made by soaking leaves in alcohol or glycerin—which extracts the herb's medicinal properties—for at least 6 weeks. Tinctures are sold in health food stores in small bottles with eyedroppers to give doses. Be sure to always store them out of the reach of children.

Give him an orange. Vitamin C after heavy exercise may reduce day-after swelling and pain, reports Dr. Clarkson. When muscles are damaged by overuse, she says, they produce free radicals. Antioxidants such as vitamin C may absorb the free radicals before they can cause too many problems, according to Dr. Clarkson. So make sure your relative is getting the Daily Value (60 milligrams a day) of vitamin C, she says. There's more than that amount in the average orange.

Encourage him to stretch. Stretching before exercising warms up the muscles, which may help prevent the tiny muscle tears that lead to morning-after pain, says Dr. Clarkson.

Before the next time your relative engages in some vigorous activity, show or read him the instructions as he tries the following all-around stretching routine from Barbara Sanders, Ph.D., chairperson of the physical therapy department at Southwest Texas State University in San Marcos. He can work this into his workout routine. Tell him to keep in mind that these stretches should be slow and gradual, not bouncy. He also shouldn't try to complete any stretch that causes pain.

- Shoulder rolls. Stand straight with your head high, chin in, and arms at your sides. Rotate your shoulders up, back, down, then forward. Repeat five times.

- Side bends. Stand with your right arm above your head, your left arm across in front of your stomach, your knees bent slightly, and your feet about shoulder-width apart. Lean to the left as far as you comfortably can. Hold for 5 seconds, stand up straight again, then repeat. Now reverse the arm positions and follow the same process, leaning to the right.

- Hip stretch. Lie on your back with your lower back snugly resting against the floor. Keeping your left leg extended, clasp your right leg with your right hand under the knee and bring it to your chest, letting your knee bend double. Hold for 5 seconds, release your leg, straighten it, and lower it to the floor. Repeat once, then do the same stretch with your left leg and left hand.

- Hamstring stretch. Sit on the floor with your right leg relaxed and your right knee bent so that your foot is flat on the floor. Extend your left leg straight in front of you. Now reach for the toes of your left leg with the fingertips of both your hands, feeling the stretch in that hamstring (the long muscle on the back of your thigh). If you can't reach your toes, grab your ankles. Stretch for 20 seconds, relax, and then do it again. Now change the position to extend your right leg and repeat the stretch.

- Calf and Achilles tendon stretch. Stand 3 to 4 feet from a wall and lean toward it, supporting yourself with your hands on the wall at roughly shoulder level. Bring your right leg forward, bending at the knee. As you lean forward, keep your left leg straight with your left foot flat on the floor, while pressing your right knee toward the wall until you feel a comfortable stretch in the straight left leg. (Don't arch your back.) Hold for 20 seconds, then repeat with your left leg forward, your left knee bent, and your right leg extended behind.

- Shoulder stretch. Stand straight with your arms extending straight behind your lower back. Grab your left wrist with your right hand and slowly pull both arms back from your spine as far as possible without causing pain, all the time staying as upright as possible. Keep your neck straight, not arched. Maintain the stretch for a few seconds, relax, then repeat with your left hand grabbing your right wrist.

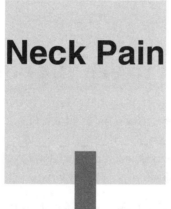

Neck Pain

Imagine a jelly doughnut that's been in the microwave oven too long. While still warm and gooey on the inside, it has lost some of its springy resilience. Now imagine a stack of these doughnuts supporting a 14-pound bowling ball on top. Doesn't sound like too promising a situation for the doughnuts or the bowling ball.

Your loved one's neck and head (and everybody else's, for that matter) have been in that situation since adolescence. The human head weighs about the same as the bowling ball and—as we get up there in years—the row of supporting disks are much too much like jelly doughnuts. As people age, disks lose a lot of the fluid that gives them their strength and shock-absorbing ability, says Karen Rucker, M.D., professor of physical medicine and rehabilitation at Virginia Commonwealth University in

Richmond. That alone can make people over 60 more prone to stiff, crampy necks.

Couple this with increases in arthritis, osteoporosis, and poor posture, and it's no wonder that neck pain tends to increase with age.

Still, you can teach your loved one to take care of her neck with the following expert advice and considerably cut down the pain, stiffness, cricks, and twinges.

Remind her with a timer. Whatever she's doing, whether it's sitting at a desk or working on a hobby, if your loved one stays in one position for a long period of time, her neck can get stiff and hurt. To prevent this, buy a kitchen timer. Set it to go off every half-hour or so, recommends Mary Ann Keenan, M.D., director of neuro-orthopedics at Al-

WHEN TO SEE THE DOCTOR

If your relative has neck pain that persists even when she changes position and is also accompanied by any of the following complaints, be sure to call the doctor immediately, says Karen Rucker, M.D., professor of physical medicine and rehabilitation at Virginia Commonwealth University in Richmond.

- Pain shooting down the arms or hands

- Numbness or tingling in the fingers or arms

- Sudden or significant muscle weakness, such as the inability to lift the legs or extend the arms

- Dizziness

- A feeling of pain when she moves her jaw, which may be a sign of an abscess or infection

- Onset of fever with a new onset of neck pain and stiffness

bert Einstein Medical Center in Philadelphia. That way, your loved one will be able to use it to remind herself to stand up, stretch a little, and take a break.

Try stretching to stop pain. If tension is causing the pain in your relative's neck, she can relieve it with a little bit of stretching. Have your relative read the following advice from Dr. Keenan for a good neck stretch: Start by tilting your head from side to side, then roll it around, first to the right and then to the left. Next, put your hand on top of your head and help the stretch by pulling your head gently halfway down toward your shoulder on each side. It's very important to perform these stretches with slow, smooth movements. "Any quick stretch is more likely to tear a muscle or ligament. You have to do it more gradually," Dr. Keenan warns.

Suggest better posture. Remember when Mom or Dad used to tell you to sit up straight? Well, now it's your turn. "When you're not using good posture—specifically, when you're slumping—all of a sudden the muscles are having to work hard to hold the head up," Dr. Rucker says. But your loved one can take some of this workload off her neck. Tell her that whenever she's sitting or standing, she should make sure that her shoulders are over her hips and her ears are over her shoulders. Her head should never be tucked under, like a horse in a bridle.

"Think about the top of the head," Dr. Rucker advises. "Try to visualize the top of your head trying to touch the ceiling. You'll lengthen, elongate your neck, and get as tall as possible."

Have her change chairs. If your relative (or you, for that matter) is still using one of those old-fashioned chairs with a seat cushion and an oval pad that can be positioned somewhere in the middle of the back, retire it in favor of a chair with a back that goes up to shoulder level. With the high-backed chair, the head, neck, and back are kept vertical, and your loved one can lean her head back periodically to give her neck a chance to relax, says Don Chaffin, Ph.D., professor in the center for ergonomics at the University of Michigan in Ann Arbor.

Apply heat or cold. You can apply a hot-water bottle or an ice pack to relieve your relative's neck pain. It's really her preference. "They both work the same way by increasing the circulation to the area," says Dr. Keenan.

Buy her an athletic bra. If your older relative with neck pain is a woman with a large bosom, she may not be getting enough support from her bra, and that can surely cause neck, back, and shoulder pain. Although it may be tough to convince her to wear it, suggest that she try an athletic or jogging bra because it gives more support and has wider straps. Athletic bras are designed to distribute weight more evenly.

Ask her to consider using a fanny pack. Carrying a weighty shoulder-strap purse can put strain on the neck, Dr. Keenan says. A better option would be to switch to a fanny pack, which fits around your relative's waist and doesn't put any strain on the neck at all. Your loved one can change to a handheld purse for more dressy occasions.

Get her a good pillow. If your relative has an old pillow that has become droopy through years of use, throw it out, advises Dr. Keenan. It's time to get a good supportive pillow, she says. You want one that will keep her head in straight alignment with her mid-back (the line from the center of the head down the back to the crease in the buttocks) and her spine when she lies on her back or side. Although pillows have firmness labels that can help, your best bet is to have your relative try them out before buying. Throw one on a bed display and have her lie down on it. Keep testing until you find the right one.

Suggest improving the way she moves. Quick, sharp movements can injure the neck or the back. But often, people are reckless about their neck movements until they start to feel pain, notes Dr. Rucker. Your relative should treat her neck gingerly. When she gets out of bed in the morning, she should roll gently onto her side first, rather than sitting bolt upright. And advise her to be careful when getting in and out of the car. She should sit on the car seat first and then rotate her body, bringing her legs around and into the car. When she gets out, she should reverse this process. We should be using those techniques all the time to minimize the daily damage that can lead to neck pain, says Dr. Rucker.

Night Vision Problems

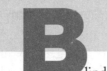

Blinded by an explosion, Charles McNider believed that his promising career as a physician and researcher had been hopelessly derailed. Then one evening as he sat alone in his darkened living room, an owl crashed through a window. McNider tore off his bandages and found that he could see in the dark!

Soon he transformed himself into Dr. Mid-nite, a 1940s comic book hero who wore special goggles to see in the light. Armed with blackout bombs that released a pitch-black cloud in which only he could see, Dr. Mid-nite battled evil foes like the Baleful Banshee and the Sky-Raider. "I am blind, yet I can see," Dr. Mid-nite declared. "The city is draped in night, but to me it is always day. There are no dark corners for evil to hide in, no shadows too deep for the ever-vigilant eyes of Dr. Mid-nite to penetrate!"

But in the real world, midnight is hardly prime time for aging eyes. "There are plenty of reasons why virtually every 20-year-old wants to go on a road trip at night and virtually every 60-year-old doesn't," says Anne Sumers, M.D., an ophthalmologist in Ridgewood, New Jersey, and a spokesperson for the American Academy of Ophthalmology. "First, as we age, the eyes need more light to work properly. Second, the lenses in the eyes aren't as clear at 60 as they were at 20. Third, as we get older, the pupils don't dilate as well as they used to. And in order to see well at night, the pupils have to get very large. So the overall result is that we have a lot more difficulty focusing on objects and seeing at night as we age."

While none of us will ever match the nocturnal prowess of the fictional Dr. Mid-nite, this chapter has plenty of simple ways to help bolster a loved one's night vision even at 60, 70, or 80. Here's how.

Let there be light. The average 60-year-old needs seven times as much light as a 20-year-old to see well in the dark, according to the

American Optometric Association. So brighten up the rooms of your home with 60- or 100-watt neodymium lightbulbs, suggests Bruce Rosenthal, O.D., chief of low-vision programs at Lighthouse International, a vision rehabilitation organization in New York City. These bulbs provide higher contrast and produce less glare than regular lightbulbs, so your loved one should be able to see better at night. Neodymium bulbs are available at specialty lighting stores and from some mail-order catalog companies.

For walking in the dark, suggest to your relative that he use a portable camping lamp to illuminate where he's stepping, says Charles R. Fox, O.D., director of vision rehabilitation at the University of Maryland School of Medicine in Baltimore. Camping lamps, which are available at most sporting goods stores, are better than flashlights because they provide a wider arc of light and make it easier to get around, he says.

WHEN TO SEE THE DOCTOR

Night vision problems could be a symptom of a serious underlying disease such as diabetes, macular degeneration, cataracts, or an inherited disease called retinitis pigmentosa, says Samuel L. Pallin, M.D., an ophthalmologist and medical director of the Lear Eye Clinic in Sun City, Arizona. So take your loved one to the optometrist or ophthalmologist if he:

- Has sudden or increasing difficulty seeing in dim light

- Can't see stars in the night sky that are visible to others

- Is limiting his activities because he is afraid to venture out after dark

- Has trouble driving at night because of glare

Bend and tilt. Adjustable floor or table lamps that swivel and bend so you can fine-tune the lighting to your loved one's needs can help overcome night vision problems, Dr. Rosenthal says.

If your relative is reading, for instance, suggest that he adjust the lamp so that it's about 12 inches from the page yet not causing an annoying glare, Dr. Rosenthal suggests. Look for lamps with built-in reflectors that will help increase illumination.

Mention trying visualization. Imagery may help improve night vision, says Robert-Michael Kaplan, O.D., an optometrist and author of books on improving vision. He suggests the following technique that you can show your loved one if he is interested: Twice a day when natural light is dim—within 2 hours of sunrise and 2 hours of sunset—take a moment to close your eyes and move your head slowly to the left and then to the right. As you do this, take 5 to 10 deep breaths and visualize beams of light streaming into your eyes and activating the portions of the vision that are responsible for seeing well at night. This exercise can be done in less than 2 minutes a day.

Get some bilberry. Some doctors think night vision problems are due to a lack of rhodopsin, a chemical produced in the rods of the eye, which are the photoreceptors that help us see in low light. If we lack rhodopsin, night sight will be less than perfect.

As the story goes, British pilots during World War II began eating jam made from bilberries, which are a type of northern European blueberry, to help counteract night blindness. Searching for the active component in these dark berries, scientists found chemical substances called anthocyanins. "Blueberries, elderberries, huckleberries, and red grapes also contain this pigment," says Robert Abel Jr., M.D., clinical professor of ophthalmology at Thomas Jefferson University in Philadelphia. In the body, Dr. Abel says, anthocyanins benefit the eyes by converting to rhodopsin.

You probably won't be able to find bilberries or bilberry jam in your local supermarket. You should be able to locate bilberry capsules at your local health food store or drugstore, however. Encourage your relative to take 100 to 500 milligrams of bilberry twice a day. Dr. Abel suggests that he try it before going out at night. He should see an effect from the capsules within 20 minutes. Your loved one can try it for a month or two to see if it helps. If so, he can continue to take one dose of 100 milligrams before going out at night.

Recommend slowing down. Many night vision problems aren't obvious until people get behind the wheel of a car, says Gary Mancil, O.D., adjunct professor at Southern College of Optometry in Memphis.

On low beam, for instance, headlights illuminate about 100 feet in front of a vehicle, says Steve Creel, a California Highway Patrol public affairs officer. And at 65 miles per hour, you're traveling at about 100 feet per second. So at that speed, even if you had perfect vision and were driving in perfect conditions, headlights wouldn't be much help. That's

Medication Alert

Pilocarpine (Isopto Carpine, Pilocar), beta-adrenergic blocking agents (Betagan), and other medications used to treat glaucoma can cause temporary night vision problems for up to 4 hours after use, says W. Steven Pray, Ph.D., R.Ph., professor of nonprescription drug products at Southwestern Oklahoma State University in Weatherford. If this dimming of vision is bothersome, ask your loved one's doctor if he can switch to another medication that might not cause this side effect. Other drugs that can affect night vision include:

- Nasal and eyedrop steroids such as beclomethasone (Vancenase)

- Antidepressants containing trazodone (Desyrel), imipramine (Tofranil), or amitriptyline (Elavil)

- Antihistamines, including over-the-counter products like doxylamine (Nyquil), diphenhydramine (Benadryl), and chlorpheniramine (Chlor-Trimeton)

why it's important to slow down at night, particularly in poor weather. To self-check his vision, your loved one could pick out an object in the distance and begin counting until he reaches the object. A 4- to 6-second count is an indication that he's driving at a safe speed. If he reaches that point in less than 2 seconds, he would not have been able to stop safely if that object were in the middle of the road, explains Creel. So advise your loved one to ease up on the throttle.

"Just because the speed limit is 55 or 65 doesn't mean you have to go that fast," says Creel. That might not be the safe speed for your loved one, particularly if he has trouble seeing at night.

Clean and be seen. Creel recommends regularly cleaning all the lights on the car, especially the headlights, because at night these lights are the only way to communicate with other drivers.

If your relative has night vision problems, he's probably driving slower than some other people on the road. So it's just as important to be seen. "One good rule of thumb is if the portions of the windshield that aren't cleaned by the wipers are covered with gunk, it's time to clean all the lights," says Creel.

Suggest looking for landmarks. Street signs are harder to read at night, so when traveling to someplace unfamiliar, your loved one should get detailed directions that include lots of gas stations, grocery stores, and other landmarks, Dr. Mancil suggests. Also, he should check out a reliable road map before leaving and take that map with him. If your loved one finds himself on darkened streets, he can always pull over, turn on the overhead light, and check the map.

Tell him to not be a deer. When he encounters oncoming traffic, advise your relative to look toward the right and follow the shoulder of the road until the other cars pass. Diverting the eyes like this will reduce the blinding glare from the approaching headlights.

Recommend that he use shades. Whenever your loved one stops at a gas station, restaurant, or other well-lighted place, suggest that he put on a pair of sunglasses before getting out of the car, Dr. Fox says. That way he'll have less trouble readapting to the darkness once he gets back behind the wheel again. Of course, he should remove the shades before driving off.

Get him a pair of night glasses. Sometimes, poor night vision is merely a sign of increasing nearsightedness, Dr. Sumers says. Ask your optometrist or ophthalmologist if a new pair of glasses specifically prescribed for nocturnal activities like driving will help your relative see better after sundown.

Get rid of the glare. Ask your vision-care specialist about getting an antireflective coating on your relative's glasses, Dr. Rosenthal suggests. These coatings cut down on glare, increase the amount of available light coming into the eyes, and can improve his night vision.

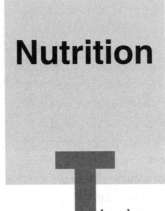

Nutrition

There's no way to get around it: Food has a lot to do with how we feel. Poor nutrition is clearly linked to several health problems, including heart disease, high blood pressure, diabetes, osteoporosis, and high cholesterol. And this fact is even more important with regard to older people, since a lot of health problems—in particular the ones just mentioned—present themselves as people age.

This chapter discusses some of the basic nutritional needs of older folks, so you can help them eat right. You'll also find some advice regarding how to get your loved ones to eat, since poor appetite can be a big barrier to good nutrition. Finally, you'll learn some "dietetic defenses" to employ in your kitchen to protect your loved ones from the most common age-related diseases.

What They Need

Here is a breakdown of the basic nutrients—and how much of them—seniors need.

Calories. People over age 55 need fewer calories per day to maintain their weight than younger adults—an average of 1,900 for women (versus 2,200 for younger adult women) and 2,300 for men (versus 2,900 for younger men). "We lose lean body mass as we age, and that's what deems how many calories we need," says Susan Saffel-Shrier, R.D., a certified gerontologist and assistant professor at the University of Utah School of Medicine in Salt Lake City. A sedentary lifestyle, she adds, can lower caloric needs even further.

Protein. A man over age 51 needs about 63 grams of protein a day. A woman in the same age group needs about 50 grams. For men and women, these protein amounts are the same as those for people between 25 and 50 years of age. Protein requirements don't change much as we age, but sometimes people's interest in protein does, says Pamela Starke-Reed, Ph.D., deputy director of the division of nutrition research coordination at the National Institutes of Health in Bethesda, Maryland. "Foods that are difficult to chew, including most meats, tend to lose some of their appeal as we get older," she says, "so we have to work a little harder to make sure we get enough protein." Lean meats and poultry are great sources, but so are eggs, soy products, and milk products. Eggs have the advantage of being what nutrition experts deem the "perfect" protein, and they are also easily incorporated into all kinds of easily digestible recipes.

Vitamins and minerals. A well-rounded diet of low fat, nutrient-rich foods can be a key to health and longevity for many older folks. Keep in mind, as you choose foods, that variety is the name of the game in ensuring that all the essential nutrients are covered in the diet. Some vitamins and minerals, especially vitamins A, E, C, and D and folic acid, have been studied for the positive influence they can have on older people's health. One study even hints that antioxidants, which include beta-carotene (the precursor to vitamin A) and vitamins E and C, may actually reverse the effects of aging on cognitive and motor function. To make sure a person in your care gets enough of these vitamins, provide plenty of fresh fruits, including oranges, strawberries, grapefruits, and blueberries, as well as dark green vegetables like spinach and broccoli.

One mineral you especially need to make sure your older loved one gets is calcium. After the age of 51, both men and women need an extra 200 milligrams of calcium in their diets each day—about 1,200 milligrams total. There are roughly 300 milligrams of calcium in 1 cup of milk. Yogurt, cheese, and canned red salmon are all great sources, too. If you are planning meals for an older person who is lactose intolerant, ask the doctor about offering a calcium supplement. Since the need for calcium increases with age, it's critical to make sure there's enough in the diet.

Fiber. There are so many different sources of protein that meeting its requirement isn't usually as big a challenge as ensuring that a diet has enough fiber, says David Reuben, M.D., professor of medicine at UCLA School of Medicine in Los Angeles. A good goal is 25 grams of fiber a day, he says, "But you really have to work at getting that much."

For lots of fiber per portion, cereals and grains can't be beat. Look at the side of the cereal box, Dr. Reuben recommends, to choose a truly high-fiber cereal. "Most cereals have between 1 and 3 grams of fiber per serving," he explains, "but some, like Fiber One and All Bran, have 9 or more grams per serving. That's a good start on the level of fiber you're looking for." Other good sources of fiber, albeit not quite as concentrated, are brown rice, oats, oatmeal, apples, avocados, blueberries, raspberries, baked beans, lima beans, and air-popped popcorn.

Fluids. Perhaps the most important concern you should keep in mind for your elderly loved one's diet isn't about food at all. Dehydration is all too common among older people because they don't feel thirsty, even when their bodies need fluids. "Any diet for an elderly person should start with ensuring they get the equivalent of 8 cups of liquids a day, at least some of it in the form of water," says Alice H. Lichtenstein, D.Sc., professor of nutrition at Tufts University School of Medicine in Boston.

When Appetite Is Flagging

Of course, knowing what foods are healthy or how many grams of each nutrient they come packed with doesn't guarantee healthy diet choices. As with most people, elderly adults are often more ruled by their hunger—or more important, the lack of it—and tastebuds than by the recommended Daily Values.

This is because one of the biggest problems facing older people when it comes to diet is a simple lack of appetite. "As people get older, their sense of smell gets weaker, and if you can't smell, you can't taste," explains Dr. Starke-Reed. "That takes a lot of the satisfaction out of foods that a person might once have enjoyed."

As if the dulled tastebuds weren't enough, other factors can cause older folks to lose their appetites as well. Dental problems like sore teeth and jaws or ill-fitting dentures, depression, indigestion, and interactions from medications can all influence appetite, says Dr. Starke-Reed.

But if you make a few small adjustments to meal planning, you can help an older family member make the most of meals.

Experiment with herbs and spices. Everyone's taste is different, so there's no single spice or herb that pleases everyone, says Saffel-Shrier. Since a dulled sense of taste affects many older people, though, choosing condiments that add to the pungency and taste of a dish can help tremendously. Garlic, pepper, basil, oregano, and cinnamon all have strong flavors that can pique the tastebuds.

Choose what's easy to chew. If you are preparing meals for a person who has dental problems or difficulty swallowing, look for recipes for easy-to-chew foods. Sometimes just the preparation of a food can make all the difference in its digestibility, says Dr. Starke-Reed. For instance, meat loaf is much easier to manage than steak. Chicken breasts cut in small pieces and cooked in a moist casserole are less daunting than they are grilled whole.

Get more for the mouthful. One of the biggest challenges in planning meals for someone with appetite or digestion problems is trying to cover all the nutritional bases *and* offer foods that are appealing enough to entice them to the table. You can make it easier to meet food requirement goals by choosing foods that meet several needs at once, says Dr. Starke-Reed. "Pick the most nutrient-positive foods you can, because all calories are definitely not created equal." A glass of milk, she points out, offers servings of protein, calcium, and vitamin D. An orange offers fiber, fluids, calcium, and several vitamins as well. A doughnut has more calories than both and doesn't fulfill any major nutritional needs.

Foods for Common Problems

Here are some common problems that people face when they age and foods you can give your loved one to help him.

Memory loss. As unlikely as it seems, memory loss and confusion often result from nutritional deficiencies and can sometimes be helped with dietary changes. "Elderly people can complain of being confused, and it could be a vitamin B_{12} deficiency," says Saffel-Shrier. Iron deficiency, too, can cause memory deficits.

If the person you are caring for has a severe deficiency, he'll need a supplement recommended by a doctor. Meat, eggs, and milk can all boost dietary B_{12}. Meat, fish, poultry, whole grains, and beans are good ways to ensure he gets more iron.

Osteoporosis. Osteoporosis is another common age-related disease. Fortunately, it's largely preventable. Getting enough calcium and vitamin D go a long way toward keeping the disease at bay. Women over 55 should get 1,200 milligrams of calcium each day—roughly the amount in four glasses of milk. In addition, vitamin D helps prevent osteoporosis. We get some vitamin D from exposure to the sun, but since our ability to make vitamin D through the skin decreases as we get older, the National Osteoporosis Foundation recommends also getting at least 400 IU of it through vitamin D–fortified dairy products. Egg yolks, dairy products, and saltwater fish are all good sources. A single egg contains 26 IU, a cup of milk has 98 IU, and a 3¾-ounce can of sardines has a whopping 250 IU.

Heart disease. Heart disease patients should have diets rich in fresh vegetables and fruits. The American Heart Association recommends that more than half of their daily calories come from complex carbohydrate foods. Those foods include fruits, vegetables, and grains. When you choose foods for a heart patient, try to pick as many natural, whole foods as you can and as few processed ones as possible. Whole foods include raw vegetables and fruits, fresh meat, poultry, and fish. Processed foods like packaged cookies, crackers, sauces, and snacks tend to be high in both sodium and sugar, and often in fat, so you should avoid giving them to your older relative. When you do choose processed foods, try to pick products that have whole foods, such as whole grains, as their first two ingredients. Since ingredients are listed by volume, products that are mostly whole foods are easy to spot by their ingredient listings.

Also, heart and stroke patients should avoid saturated fats, cholesterol, and sodium. The American Heart Association recommends that no more than 30 percent of calories come from fats, with less than 10 percent from saturated fat. It's not hard to judge how many calories in a diet are coming from fat if you keep an eye on product labels. Look at the total number of calories per serving, then at the "calories from fat" number. If more than a third of the calories in any product come from fat, you'll need to either skip it or choose some other lower-fat foods that day. Foods containing or made with animal fats—like whole milk, eggs, butter, cheese, and meats—are the highest in saturated fats and cholesterol.

So to help your older loved one, you should switch to fat-free dairy products. Use water, broth, cooking wine, or cooking sprays to substitute for high-fat oils and butter. Bake or steam foods instead of frying them. Limit servings of red meat to no more than 3 to 5 ounces and substitute fish or poultry when you can.

Arthritis. Arthritis strikes people of any age, but a third of all patients are age 65 or older. Through experience, people with this sometimes very painful disease learn what aggravates and what eases their discomfort. Milk products and fish oil can sometimes aggravate sore joints. Since dairy products and fish are great nutrition sources, though, it's important to make sure a person with the disease makes up his calcium and protein with other foods. Meats, chicken, tofu, and beans are all good substitute protein sources. Though calcium is found in some of those foods, talk with your loved one's doctor about giving a calcium supplement to ensure he gets enough.

To reduce arthritis pain, try giving your loved one oranges, grapefruits, strawberries, and other fresh fruits. They contain vitamin C, and in at least one study vitamin C has been shown to ease arthritis pain. Vitamins A, E, and D have also been studied because they seem to help relieve arthritis pain. Fresh fruits and vegetables are rich in both vitamin A and vitamin E, and fortified milk contains plenty of vitamin D. Spinach is such a great source of both vitamins A and E that it's worth working it into your family's diet. Aside from including it in salads and as a vegetable side dish, spinach added to sauces, spaghetti, chili, and casseroles has very little flavor or texture, but loads of vitamins.

Osteoporosis

Drink your milk, then go outside and play." Good advice when we're 6. Good advice at 46. Turns out, that's even good advice at 60 or 86 if you want to stave off osteoporosis.

Osteoporosis, which literally means "holes in the bones," occurs when the loss of bone tissue exceeds its replacement, a process that begins when we're in our thirties. A silent disease in that there are no symptoms or pain until a fracture occurs, osteoporosis robs bones of their strength over many years. Once this silent thief has done its work, bones can be so fragile that everyday actions like sneezing or lifting a bag of groceries can cause a fracture.

While women are four times more likely to develop the disease, men also suffer from osteoporosis. Women lose bone mass rapidly in the years following menopause, because their bodies produce less estrogen; yet by age 65 or 70, women and men lose bone mass at the same rate, experts say, and calcium absorption decreases in both sexes. Osteoporosis in men has been recognized as an important public health issue, given that the number of men over 70 is estimated to double between 1993 and 2050.

Fractures resulting from osteoporosis typically occur in the hips, spine, and wrists, frequently costing people their independence. Yet although it affects nearly half of all people over the age of 75, doctors say that osteoporosis is not an inevitable part of aging.

Bone tissue renewal continues throughout life. So with proper diet and lifestyle changes, you can help your loved one slow, or even stop, osteoporosis, says James Webster, M.D., director of the Buehler Center of Aging at Northwestern University in Chicago. The time to combat osteoporosis, he emphasizes, is before the bones start to break.

Make sure she gets plenty of calcium. Your loved one might not like milk, but she does need enough calcium. Up to age 65, doctors recommend 1,000 milligrams of calcium a day for women on estrogen replacement therapy (ERT) and for all men. Women who are past menopause but who are not receiving ERT should consume 1,200 milligrams of calcium daily, as should everyone over age 65.

To reach or surpass the goal of 1,000 milligrams through diet alone, encourage your relative to drink 2½ to 3 eight-ounce glasses of fat-free milk a day. She'll get that through a healthy, balanced diet, says Robert P. Heaney, M.D., professor of medicine at Creighton University in Omaha, Nebraska.

Milk is fortified with vitamin D, which the body needs to assimilate calcium, so it's really the best calcium source. But there are other foods that supply calcium alone. Your loved one can get 1,000 milligrams from eating 2½ cups of fat-free yogurt or 5 ounces of Cheddar cheese. Other good sources of calcium are sardines (with bones), collards, tofu, and calcium-fortified orange juice.

WHEN TO SEE THE DOCTOR

To make sure your loved one avoids becoming one of the people who first learn that they have osteoporosis while their doctors are setting their broken bones, take her to the doctor for DEXA (dual energy x-ray absorptiometry). This simple 15-minute test will measure bone density and determine whether your loved one is at risk for osteoporosis.

In general, people are especially at risk for osteoporosis if they:

- Are thin and small-boned

- Have a history of eating disorders

- Have family members with osteoporosis

- Have generalized bone pain and tenderness

- Take corticosteroids, anticonvulsants like phenytoin (Dilantin), thyroid medication, or blood thinners

Consider supplements. It's best to get calcium through food, but if your loved one can't get enough in her diet, supplements offer the elemental calcium that the body needs, says Dr. Webster. If your relative is ill or has had kidney stones, however, talk to her doctor before giving any supplements.

For best absorption, have her take supplements in divided doses of 500 to 600 milligrams at a time, and 1,000 to 1,200 milligrams per day, advises Elizabeth Lee Vliet, M.D., professor of family and community medicine at the University of Arizona in Tucson. "The body will absorb a smaller amount better than taking the daily dose all at one time."

Calcium carbonate and calcium citrate are two common supplements available over the counter. Dr. Vliet says that calcium carbonate can cause bloating or gas; calcium citrate doesn't, but these tablets contain less calcium, so your loved one will have to take more. Don't buy bonemeal or dolomite supplements, she warns, because they may contain lead and other toxic metals.

Suggest maximizing her magnesium intake. Magnesium is another crucial mineral to help build strong bones as well as aid bowel function, prevent leg cramps, and improve sleep, according to Dr. Vliet. "But the sad fact is that most American women's diets are seriously deficient in magnesium." She recommends consuming 250 milligrams in the morning and another 250 milligrams at night. Encourage your relative to try a capsule formulation since it's better absorbed. For women with significant bone loss, problems with constipation, or nighttime leg cramps, the dose may need to be increased to 400 milligrams twice a day, suggests Dr. Vliet. Talk to the doctor first before giving your loved one supplemental magnesium. It may cause diarrhea. Also, people with heart or kidney problems should not take it.

Defend with D. As mentioned earlier, to absorb calcium and build strong bones, the body needs vitamin D. Several studies have shown that when vitamin D and calcium are taken together, bone mineral density increases and the number of fractures decreases. Unfortunately, there aren't many good sources. Milk is fortified, and so are some cereals. It is important to read labels to see how much of the Daily Value your loved one is getting. Apart from that, the best source is sunlight, which triggers vitamin D production in the body. As little as 10 minutes of summer sun exposure on the hands, face, and arms is enough, says Dr. Vliet. Sunscreens with an SPF of 8 or above prevent vitamin D synthesis, so tell her to apply one immediately after the 10 minutes are up.

If your loved one can't get outdoors, dietary vitamin D intake should be at least 400 IU but not more than 600 IU a day, recommends Dr. Vliet. One cup of fortified milk, whether it's whole, low-fat, or fat-free, has 100 IU, and most multivitamins provide 400 IU. Too much vitamin D, however, can have harmful effects, including kidney damage, so don't give her supplements above the Daily Value of 400 IU without first consulting the doctor.

Try low-profile vitamins and minerals. Vitamin K is a bit of a forgotten vitamin. It certainly doesn't get much mention in the media, but it's very important for maintaining bone health. It helps reduce the amount of calcium lost through urine, says Lorilee Schoenbeck, N.D., a naturopathic physician in Middlebury, Vermont.

Vitamin K is also crucial to the formation of osteocalcin, a protein that is the matrix upon which calcium is put into the bone. "Vitamin K is kind of like the foundation that calcium builds on," Dr. Schoenbeck says.

The Daily Value for vitamin K is 80 micrograms. Since this vitamin is abundant in green leafy vegetables and whole grains, a diet rich in these foods may supply your relative with the daily dose.

Boron, a trace mineral found in many vegetables and fruits, helps reduce the amount of calcium and possibly magnesium that are excreted in urine. It may also help to slightly raise estrogen levels, which could prevent bone loss as well, says Dr. Schoenbeck. Because of that same estrogen-increasing property, however, women with breast cancer should avoid it. A safe daily amount for women with no breast cancer history is 3 milligrams, she adds.

Encourage activity. Weight-bearing exercise helps bones grow stronger. Your relative should start doing any exercise—walking, running, aerobics, pumping iron—that forces the bones and muscles to work against gravity.

Exercise stimulates bones to lay down new tissue, says Dr. Webster. Ideally, everyone should follow the American College of Sports Medicine's suggested minimum of 20 minutes of aerobic exercise a day at least three times a week, but for some older people that much exercise at one time is not realistic, he explains.

If your relative can't handle 20 minutes of walking or weight lifting, Dr. Webster recommends breaking it down into "movement moments."

Any exercise that makes your loved one carry her own body weight, like lifting weights or pressing against some resistance, is going to help. For example, among the movement moments she can try are a 10-minute stroll around the block or 5 minutes of biceps curls using 1-pound weights. All she has to do is make sure these movement moments add up to a total of 20 minutes of aerobic exercise.

But she shouldn't take it too easy either. Doing as much as she can handle is going to get the best results. Walking will strengthen the bones of the hips and lower back, says Dr. Webster, but if she can add light leg weights, that's even better.

Discourage overdoing it. Exercising too lightly isn't good because your loved one won't challenge her body enough. But she has to strike a careful balance and not challenge her body too much, or she'll get hurt. So encourage her to exercise, but make sure she chooses an activity that doesn't put any sudden or excessive strain on her bones.

Dr. Webster says your loved one should take care when lifting heavy objects and should avoid exercises that cause bending forward or twisting the spine. These movements tend to encourage compression fractures in the spine. Instead, she should lift with the thigh muscles by squatting.

Not surprisingly, doctors often suggest that patients with brittle bones give up golf, tennis, and basketball because of the twisting motions associated with these sports and their impact on joints. Ask the doctor what type of exercises your loved one can do safely to preserve bone, or ask for a referral to a physical therapist who specializes in osteoporosis.

Whatever activity your relative chooses, make sure she does something that minimizes the chances of breaking a bone. And remember, says Dr. Webster, that the benefits of exercise last only as long as she sticks with it.

Protect with proteins. Bones are not made of calcium alone. In fact, the bone matrix—the close weave of tissue that holds the calcium—incorporates a great deal of protein. Too often, experts say, the diets of older Americans are short on protein, which adds to the osteoporosis risk.

Dr. Webster suggests adding a packet of instant breakfast or another protein supplement to a glass of low-fat or fat-free milk twice a day to increase bone strength. Protein should make up 30 to 40 percent of your loved one's diet, he says, noting that skinless chicken breasts are a good source of inexpensive protein.

Take fall-safe measures. With osteoporosis, bones break more easily when someone takes a tumble. If you want to decrease your loved one's risk of debilitating fractures, you have to prevent falls, say doctors.

Remedying unsafe situations is an important part of changing the way your loved one does things, says Kay Solar, M.D., an obstetrician/gynecologist in Baton Rouge, Louisiana. The best way to do this is to suggest that she evaluate her everyday routine. Your loved one should think about what she is about to do, whether it's washing dishes or getting the newspaper, and consider if it may cause extra stress on her bones. She should avoid sudden movements and learn to move slowly and wisely.

Also, think about your loved one's surroundings at work or home. Is there anything that could cause her to trip or fall? If so, correct the problem, says Dr. Solar. In the kitchen, store frequently used items within easy reach. Avoid using step stools. Put handrails on both sides of a staircase. Get rid of throw rugs.

Control the calcium flushers. If your loved one drinks coffee, tea, or soft drinks with caffeine, she should limit herself to 2 to 3 cups per day, says Dr. Solar. Beyond that, caffeine acts as a diuretic, flushing calcium from the body.

Hold the salt. As with caffeine, too much salt causes the body to excrete calcium. Check food labels, advises Dr. Solar. Your loved one should avoid products with more than 300 milligrams of salt per serving and limit daily sodium intake to 2,400 milligrams a day.

Parkinson's Disease

There was a time when the only images conjured up by thoughts of boxing great Muhammad Ali were those of sweat, blood, and knockouts in the ring. That changed, though, when the former heavyweight champ began making public appearances in the 1990s with visibly shaking hands, a tightly muscled face, and the slow, shuffling gait that are the hallmarks of advanced Parkinson's disease. Not all people with Parkinson's have all the symptoms or the severity of Ali's case, but most can relate to the frustration of having a body that doesn't follow the mind's directions and the challenges of having such a visible illness.

Parkinson's disease affects about 1½ million Americans, with most people becoming ill when they are 50 or older. Unfortunately, after decades of study, researchers still don't know for sure what causes it. One study suggests that toxins, including some pesticides and a chemical used in oil refineries, may influence Parkinson's, but nothing has been proven.

Parkinson's affects movement and balance by progressively attacking and killing the cells that produce dopamine, a chemical transmitter that activates the brain cells that control motor function. Because those cells are dying, the brain doesn't produce enough dopamine and eventually doesn't produce any at all in people with Parkinson's. Without dopamine, they may experience tremors, rigidity, and slowness or lack of movement.

The major medical treatments for Parkinson's focus on stimulating the brain to make dopamine or simulating dopamine so that a person's system thinks that the chemical is there when it's not, explains Rosabel Young, M.D., director of the movement disorders and neuromuscular diseases program at King-Drew Medical Center in Los Angeles. The most common medication, Sinemet (a combination of carbidopa and levodopa), fools the brain into making dopamine on its own. When brain cells lose the capability to make dopamine, medications from a group called dopamine agonists can stimulate the brain somewhat like natural dopamine would.

In addition to medications, some people with Parkinson's are also treated with surgery to implant a pacemaker-like device in the brain that can stimulate motor centers, Dr. Young explains. Your loved one should speak with his doctor about surgical options that may be appropriate for his condition.

How You Can Help

Unfortunately, Parkinson's medications have possible side effects that caregivers should know about. Some of the side effects can be prevented or better managed if you carefully time the medications and make certain dietary adjustments. Here are doctors' suggestions.

Stick to the schedule. "If you are going to do one thing for a person with Parkinson's, be compulsive with the medication schedule," says James Tetrud, M.D., a movement disorders specialist at the Parkinson's

Institute in Sunnyvale, California. The steady flow of Sinemet and dopamine agonists helps people maintain the most even control of their movements and balance.

Give medications with high-carb foods. Giving Parkinson's medications with food helps reduce side effects, especially nausea, says Dr. Tetrud. He recommends giving meds with carbohydrate-heavy foods like breads, cereals, or applesauce.

Don't give Sinemet with protein. Sinemet, the most frequently prescribed medication, is derived from amino acids. When taken with proteins, both vie for the same transport system to get from the stomach to the bloodstream. The upshot of that competition, says Dr. Young, is that the medication gets absorbed too slowly to give much relief. She recommends eating protein foods 30 to 60 minutes after a medication dose.

Talk with the doctor about timing. If one of your relative's medications is causing sedation or insomnia, talk with the doctor about changing the timing of the dose, suggests Dr. Young. Often, doses can be shuffled so that an insomnia-inducing medication is taken in the morning or one that causes sedation is taken just before bedtime.

Help him steer clear of saturated fats. Animal fats, like those in red meat, eggs, and butter, promote cell oxidation. This process occurs naturally, even without the animal fats: When we breathe, we take in oxygen, which combines with certain natural compounds in our bodies and produces oxygen molecules that are missing an electron. These molecules become what scientists call free radicals. They roam around the body looking to make up for the electron they lost, so they steal an electron from another molecule. Then that molecule turns into a free radical, which goes out and steals an electron from another molecule.

It's kind of like what happens in vampire movies: One vampire bites a human, who then becomes a vampire and bites somebody else, who becomes one as well, and so on, until everybody in town is a vampire. This chain reaction of molecules stealing electrons and producing more "vampire" molecules leads to many diseases, scientists suspect. If you want a real-life example of how this process works, look at a piece of metal rusting. That is essentially what's happening to us with these nasty little free radicals. We're rusting.

Smoking and eating certain animal fats, like the kind you find in lard and red meat, also worsen oxidation. This is a big problem for people with Parkinson's because this rusting can destroy the brain cells that naturally produce dopamine. Eating a minimum of these foods can help preserve for as long as possible the dopamine-producing ability that these people still have, states Dr. Young.

To help lower the saturated fat in meals, you can use more egg whites in cooking and fewer whole eggs, or for egg dishes and omelettes, you can use a commercial product like Egg Beaters, which has reduced fat. Also, choose lean cuts of meat—or better yet, opt more often for poultry and fish. Another trick is to use nonstick cookware and cooking spray rather than cooking with butter. Or sauté foods in broth or cooking wine—they taste just as good as those cooked in butter. Finally, at the table, try substituting a reduced-fat vegetable oil spread for real butter.

Pile plates with antioxidants. Just as some foods promote cell oxidation, others prevent it. There are nutrients called antioxidants in foods that scientists believe act kind of like the rust-proofing liquid you put on metal. The three main antioxidants are vitamin C, vitamin E, and beta-carotene. So make sure your loved one with Parkinson's gets plenty of spinach, which has beta-carotene; broccoli and oranges, which have plenty of vitamin C; and wheat germ, which is an excellent source of vitamin E.

Some Natural Helpers

If your loved one has already been diagnosed with Parkinson's, you should know that none of the following remedies are substitutes for any medication his doctor may prescribe. If started early enough, however, some medical professionals believe these supplements can help prolong the time before medication becomes necessary. If your loved one is already taking prescription drugs, adding supplements like these is a safe and effective way to help keep symptoms from getting worse. Even so, be sure to inform the doctor about any supplements that your loved one is taking, since some can interact with prescription medicines.

Get him on guard with ginkgo. Ginkgo, the popular "memory herb," boosts blood circulation to the brain, but it appears to have additional positive effects on gray matter. In particular, it may offer hope for people with Parkinson's. Studies have shown that animals exposed to a neurotoxin called MPTP will develop symptoms that are identical to those of Parkinson's disease. When they are pretreated with ginkgo extract, however, they don't develop the symptoms, says David Perlmutter, M.D., a neurologist in Naples, Florida.

Ginkgo performs its guardian gig through a process of membrane stabilization. By stabilizing nerve cell membranes, it helps prevent a breakdown of communication between the nerve cells. "It allows neurons to communicate with each other more readily," concludes Dr. Perlmutter.

Ginkgo has antioxidant properties that come in quite handy as well. "Ginkgo blocks the formation of free radicals that would otherwise be stimulated into destroying brain cells," says Dr. Perlmutter. Give your loved one 60 milligrams of ginkgo extract twice a day.

Care for him with coenzyme Q_{10}. Coenzyme Q_{10} is a chemical with a dual personality. Not only does it help generate energy inside the microscopic cell bodies called mitochondria, it also functions as a powerful antioxidant. Coenzyme Q_{10} is most often associated with treating heart disease, but people with Parkinson's should take note as well, says Carl Germano, R.D., a registered/certified nutritionist in New York City. A study by Harvard Medical School researchers showed that coenzyme Q_{10} protects certain neurons in the brain from the substance that produces Parkinson's damage, according to Germano. Try giving your loved one 200 milligrams of the supplement once a day with a meal.

Try to help in a different way. Parkinson's disease is often regarded as strictly a brain disorder, but addressing only the brain may mean missing out on other ways to ease the disease. "You need to look at the entire picture," says Germano. "There are many pathways to this disease." That means that there are many paths to healing as well.

When the body is dealing with the negative effects of a possible overload of toxins such as pesticides, liver function is crucial. In fact, Dr. Perlmutter believes that healing the liver can bring dramatic improvement to people who have Parkinson's. "I have patients diagnosed with this disease in their thirties who respond beautifully to liver detoxification," he says.

One herb that's linked to liver health is milk thistle. This herb, and the extract it yields, silymarin, are said to be powerful liver protectors. For anyone who regularly deals with pollutants like pesticides and who may thus be at higher risk for Parkinson's, milk thistle is one of several herbs recommended by Germano. Give your loved one up to 300 milligrams of standardized milk thistle extract daily.

Lifestyle Strategies Can Help

Dietary and medication considerations aside, Parkinson's is a disease that primarily affects the way people move, and so one of the most important things you can do to help someone with the disease is to encourage physical activity.

Get him moving. "Exercise is vital," says Dr. Tetrud. "Stretching to keep muscles flexible and aerobic exercise to increase bloodflow can help slow the progress of the disease *and* make patients more comfortable." For example, Dr. Young recommends that patients stretch and extend their legs while watching television and start their mornings with stretches.

Other ways for Parkinson's patients to get exercise include:

- Performing everyday tasks. Buttoning a shirt, for example, will strengthen and train the muscles needed for that task and make it easier.

- Wiggling the toes. People with Parkinson's disease sometimes find that their muscles "freeze up" on them, even when they are up and walking. Wiggling the toes can often give other muscles a start and help your loved one get moving again.

- Walking. Sometimes just walking across the room can seem daunting to a person with Parkinson's. Have your loved one practice walking in small steps with his feet spread about 10 inches apart. Having the feet set wide apart will improve his balance. And if your loved one lists to one side when he is walking, give him something to carry in the opposite hand to help bring him into alignment and improve balance, suggests the Parkinson's Disease Foundation.

Plan to prevent falls. Since people with Parkinson's often have trouble maintaining their balance, Dr. Young recommends choosing shoes with leather soles that grip rather than rubber ones that tend to stick. She also suggests removing any small area rugs that aren't tightly affixed to the floor. Removing doorsills can help prevent falls as well.

Mark halls and stairways with stripes. Marking hallways and stairwells with perpendicular stripes may seem like an unusual way to assist a person with Parkinson's, but long vertical spaces have been proven to be slowing and disorienting for them. Dr. Young suggests using a striped rug in halls, marking stripes with masking tape, or even painting stripes on the floor to help make navigating the length easier for Parkinson's patients. On stairwells, mark the outer edge of each step with tape that's a different color than the carpet or wood to help the patient spot the step edges and prevent falls.

Be patient. One of the most frustrating elements of Parkinson's disease is the amount of time it takes to do things that used to be simple. Getting dressed, bathing, and even eating are all more time-consuming for a person with Parkinson's. To help ease the frustration—both yours and your loved one's—allow plenty of time for him to take care of routine tasks without feeling rushed, says Dr. Tetrud. A good guideline is about four times as long for any task. For example, if a person used to get dressed in 15 minutes, give him 60. For a 10-minute meal, allow 40 minutes.

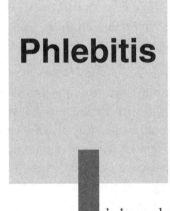

Phlebitis

It's been dubbed "economy-class syndrome" by British researchers studying airline travelers, but you may know it by its more common name: phlebitis (an inflammation of veins, usually in the legs). It tends to happen to a lot of healthy people who sit through long flights or travel by car, says Gabriel Goren, M.D., a vascular surgeon and director of the Vein Disorders Center in Encino, California.

With little leg room, leg circulation is constricted, and that impedes bloodflow. "When blood is pooling and stagnating in veins, it can clot," says Dr. Goren. "The clot triggers the inflammation, and phlebitis is born."

But a person doesn't have to fly coach to spark a phlebitis attack. Any period of immobility can trigger an episode, and that includes time spent recovering from an injury, illness, or surgery. As people get older, especially during episodes of debilitating diseases, their risk of developing phlebitis increases.

"There are two types of phlebitis: superficial, and deep-vein phlebitis or thrombosis (DVT)," says Dr. Goren. Superficial phlebitis is generally seen in people who have varicose veins. Just beneath the skin of the leg, you may notice a red cordlike vein that feels hard, warm, and painful to the touch and is accompanied by redness of the skin around the affected vein. In the case of DVT, you may feel an overall heaviness in the leg, mainly in the calf, and occasionally ankle swelling.

An estimated 30 percent of DVT cases go undiagnosed and go away on their own, says J. A. Olivencia, M.D., a vascular surgeon and medical director of the Iowa Vein Center in West Des Moines. But if the doctor detects this kind of thrombosis, he'll surely give the patient some sort of treatment.

WHEN TO SEE THE DOCTOR

Any type of phlebitis needs to be seen by a doctor to determine how serious it is. If your loved one has been diagnosed with superficial phlebitis, call your doctor if he still has symptoms after 7 to 10 days or if the condition recurs. If you notice lumps, high fever, or overall pain and swelling in the limb, your relative may have developed deep-vein phlebitis and will need immediate medical attention, says Gabriel Goren, M.D., a vascular surgeon and director of the Vein Disorders Center in Encino, California.

If your loved one has deep-vein thrombosis and is taking anticoagulant drugs, take him to the hospital if he experiences any unusual bleeding or signs of an internal hemorrhage, such as difficulty breathing, unexplained swelling, or chest, abdominal, or joint pain.

Regardless of how the doctor decides to treat this problem, there are things you can do to help a loved one with superficial phlebitis. Our experts offer the following strategies.

Beat it with heat. Help your loved one apply moist heat to the affected area to soothe discomfort and speed healing. The heat especially improves circulation, which will help the body absorb the clot faster, says Dr. Olivencia. Cover the inflamed area with a towel that has been dipped in hot water and wrung out. Then cover the towel with a heating pad or hot-water bottle to maintain the temperature. Do this for 20 to 30 minutes at least twice a day.

Get it up. Elevate the affected leg, which also will promote increased circulation and speed healing, says Dr. Olivencia.

Forget aspirin. To relieve pain and inflammation, give him ibuprofen instead of aspirin. It works better than aspirin in two ways. A more effective pain reliever, ibuprofen also helps counteract the inflammatory reaction that generates pain and swelling in the vein, says Dr. Goren. Each over-the-counter tablet contains 200 milligrams, which is a relatively small dose. To control the pain and inflammation during an episode of phlebitis, give 400 milligrams, or two pills, three times a day after meals.

Try stockings. Compression stockings help reduce the swelling and alleviate some of the discomfort caused by phlebitis, because they squeeze the veins and minimize the buildup of fluid in the leg. If you look on the package of compression stockings sold in drugstores, you'll find that the compression is rated from light to extra-strong on a scale of one to four. Go with grade two, a moderate level of compression, to relieve superficial phlebitis symptoms, says Dr. Olivencia. "The stockings may be very uncomfortable if a person has a clot behind the knee or if he has large legs." But if the stockings are too uncomfortable, you shouldn't force your loved one to wear them.

Encourage him to keep circulating. To reduce your older relative's risk of developing phlebitis, advise him to keep circulation moving whenever he's sitting for more than a few hours, says Dr. Goren. Whether flying coast to coast or taking a long drive in the car, he should take a stretch break.

Once an hour, your loved one should walk around for at least 3 to 4 minutes to return the blood in his legs back to his heart. While seated, he should flex his calf muscles every 10 minutes by moving his feet up and down.

Make sure he takes B vitamins. Vascular diseases are more common in people with high levels of the amino acid homocysteine. Research has shown that the B vitamins folate, B_6, and B_{12} can reduce elevated homocysteine levels, says James Finkelstein, M.D., professor of medicine at Howard, George Washington, and Georgetown Universities, all in Washington, D.C.

To maintain optimum health of both the veins and the arteries of your loved one, Dr. Finkelstein recommends giving him supplements of 400 micrograms of folic acid (the synthetic form of folate) and 25 milligrams of B_6 daily. Because older people are at risk for vitamin B_{12} deficiency, they should also take 100 micrograms of B_{12} daily, he says. Folate-packed food sources include orange juice, spinach, asparagus, lentils, and navy beans. Bananas, lean chicken, potatoes, and watermelons are good sources of vitamin B_6. Vitamin B_{12} is found in animal products such as meat, milk, cheese, and eggs. But because people older than 50 years of age may not adequately absorb this vitamin from food, the National Research Council advises that they eat foods fortified with vitamin B_{12}, such as ready-to-eat cereals, or use a supplement.

Note: If your relative has been diagnosed as not having the intrinsic factor, which aids in the absorption of B_{12}, you should talk to the doctor about your loved one getting regular B_{12} injections.

Suggest trying this clot stopper. Several studies indicate that vitamin E helps protect against clots, according to Joseph Pizzorno Jr., president of Bastyr University in Bothell, Washington. Vitamin E helps prevent platelets (components of the blood involved in clotting) from sticking to each other and to the walls of the blood vessels. To reduce platelet stickiness, give your relative 200 to 600 IU a day.

Note: If your loved one is taking anticoagulants, he should not take vitamin E. Although vitamin E is generally sold in doses of 400 IU, one small study showed a possible risk of stroke in dosages higher than 200 IU. Consult with your doctor if your relative is at high risk for stroke.

Apply a cream to cut down on swelling. "Horse chestnut is a very good and very well-established anti-inflammatory for the veins," says British herbalist Christopher Robbins, a member of Britain's National Institute of Medical Herbalists who practices herbal medicine in Ross-on-Wye, Herefordshire, England. Studies have shown that horse chestnut extract significantly reduces the sensation of heaviness and swelling in the legs of people with phlebitis. Calendula is known for its anti-inflammatory properties.

To make the cream, mix together 4 parts calendula cream (which you can find in most health food stores) and 1 part horse chestnut tincture, and store the cream in a jar with a tight-fitting lid. Smooth this herbal cream directly onto the inflamed area two or three times a day. When you buy the calendula cream, check the label to be sure it's herbal cream, not the homeopathic version.

Note: A tincture is a highly concentrated herbal liquid. It's made by soaking leaves in alcohol or glycerin—which extracts the herb's medicinal properties—for at least 6 weeks. Tinctures are sold in health food stores in small bottles with eyedroppers to give doses. Be sure to always store them out of the reach of children.

Help reduce the inflammation with arnica. Germany's Commission E, which evaluates herbs for safety and effectiveness, gives arnica its seal of approval for treating phlebitis. Arnica's bright yellow flowers contain anti-inflammatory and pain-relieving compounds. This herb also keeps the blood moving by stimulating the circulation, says Roy Upton, executive director of American Herbal Pharmacopeia, an herbal education foundation based in Santa Cruz, California. Arnica lotion, generally sold as a remedy for soothing bumps and bruises, is easy to find in health food stores. Smooth cream or lotion onto your loved one's swollen vein up to four times daily until the pain subsides.

Treat him with tinctures. The Australian naturopath Andrew Pengelly, N.D., who runs the Valley Herb Clinic in Hunter Valley, New South Wales, recommends the following formula that combines tinctures of three herbs: calendula, an anti-inflammatory; yarrow, a vein toner; and echinacea, an infection fighter.

Mix 2 milliliters of each tincture and add 3 to 5 milliliters of the blend to 2 ounces of water. Mix this slightly bitter-tasting brew with a small glass of juice and give it to your relative three times daily. As long as your relative has periodic checkups with a qualified practitioner who knows that he is taking this remedy, Dr. Pengally says that it is safe to use as long as needed for pain and inflammation.

Brew some bark to ban the pain. To ease the pain of an inflamed vein, mix 3 tablespoons of white oak bark powder (which you can buy at health food stores) with 1 cup of water in a saucepan, bring it to a boil, and simmer for 10 minutes, says Upton. Let the liquid cool just a little, until it's comfortable to the touch. Soak a cloth in the tea, then press it gently onto the tender area. Leave it in place for 20 minutes with your relative's legs elevated. You can do this treatment three times a week until the pain subsides.

Buy bromelain. The blood-thinning and anti-inflammatory properties of bromelain, an enzyme derived from pineapple, work together to help prevent a recurrence of phlebitis, says Decker Weiss, N.M.D., a naturopathic physician at the Arizona Heart Institute in Phoenix. In a study of 73 people with a severe kind of phlebitis who took bromelain along with a pain reliever, researchers found that all symptoms of inflammation decreased, including pain, swelling, and elevated skin temperature.

Dosages of bromelain typically range from 500 to 1,000 milligrams a day, says Dr. Weiss. To get the best effect, give him a divided dose four times a day on an empty stomach, he advises. If it's taken with food, bromelain will simply act as a digestive enzyme rather than helping to prevent clotting.

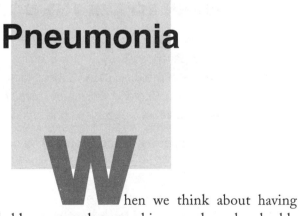

Pneumonia

When we think about having pneumonia, we probably see ourselves coughing up a lung, barely able to breathe, and with a fever hot enough to cook an egg.

But for older people, pneumonia may look a bit different if it takes hold of them. It doesn't manifest the way one thinks it would, with the classic symptoms of fever, heavy sweating, coughing, sputum production, chest pain, and chills, says Henry Gong Jr., M.D., professor of medicine at the University of Southern California School of Medicine in Downey.

Instead, pneumonia shows itself in ways you'd never expect and with symptoms that may seem completely unrelated. Some people seem suddenly confused or less aware of others or of their surroundings. Others exhibit weakness and fatigue. Rapid breathing, rapid pulse, or shortness of breath may also be signs of pneumonia. Some people have symptoms like nausea and diarrhea, which we normally associate with intestinal problems. In fact, someone with pneumonia who has some or all of these symptoms may never utter a single cough.

If you notice these atypical symptoms in a loved one, he should see a doctor. Although the advent of antibiotics knocked out pneumonia as the leading cause of death back in the 1940s, the disease is still dangerous, especially to people over age 65.

The cause of pneumonia is still the same, no matter what age a person is. It is an infection of the lungs caused by bacteria, viruses, or

WHEN TO SEE THE DOCTOR

The symptoms of pneumonia in older persons are often different from those experienced by younger persons, says Bruce Leff, M.D., professor of medicine at the Johns Hopkins Bayview Medical Center Geriatric Center in Baltimore. Therefore, watch for these symptoms and contact a physician right away.

- Cough (especially if accompanied by colored phlegm)
- Fever
- Shortness of breath
- Chest pain
- Confusion

other organisms. Although the disease has more than 30 different causes, bacterial pneumonia is the most common. In this version, bacteria that's normally present in the throat when a person is healthy starts multiplying in the lungs when immunity is down. In viral pneumonia, a virus takes hold in the lungs and multiplies. A weakened immune system is also a common risk factor for contracting viral pneumonia.

In all kinds of pneumonia, the air sacs in the lungs fill with pus and liquid, which prevents oxygen from reaching the blood. Without enough oxygen in the bloodstream, the body's cells can't work correctly.

The well-traveled myth that a cold can turn into pneumonia simply isn't true. But it is so ingrained that Bruce Leff, M.D., professor of medicine at the Johns Hopkins Bayview Medical Center Geriatric Center in Baltimore, can't even convince his mother it's false.

People believe that a cold can directly lead to pneumonia because the first sometimes precedes the second. But a cold just lowers the immune defenses, and when the defenses are down, a person is more susceptible to another infection such as pneumonia. Both colds and pneumonia are more common during the winter months, says Dr. Leff.

Once your loved one gets pneumonia, he *must* be under a doctor's care. Home treatment can be dangerous, especially for older people, and it's important to remember that pneumonia can be deadly.

But rather than fight pneumonia just when it arrives, the better course of action is to prevent it. Pneumonia usually strikes when the defenses are already down because of another illness. So the best defense against pneumonia is to keep the immune system in top shape. Read the following tips, so you can keep your older loved ones healthy.

Make sure he gets stuck. Ask your doctor to give your loved one the pneumococcal vaccine, Dr. Leff says. Given the seriousness of pneumonia, you don't want to neglect this important form of prevention.

This vaccine, which protects people from certain strains of bacterial pneumonia, is recommended by the Centers for Disease Control and Prevention (CDC) for everyone who is over the age of 65, chronically ill, or at risk for infection due to a weakened immune system.

Despite that recommendation, only about 28 percent of the over-65 population has ever received a pneumonia vaccine. A study by the CDC at a nursing home in Oklahoma observed that the vaccine probably could have prevented a pneumonia outbreak there that killed three people. If your loved one is over 65, the CDC recommends that he get a booster shot if it has been over 5 years since the original vaccine.

Just one warning about getting a vaccine: Don't assume that because your loved one got the injection, he can't get pneumonia. He can still catch a different strain of bacterial pneumonia or catch viral pneumonia, which isn't affected by the vaccine, says Dr. Gong. So if you suspect that your loved one has pneumonia, get him to a doctor even if he has been vaccinated in the past.

Make sure he gets plenty of C. Deirdre O'Connor, N.D., a naturopathic physician in Mystic, Connecticut, tells all her older patients who seem vulnerable to upper respiratory problems to increase their vitamin C intakes during the winter months. She recommends a supplement of between 1,000 and 3,000 milligrams a day. In addition to supplementation, make sure your relative piles his plate with foods high in vitamin C, such as broccoli, brussels sprouts, red peppers, sweet potatoes, and citrus fruits.

Vitamin C is necessary for a healthy immune system, Dr. O'Connor reports. In studies, it has been shown to help older people who have severe respiratory infections, she says. Excess vitamin C may cause diar-

Medication Alert

For the treatment of bacterial pneumonia, doctors will prescribe antibiotics. Some people are allergic to certain antibiotics, so talk to your doctor if your relative has had an allergic reaction before, says Bruce Leff, M.D., professor of medicine at the Johns Hopkins Bayview Medical Center Geriatric Center in Baltimore. Also, check with your doctor before your loved one mixes antibiotics with anticoagulants such as warfarin (Coumadin). If your relative is given an antibiotic, be certain that he takes the full course of treatment.

rhea in some people, so your relative may need to cut back on his dosage until he finds a comfortable level.

Put some muscle in his immunity. Your loved one's daily multivitamin should have 15 milligrams of zinc in it, Dr. O'Connor says. In older people, this mineral isn't always absorbed properly from diet alone, so some people develop deficiencies. Immune cells are so dependent on zinc that they can't fight off infection unless they have this mineral. You'll also find zinc in meats, poultry, eggs, dairy products, and oysters.

Make some "carotene soup." Start with a basic vegetable broth, then toss in red peppers, winter squash, carrots, garlic, onions, and any other colorful vegetables. Serve this tasty meal to your loved one frequently during the winter and especially when he's sick, suggests Dr. O'Connor. She calls this carotene soup in honor of beta-carotene and other carotenoids that enhance the work of the immune system.

Carotenoids are especially prevalent in brightly colored vegetables such as carrots and squash. It's best to get carotenoids from foods, says Dr. O'Connor, because natural carotenoids are better absorbed and work better than synthetic supplements.

Get some garlic and onions. During the winter, Dr. O'Connor urges people to cook with lots of garlic and onions. These two related foods may have antiviral and antibiotic properties, she says, so they can help the immune system fight off both viral and bacterial pneumonia. Garlic and onions go with everything from mashed potatoes to meat or fish, and they're especially good in soups.

Now, you and your loved one may love the taste of garlic and onions but could do without the bad breath they cause, especially because they seem to come out of your pores when you eat them. And they actually do. Some powerfully pungent foods are absorbed into the bloodstream, explains F. Michael Eggert, D.D.S., Ph.D., professor of dentistry at the University of Alberta in Edmonton, Canada, and the smell comes out through the pores and through the lungs to the breath. But the volatile oils of peppermint do the same thing. Not only do they help kill stinky bacteria in the mouth, but the oils also travel to the bloodstream and come out through the same avenues as the onions and garlic.

Fresh peppermint is available at some produce stands and supermarkets. All your relative has to do is break off a few leaves, chew them slowly, and swallow. He should repeat as often as necessary, recommends Dr. Eggert. If your loved one prefers a warm alternative, buy any of the commercially available peppermint teas and follow the package instructions.

Suggest staying active. Encourage your loved one to take a brisk daily walk for ½ hour a day. There's no guarantee, but daily walks may help keep pneumonia at bay. "Regular exercise keeps the immune system functioning very well," Dr. O'Connor says.

If your relative prefers other activities such as cycling or swimming, he should go ahead and enjoy them, she says. Any daily or regular exercise will keep the immune system strong. She also recommends trying different workouts like yoga.

Poor Concentration

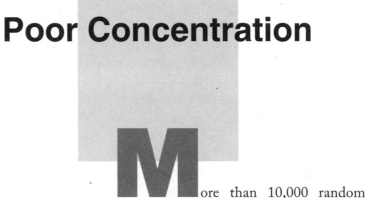

More than 10,000 random thoughts and fleeting images zip though an average person's mind every day. They could include a snippet of a song, a momentary image of an old friend, or a fragment of a joke.

In most cases, these intruders are quickly banished from the mind so the person can concentrate on the task at hand. But as people get older, it becomes harder to filter out these distractions and stick to a project, organize thoughts, or follow the flow of a conversation, says Richard Restak, M.D., clinical professor of neurology at George Washington University School of Medicine and Health Sciences in Washington, D.C. Poor concentration also can affect memory. So if a woman is doing the laundry, for instance, she can forget a boiling tea kettle in the kitchen until the smoke alarm goes off.

"It's just a natural part of aging," Dr. Restak says. "As people get older, it is simply going to take more effort to concentrate on complicated tasks like reading. It doesn't mean it can't be done, just that they need to develop some new strategies." Here are a few tips you can share with an older loved one who has trouble concentrating.

Encourage her to work for short periods. Your loved one should take a 5- to 10-minute rest every 30 minutes when working on a project. It will help her stay focused, Dr. Restak suggests. "As we get older, marathon work sessions become more difficult," he says. Your loved one simply needs to take more frequent breaks in order to maintain good concentration.

Suggest doing one thing at a time. It's easier to get distracted if you're doing several things at once, says Michael Chafetz, Ph.D., a clinical psychologist in New Orleans.

Advise her to focus on the main things. Your loved one needs to

WHEN TO SEE THE DOCTOR

Seek medical care if you notice a significant drop in your relative's attention span or ability to concentrate, says Richard Restak, M.D., clinical professor of neurology at George Washington University School of Medicine and Health Sciences in Washington, D.C. If your relative finds herself losing track of the subplot in a movie or if she discovers that filing her income tax suddenly takes her twice as long, she shouldn't simply assume that her mind is going. A number of correctable medical problems could be interfering with her ability to concentrate, including:

- Hearing loss

- Vision changes

- Poor circulation

- Thyroid disease

- Severe depression

learn to resist the temptation to get distracted. For instance, if she is paying bills and has to go to another room to get some stamps, she should do that and immediately go back to paying the bills. If she finds that she gets distracted while hunting down the stamps, she should pause, take a deep breath, and ask herself: "What am I really here for?" Doing that will refocus her attention on what she really needs to get done, Dr. Chafetz says.

Give her some ginseng. One of the biggest enemies of concentration is fatigue. "A person who's tired all the time can't concentrate," says William Warnock, N.D., a naturopathic physician and director of the Champlain Center for Natural Medicine in Shelburne, Australia. Ginseng has been used for centuries to address just that problem, among others. Give her an extract that provides 10 to 15 milligrams of ginsenosides, the active ingredients, three times a day.

If you want to use ginseng to help your loved one for more than 6 to 8 weeks at a time, it would be better to stop giving it to her for a week, then start giving it again for 6 to 8 weeks. Continue cycling on and off in this way if your relative needs to continue taking it.

Assist her with an Ayurvedic aid. A staple of Ayurveda, India's ancient form of medicine, brahmi is the perfect herb for people who have problems concentrating because they're nervous, says C. Leigh Broadhurst, Ph.D., a nutrition consultant and herbal researcher based in Clovery, Maryland. The botanical name for brahmi is *Bacopa monniera*, but in some parts of India, gotu kola (*Centella asiatica*) is also called brahmi, so check the label to be sure you're getting the right herb.

Tension can cause changes in brain chemistry that interfere with the brain's ability to retain and access information. In extreme cases, the brain "freezes up" in trying situations. According to Ayurvedic medical tradition, brahmi helps thaw that freeze, Dr. Broadhurst says.

Tests have shown that anxiety-prone people significantly increased their performance on memory tests after taking brahmi for at least 2 weeks, she says. The improvement was even greater after 4 weeks. That's not to suggest that there's any reason to exceed the 100- to 200-milligram recommended dose, however.

Encourage your loved one to take 100 to 200 milligrams of standardized extract daily. But Dr. Broadhurst warns that this isn't an herb that will give more benefit the more she takes. "A little too much may produce anxiety, restlessness, or, alternatively—with drastic overdose—

Medication Alert

Any medication that causes drowsiness can decrease concentration, says W. Steven Pray, Ph.D., R.Ph., professor of nonprescription drug products at Southwestern Oklahoma State University in Weatherford. In particular, you and your loved one should be wary of:

- Over-the-counter sleeping tablets that contain diphenhydramine (Nytol, Unisom)

- Over-the-counter antihistamines with diphenhydramine (Actifed, Benadryl)

- Antipsychotic medications such as risperidone (Risperdal) or haloperidol (Haldol)

- Tranquilizers like hydroxyzine (Atarax, Vistaril)

- Antidepressants such as imipramine (Tofranil)

- Antianxiety medications like diazepam (Valium), chlordiazepoxide (Librium), and other drugs known as benzodiazepines

sedation," she explains. Once she's experienced relief from the acute symptoms of anxiety, she may want to cut back to just once every 3 days, she says. That seems to do the job for most people.

Offer her some ashwaganda. This herb is another staple of Ayurvedic medicine—it's called the Indian ginseng, according to Dr. Broadhurst. Like brahmi, ashwaganda is thought to help the neurons of the brain remodel themselves so that they can "learn" and retain new memories, although even prior to modern research, it had been used for centuries to help counteract concentration problems.

As exotic as it may sound, ashwaganda has very familiar relatives. It's a member of the nightshade family, Dr. Broadhurst says, as are tomatoes, potatoes, and peppers. It's widely available and safe for regular use. Give your relative one 500-milligram capsule two or three times a day for as long as needed.

Look for more help from India. Gotu kola has long been popular in India, says Andrew Chevallier, an English herbalist. There, it's used as a revitalizing herb that's useful for strengthening nervous function and memory.

FOCUS ON THIS SCENTED BLEND

Here's an aromatherapy formula to help with concentration problems, designed by aromatherapist Victoria Edwards, owner of Leydet Aromatics in Fair Oaks, California. She named it Cassandra's Blend, after her daughter.

Edwards came up with this formula to help her study for a chemistry final, which she says it helped her pass. She describes the aroma as spicy and lemony, with an "energetic and stimulating" effect, particularly for those who tend to be nervous when they're on the spot.

Your loved one can either sniff the formula directly from the bottle or place a few drops in a diffuser. Do not apply it to the skin, because the black pepper can cause irritation.

4   drops black pepper essential oil
2   drops cistus essential oil
6   drops may chang essential oil

Mix the pepper, cistus, and may chang oils in a clean glass dropper bottle. Shake well before using.

Cistus (*Cistus ladaniferus*) and may chang (*Litsea cubeba*) may be difficult to find, but you should be able to locate them at well-stocked health food stores and through some mail-order suppliers.

Gotu kola helps people concentrate by easing anxiety, but its effects are subtle. "It doesn't lead to the drowsiness or relaxation that kava often does," Dr. Warnock says, "but for some people, it seems to be able to clear the mind equally well."

Give your loved one 100 milligrams twice a day. Dr. Warnock recommends taking an extract standardized for 40 percent asiaticosides, the active ingredients. If you want to give it to your loved one for more than 6 to 8 weeks at a time, it's better to stop giving it for a week, then start up again for 6 to 8 weeks. You should keep cycling on and off in this way if your loved one needs to continue taking it.

Suggest meditation to quiet things down. Meditation is a simple and terrific way to boost the powers of concentration, says Laura Slap-Shelton, Ph.D., a clinical psychologist with a specialty in neuropsychology at Jeanes Hospital in Philadelphia. "The mind is a noisy place, talking to itself and responding to all sorts of stimulation in the world around it," she says. "Meditation quiets the mind and can help filter out all the annoying distractions that make concentration difficult."

To try it, your loved one should sit in a comfortable chair and begin to slowly breathe in for a count of 4 to 8 seconds, allowing her diaphragm to expand fully, Dr. Slap-Shelton says. She should hold her breath for several seconds, and then slowly breathe out as much air as possible. To make sure she's breathing with the diaphragm, she should put her hand over her stomach and feel it expand and contract while she breathes. Whenever a distracting thought pops into her mind, she should note it and forget about it, always focusing on breathing. If she does this simple exercise twice a day, her ability to concentrate may improve, Dr. Slap-Shelton says.

Have her play with her mind. Your loved one should "exercise" her brain with chess, checkers, crossword puzzles, or board games like Scrabble at least twice a week. These fun, mind-stretching activities can help keep concentration in tip-top shape.

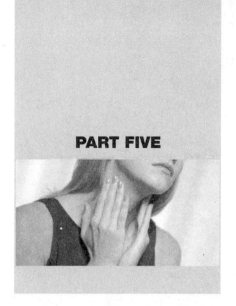

PART FIVE

Mom's Medicine for Mom Herself

Anemia

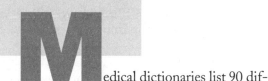

edical dictionaries list 90 different kinds of anemia. Various and sundry factors—such as bacterial or viral infections or nutritional deficiencies, among others—can deplete your total blood volume and reduce your red blood cell count. Red blood cells contain hemoglobin, the protein that carries oxygen through the blood. Oxygen gives you energy. So anything that disturbs the quality and quantity of your red blood cells leaves you feeling lousy. Tired all the time. Pale. Cold. Lifeless.

That's where iron (or lack of it) comes into play. Embedded in every hemoglobin molecule are iron atoms that bind with oxygen in the lungs and transport it to the heart, muscles, and body tissues. If iron stores are low, your body makes fewer and smaller red blood cells, with less hemoglobin.

In conversation, we use *anemic* as an adjective to describe someone who lacks energy or vitality. No wonder: Iron-deficiency anemia leaves you exhausted.

Iron-deficiency anemia is the most common type of anemia among reproductive-age women. When you menstruate, you lose blood and hemoglobin, and with blood, iron. If your periods are heavy, you lose a lot of iron on a regular basis. Women can also become anemic during pregnancy because blood is diverted to the fetus, and a considerable amount is lost during childbirth. Women who crash-diet or chronically watch their weight often don't eat enough to have sufficient iron in their blood. Iron-deficiency anemia is rare, however, in women past menopause. At that time, too much iron can be a problem.

Less often, anemia is caused by a deficiency of the B vitamin folate, vitamin B_6, or vitamin B_{12}.

Upping Iron Intake in the Kitchen

If blood tests show that you have iron-deficiency anemia, your doctor will probably recommend a strategy geared toward improving the quality and quantity of iron consumed. Here are some ways to do it with diet.

Beef up your blood. Eat one 3-ounce serving of beef a day, says Barry Skikne, M.D., associate professor of hematology in the department of medicine at the University of Kansas Medical Center in Kansas City.

Buy lean cuts, such as ground sirloin, flank steak, or top round. Three ounces of broiled top round supplies 2.5 milligrams of iron, for example. Or buy cheaper cuts of beef such as strip or chuck steak and trim the fat, suggests Fergus Clydesdale, Ph.D., head of the department of food science at the University of Massachusetts at Amherst.

Combat it with this combination. Have minestrone made with ground beef and spinach. Aside from supplying a hefty amount of highly absorbable heme iron, meat enhances the absorption of nonheme iron, found in vegetables such as spinach, says Dr. Skikne.

Eat shish kebabs. Combining meat with vegetables that are high in vitamin C, such as peppers and tomatoes, enhances iron absorption.

If you're a vegetarian, get plenty of legumes and soy. Vegetarians can get enough protein to ensure their iron count is high enough, says

WHEN TO SEE THE DOCTOR

See a doctor immediately if you have abnormal blood loss for any reason, such as blood in your stool or urine, which may indicate a more serious condition than anemia, says Barry Skikne, M.D., associate professor of hematology in the department of medicine at the University of Kansas Medical Center in Kansas City.

Also, consult your doctor if you are taking iron supplements for fatigue or other symptoms of anemia and your energy levels don't improve within 2 to 3 months, he says.

Allan Magaziner, D.O., president of Magaziner Medical Center in Cherry Hill, New Jersey. Three ounces of tofu, a soy food, supplies 8.5 milligrams of iron, for example. And ¾ cup of hot and healthy Cream of Wheat cereal provides 7.7 milligrams. You may also want to try quinoa, a plant protein that is similar to rice. It's available in health food stores.

Juice up. If you drink orange juice with your food, the vitamin C it contains also helps the body absorb iron, says Dr. Clydesdale. For maximum iron intake, try drinking it with tofu, vegetables, or iron-fortified ready-to-eat breakfast cereals.

Use Iron Pills Cautiously

Most experts don't recommend taking iron supplements unless your doctor confirms the need with a blood test. If your doctor concurs that extra iron is appropriate for you, you may consider taking 300 milligrams of ferrous sulfate daily for 7 days during menstruation only.

Ferrous sulfate (an inexpensive supplement available without a prescription) ensures that you get the iron you need when you need it most, without risking toxic buildup, says Allan Erslev, M.D., professor of medicine at Thomas Jefferson University Hospital in Philadelphia. If you do decide to take iron tablets, be sure to take them on an empty stomach with orange juice at bedtime; taking them with milk or food inhibits iron absorption, explains Dr. Skikne.

Some women take calcium supplements to protect against osteoporosis. If you're one of them and you need to take iron pills, listen up: Calcium supplements may impede iron absorption, says Dr. Clydesdale. So make sure you space these supplements 3 hours apart.

Options from Nature's Medicine Chest

As we indicated earlier, if your doctor confirms that you have iron-deficiency anemia, he'll probably give you a prescription for iron supplements in the form of ferrous sulfate. An herbalist, however, is likely to take a different tack. For one thing, herbalists and other experts question how well inorganic iron supplements like ferrous sulfate (from chemical rather than plant or animal sources) are absorbed by the body. They also point out that iron supplements may cause side effects, in-

The Best Sources of Iron

To achieve and maintain a healthy blood level of iron, it's important eat more iron-rich foods. The following chart highlights some of the best dietary sources of the mineral. "DV" stands for the Daily Value of each food.

Food	Portion	Iron (mg)	% DV
Pumpkin seeds, hulled, dried	⅔ cup	13.8	77
Clams, steamed	About 20	11.9	66
Oysters (eastern), steamed	About 6 medium	10.2	57
Tofu, firm, uncooked	¼ block	8.5	47
Quinoa, raw	½ cup	7.9	44
Cream of Wheat, cooked	¾ cup	7.7	29
Soybeans, boiled	½ cup	4.4	25

cluding diarrhea and constipation. What's more, evidence suggests that high levels of iron taken for an extended period of time may fuel the formation of free radicals, oxygen-stealing molecules that contribute to diseases such as colon cancer and heart disease.

"There are questions about toxicity and whether inorganic iron aggravates the condition it's supposed to cure," says Cascade Anderson Geller, an herbal educator and consulting herbal practitioner in Portland, Oregon.

Instead of prescribing iron supplements, an herbalist may tell you to eat more dark leafy greens and other iron-rich foods. And he may suggest some herbal remedies. Here are a few you can try.

Food	Portion	Iron (mg)	% DV
Quail	1 bird	4.2	23
Cassava (tapioca)	4 oz	4.1	23
Venison, roasted	3 oz	3.8	21
Pot roast, lean, braised	3 oz	3.2	18
Spinach, chopped, cooked	½ cup	3.2	18
Flank steak, lean, braised	3 oz	3.0	16
Potato, baked	1	2.8	15
Kidney beans, boiled	½ cup	2.6	14
Sirloin steak, lean, broiled	3 oz	2.6	14
Top round steak, lean, broiled	3 oz	2.5	14
Ground beef, extra lean, broiled	3 oz	2.0	11
Parsley, raw, chopped	½ cup	1.9	10
Pumpkin, canned	½ cup	1.7	9
Apricots, dried	¼ cup	1.5	9
Spaghetti, enriched, cooked	½ cup	1.0	5
Raisins, seedless	¼ cup	0.85	5

Defeat it with dandelion. "Dandelion is a great herbal ally for treating anemia," says Ryan Drum, Ph.D., an herbalist from British Columbia, Canada.

"Dandelion is a good source of iron and magnesium, which may help your body utilize iron better," he says. "But dandelion also seems to pamper the liver, and it enhances the production of bile, an essential substance that helps your body absorb nutrients."

"Turn a dandelion into a delicious salad dressing," suggests Dr. Drum. Cut the dandelion leaves off right at the crown of the plant, rinse thoroughly to remove any dirt, and toss a few handfuls into a blender. Add some oil and vinegar (use the same proportions as for your favorite salad dressing), then season to taste with your choice of herbs and spices. Blend until the dandelion is pureed. Pour freely over a salad of dark leafy greens like kale, spinach, and parsley. (Make sure, however, that the dandelion you pick comes from a pesticide-free yard.)

Disguise some yellow dock. "Yellow dock root banishes anemia quickly," says Dr. Drum. But, he adds, its bitter taste can be a challenge to conceal. So try this: Grate about 1 teaspoon of dried yellow dock root and add it to dishes flavored with curry, ginger, or cumin. The spices will completely cancel out the herb's bitterness, he says. Another option is to fill two or three gelatin capsules (size "00") with grated yellow dock root and take daily. Or simply take commercially made capsules according to label directions. "In my experience, you can end anemia in about a month by taking yellow dock regularly," says Dr. Drum.

Breast Discomfort

For most women who menstruate, breast discomfort waxes and wanes with each monthly cycle. When levels of the female hormone estrogen are highest, which they are just before and during menstruation, your breasts may swell and ache or be tender. They can pull at your neck and back and hurt at the slightest bump. They can make running, jumping, and even rolling over in bed pure agony. "Some women demand breast reduction surgery because they have such pain," says Bernard Ginsberg, M.D., a doctor in Santa Monica, California.

Breast discomfort usually occurs just prior to menstruation, when hormones stimulate fluid retention in breast tissue, says David P. Rose,

M.D., D.Sc., Ph.D., chief of the division of nutrition and endocrinology at the Naylor Dana Institute of the American Health Foundation in Valhalla, New York. Breastfeeding can also cause pain.

Women sometimes hesitate to seek treatment for breast discomfort because they fear the worst. Yet doctors say that premenstrual breast changes such as swelling and lumpiness are pretty much normal. Moreover, having lumpy breasts does not in itself put you at greater risk for breast cancer, says Dr. Ginsberg.

So if you're bothered by breast pain, you should know that you can do something about it. Here's what experts recommend.

Actions That Alleviate

When your breasts hurt, you want to make them as comfortable as possible, as quickly as possible. The following remedies provide prompt, effective relief.

WHEN TO SEE THE DOCTOR

If you try dietary and lifestyle changes for 3 months and your breasts still hurt, or if your breasts become tender and swollen over the course of a day or two, see your doctor, advises David P. Rose, M.D., D.Sc., Ph.D., chief of the division of nutrition and endocrinology at the Naylor Dana Institute of the American Health Foundation in Valhalla, New York. You may have a hormonal problem that requires medical treatment.

Also see your doctor if your breasts become painful after you start taking oral contraceptives or hormone-replacement therapy. Your dosage may need adjustment, or you may need to switch to a different type of drug. And, of course, consult your doctor if you notice anything unusual during your monthly breast self-examination.

Take 20. Soak in a bathtub filled with comfortably hot water for at least 20 minutes. "Settle back into the tub so that your chest is submerged," suggests Rosalind Benedet, R.N., a breast health nurse specialist with the California Pacific Medical Center in San Francisco. "The water soothes your breasts and relaxes your entire body."

Chill out. As an alternative to heat, apply a cold pack to sore breasts for up to 20 minutes at a time whenever you need relief. Use either crushed ice or a bag of frozen peas, since either will conform to the shape of your breasts, says Benedet. And remember to wrap the ice or bag of peas in a thin towel so that the extreme cold doesn't injure your skin.

Supplement with this soother. Evening primrose oil is an anti-inflammatory that has the ability to soothe pain and help shrink lumps, says Jill Stansbury, N.D., a naturopathic physician and chairperson of the botanical medicine department at the National College of Naturopathic Medicine in Portland, Oregon. To reduce harmless but bothersome lumps, Dr. Stansbury suggests taking one or two capsules, either 500 or 1,000 milligrams (she prefers 1,000 milligrams), of evening primrose oil three times a day for several months.

Discover a new use for an old standby. You may know this less-than-tasty remedy best because your mom gave it to you as a kid when you had stomach trouble. Today you can try a new twist on castor oil. Herbalists recommend castor oil packs for reducing the pain and inflammation of lumpy breasts. Castor oil has been employed for hundreds of years in India, Egypt, and China as an external remedy for sores and abscesses.

To make a castor oil pack, sprinkle 2 ounces of castor oil on a piece of flannel that's wide enough and long enough to cover both breasts, say herbalists (or you can rub the castor oil directly onto your breasts). Cover with plastic wrap and a thin towel. Keep the pack warm with a heating pad set on low or a hot water bottle. Bundle yourself up in a warm robe or just get under the bedcovers to hold the wrap in place, suggests Dr. Stansbury. This wrap will soothe your breasts with warmth for about 45 minutes, she says. You can relieve sore breasts with this pack once a week or more often as needed.

Help your liver. It may seem as if one has nothing to do with the other, but "I've found in my practice that breast problems are often a sign of poor liver function," says Dr. Stansbury. Herbalists believe that the same bitter roots that stimulate digestion and support liver function can ease breast pain and lumpiness by normalizing levels of circulating hormones in your body. "When the liver is working properly, it removes hormones from the bloodstream so they can be eliminated," she adds.

Help your liver with this tea: Combine equal parts (1 teaspoon each) of dandelion root, burdock root, Oregon grape root, and yellow dock root; then, for flavor, add equal parts of licorice, fennel seed, organic dried orange peel, dried gingerroot, and broken pieces of cinnamon sticks. To brew the tea, gently simmer 1 teaspoon of the herb mixture in a cup of boiling water for 15 minutes. Strain and enjoy three or more cups a day, Dr. Stansbury suggests.

Wear a larger-size bra while your breasts hurt. Select one that keeps your breasts secure without being uncomfortably constricting, suggests Benedet. "A sports bra with a wide elastic band may be your best bet," she says. "But every woman is different, so shop around to find the bra that's just right for you."

You may even want to plan to shop when your breasts are most swollen. When you try on the bra, move around to make sure it gives you comfortable support while you are moving.

Nutritional Neutralizers

Whether or not you experience breast discomfort depends to some degree on your eating habits. Some foods can prevent breast symptoms, while others can make those symptoms worse. To shape a more breast-friendly diet, give the following tips a try.

Take a vitamin E supplement every day. Doctors have yet to determine why, but vitamin E seems to help some women with breast pain, according to Michael DiPalma, N.D., a naturopathic physician in Newtown, Pennsylvania. He starts his patients with 400 IU of vitamin E a day, then increases the dosage by 100 IU monthly until the women report that their breasts feel better. Dr. DiPalma sometimes prescribes up to 1,600 IU a day, but no more than that. Women who require such a high dosage may find that after a few months they can cut back without experiencing a flare-up in their symptoms.

If you plan to take more than 600 IU of vitamin E a day, you should talk to your doctor first.

Consume at least 30 grams of fiber a day. Both kinds of fiber—soluble and insoluble—help escort excess estrogen from your body. This prevents the hormone from stimulating breast tissue and causing discomfort, explains Dr. Rose. Unfortunately, most women get less than half the amount of fiber that Dr. Rose recommends. To boost your intake, fill your meals with whole grains, beans, fruits, and vegetables. For example, ½ cup of cooked barley contains almost 3 grams of fiber. One-half cup of boiled lima beans provides more than 6 grams. And ¼ cup of dried figs supplies more than 4 grams.

Drink at least eight 8-ounce glasses of water a day. Paradoxically, the more water you drink, the less likely your breasts are to swell before your period. Water flushes salt out of your body, so you retain less fluid, says Benedet.

Restrict your salt consumption. Salt makes your entire body retain fluid—including your breasts, which can swell up like water balloons. "Lots of women crave salty foods such as potato chips and pickles right before their periods," notes Benedet. "But these foods just make matters worse."

If you feel that you can't resist them, Dr. DiPalma advises, don't even bring them into your home.

Cool it with the caffeine for a while. Caffeine—which is found in coffee, black tea, cola, and chocolate—seems to increase the sensitivity of breast tissue to estrogen. Although this remains controversial, some people do find that their pain decreases if they eliminate caffeine sources from their diets for a month or two. One study, conducted at Michigan State University College of Human Medicine in East Lansing, found that women who consume more than 500 milligrams of caffeine a day (the amount in about four cups of coffee) have more than double the risk of lumpy, painful breasts compared with those who abstain. Women who eliminate caffeine from their diets experience a 60 to 65 percent reduction in their symptoms.

Take notice if your breast pain improves during the month you abstain from caffeine. "Some women can then go back to drinking one cup a day without problems," says Dr. DiPalma. "Others may need to give up caffeine only during the second half of their menstrual cycles."

"If you are a big coffee drinker, restricting or eliminating caffeine may be all you need to do to end your breast pain," adds Benedet.

Strategies for Long-Term Care

To reduce breast pain or even get rid of it for good, some women may need to look beyond good nutrition to other aspects of their lifestyle. "You may have to make some changes, but once you get through them, your whole body feels better, not just your breasts," Benedet says. Consider the following tactics for maintaining healthy, pain-free breasts.

Maintain a healthy weight. If you carry too much body fat, you may have more estrogen circulating in your system than is good for you. "In women, body fat acts like an extra gland," explains Dr. Rose. "It produces and stores estrogen, which stimulates breast tissue." Also, research has established a link between weight gain after menopause and an increased risk of breast cancer.

While there are a number of complex formulas for figuring out your ideal weight, one simple formula used by some experts can tell you if you are close: If you are 5 feet tall, you should weigh 100 pounds. If you are taller, add 5 pounds for each additional inch of height. Then to that number, add 10 percent if you have a large frame, or subtract 10 percent if you have a small frame. (For more information on how to lose weight, see the Overweight chapter on page 445.)

Exercise for at least 30 minutes every day. Women who regularly engage in aerobic workouts (the kind that elevate your heart and breathing rates) are less likely to have premenstrual symptoms, including breast pain, according to Dr. Rose.

If exercise seems to worsen premenstrual breast pain, switch to a low-impact activity until you feel better. Running, in particular, may aggravate your symptoms, says Benedet. Try swimming, walking, or bicycling instead.

Cancer Prevention

It's probably the last thing in the world anyone wants to think about. But we still do every now and then, particularly when someone we know gets cancer. Each of us wonders: Could cancer be silently growing somewhere inside *my* body?

But is worrying about cancer so bad if it induces us to take action to avoid it, perhaps even prevent a recurrence?

In fact, the major cancer killers of women—lung, breast, and colon cancers—are pretty much avoidable. "People need to realize that cancer is a preventable illness, just like heart disease," says Graham Colditz, Dr.P.H., professor of medicine at Harvard Medical School. "Nearly two-thirds of cancer deaths in the United States can be linked to tobacco use, diet, and lack of exercise. If people simply applied in their own lives the knowledge that we now have about preventing cancer, we could cut its incidence way back."

Some people, apparently, are confused about the best ways to prevent cancer. Should they eat that carrot, even if it's not organically grown? Drink only bottled water? And what about things like green tea and ginseng?

"The truth is that although these things may one day prove to be helpful, there are a lot more prosaic things already proven to help prevent cancer," says Dr. Colditz. So they appear below—the things that experts say every woman should do, all the time, to reduce her risk for cancer.

Sidestepping Strategies

These cancer-dodging tactics offer the most protection in exchange for your efforts, experts say.

If you smoke, quit. Cigarette smoking causes nearly all cases of lung cancer, the current top cancer killer in women. It has also been directly linked to one-third of all other cancers, including cancers of the throat, mouth, cervix, colon, bladder, kidney, and pancreas, says Peggy O'Hara, Ph.D., professor of epidemiology and public health at the University of Miami School of Medicine. Once you stop smoking, your risk for many of these cancers begins to drop until, in 10 to 15 years, it's comparable to the cancer risk of someone who has never smoked.

The best time to kick the habit is during the first half of your menstrual cycle. That's when high levels of female hormones can counterbalance withdrawal symptoms such as irritability and depression, recommends Dr. O'Hara.

Realistically, quitting smoking is easier said than done. (For more information, see the Smoking chapter on page 236.)

Keep it to one drink a day. "Consuming more than that increases your risk for esophageal cancer and, possibly, breast cancer," Dr. Colditz

WHEN TO SEE THE DOCTOR

Cancer takes many forms, and so do its symptoms. The American Cancer Society recommends that you see a doctor promptly if you have any of these symptoms: a persistent cough, bloody phlegm, chest pain, recurring pneumonia, or bronchitis; rectal bleeding or a change in bowel habits; a lump, thickening, dimpling, or irritation in a breast, or nipple tenderness or discharge; enlarged lymph nodes, itching, fever, night sweats, anemia, and weight loss; fatigue, repeated infections, frequent bruising, and nosebleeds; abdominal pain or swelling or jaundice; headaches, nausea, and vomiting; vision or hearing loss; difficulty speaking or swallowing; or a change in the shape, color, or size of a mole.

says. A drink, by the way, is one 12-ounce beer, one 5-ounce glass of wine, or a mixed drink made with 1½ ounces of liquor.

Stay at a healthy weight. If you exceed your optimum weight by 35 percent or more, you raise your risk for cancer of the breast, cervix, endometrium, uterus, and ovaries, Dr. Colditz says. So for a woman whose optimum weight is 135 pounds, for instance, carrying an extra 47 pounds—or 182 pounds total—would put her in the danger zone. While there are a number of complex formulas for calculating your ideal weight, one simple formula used by some experts can let you know if you're close: If you are 5 feet tall, you should weigh 100 pounds. If you are taller, add 5 pounds for each additional inch of height. Then to that number, add 10 percent if you have a large frame, or subtract 10 percent if you have a small frame. (For more information on how to lose weight, see the Overweight chapter on page 445.)

Exercise for at least 30 minutes every day. "Even moderate levels of activity, such as brisk walking, for a total of 3 hours a week could substantially lower your risk of cancer," Dr. Colditz says. "So figure on ½ hour almost every day." More active women—those who run or jog for a total of 5 hours or more a week—probably cut their risk by more than half, he adds.

"Exercise decreases bowel transit time, so it reduces the amount of time that potential carcinogens in the stool may be in contact with the intestines," explains David P. Rose, M.D., D.Sc., Ph.D., chief of the division of nutrition and endocrinology at the Naylor Dana Institute of the American Health Foundation in Valhalla, New York.

It also reduces insulin levels, and there's some evidence that high circulating levels of insulin promote tumor growth, Dr. Colditz says. In the case of breast cancer, exercise may change levels of hormones, such as estrogen, in a way that makes them less cancer-promoting.

Identify the enemy. Pinpoint all of the hazardous materials that you are exposed to at work and learn how to handle them safely. If you are a hairdresser, electronics assembler, or x-ray technician, for instance, or if you are exposed to glues, solvents, paints, radioactive materials, wood dust, pesticides, or other chemicals, know the names and chemical compositions of all potentially hazardous substances with which you work, Dr. Colditz recommends. "Get a copy of the 'Material Safety Data Sheet' for the material you're handling and read it," he says. By law, your employer is obligated to provide this to you. Wear personal protective equipment where indicated. Insist that your work environment be designed and ventilated to prevent exposure to toxic substances.

Dietary Defenders

Good nutrition is absolutely essential to a cancer-combating lifestyle. In fact, certain foods contain nutrients and other compounds that appear to reduce cancer risk. Based on what research has shown so far, experts suggest the following guidelines for creating your own anticancer eating plan.

Value veggies. You should eat a cup or two of dark green leafy vegetables each day. Kale, spinach, mustard greens, beet greens, and romaine lettuce are your best sources of folate, a B vitamin that helps protect cells against cancer-inducing genetic damage from chemicals and viruses. To prepare greens, try lightly steaming or braising them, then sprinkling them with olive oil and sesame seeds.

Combat cancer with carotenoids. Eat at least ½ cup of orange-colored produce every other day. Try rich sources such as carrots, sweet potatoes, and pumpkin to boost your intake of carotenoids, which have shown promise as cancer-fighting compounds. Research has suggested that carotenoids may slow the development of precancerous lesions and even reverse precancerous cell changes. Try adding shredded carrots to tomato sauce and meat loaf, serving mashed sweet potatoes or baked sweet potato fries, or baking a low-fat pie using pumpkin and fat-free evaporated milk.

Eat more cruciferous veggies. Cruciferous vegetables include broccoli, brussels sprouts, cabbage, and cauliflower. Eat these at least every other day because they contain compounds that stimulate your body's production of cancer-blocking enzymes. Enjoy low-fat coleslaw or steamed broccoli in garlic sauce.

Eat tomatoes every day. Tomatoes are rich in lycopene, a member of the carotenoid family with similar cancer-fighting properties. Italian researchers found that people who ate seven or more servings of tomatoes a week were 60 percent less likely to develop cancer of the stomach, colon, and rectum than were people who ate two or fewer servings a week. If tomatoes don't tempt your tastebuds, then try red grapefruit and sweet red peppers, which also have abundant supplies of lycopene.

Get some garlic in you regularly. Research suggests that garlic and other members of the onion family, known as alliums, cut your odds of developing cancer. In one study, women who ate garlic at least once a week cut their colon cancer risk by one-third compared with women who never ate the stuff.

Reduce your intake of red meat. Harvard University researchers have shown that restricting your consumption of red meat to just one serving a month can cut your risk for colon cancer in half compared with that of women who normally eat beef, pork, or lamb every day. Instead, get more seafood and vegetables on your plate. Seafood is a rich source of omega-3 fatty acids, which have been shown in clinical and epidemiological studies to decrease the incidence of both colon and breast tumors. Vegetables also provide a healthy dose of cancer-fighting compounds such as genistein and other isoflavones.

Substitute olive oil for saturated fats. Scientists have yet to establish a definite link between a high-fat diet and cancer. But they do know that eating more monounsaturated fats, such as olive oil, and fewer saturated fats, such as butter and lard, can protect against breast cancer, according to Dr. Colditz.

Get your daily dose. Take a daily multivitamin that contains 500 to 1,000 milligrams of vitamin C, 200 to 400 IU of vitamin E, and 800 micrograms of folic acid (the synthetic form of folate), along with other essential nutrients. "I believe that women need this extra protection against cancer—even if they eat healthfully," says Dr. Rose. However, doses of folic acid exceeding 400 micrograms per day should be taken only under the supervision of a doctor. In large amounts, the nutrient can mask signs of a vitamin B_{12} deficiency.

Caregiver Stress

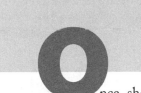

Once, she fed you, diapered you, clothed you, nursed you, loved you, and protected you from harm. Now, decades later, it's your turn.

"Caregiving is largely about women caring for women," says Thomas Humphrey, executive director of Children of Aging Parents (CAPS), a not-for-profit foundation based in Levittown, Pennsylvania. "Today's caregiver is typically a 34- to 49-year-old woman who is likely to spend more years taking care of an aging relative than she did raising her children."

You know you have become a caregiver when:

- A little old lady who looks a lot like your mom is permanently ensconced in your guest room.

- You've had to childproof your home—though your kids are long past puberty.

- Instead of buying Pampers for your infant, you're buying Depend incontinence garments for your father.

- You consider it a good day when your live-in mother-in-law remembers your name.

- You can't remember the last time you went to a movie, read a book, or took a bubble bath.

"It's good to be needed, to give love, and to perform worthwhile tasks," says Barbara Wich, M.D., a physician at the William F. Middleton Veterans Administration Hospital in Madison, Wisconsin. "But caregivers can suffer from severe burnout—it's a relentless, 24-hour-a-day occupation."

Burnout isn't the only problem that can bedevil caregivers, says Dale

A. Lund, Ph.D., professor of gerontology at the University of Utah College of Nursing in Salt Lake City. "Caregiving can lead to depression, marital troubles, health problems, and lots of guilt, anger, and resentment."

Caregivers must realistically balance their own needs with the needs of the person they are caring for, says Dr. Wich. If that sounds nearly impossible, read on.

Plan Ahead

If you have parents or other beloved elders, it is likely that at some point in time you will become their caregiver. You could become a long-distance caregiver, a full-time caregiver, a part-time caregiver, or just an occasional caregiver. No matter which caregiving hat the future holds for you, start planning now to make sure that the hat fits comfortably when your time comes to wear it.

Tackle the tough issues. The time to talk to your beloved elders about the future is now, before your care is needed, says Dr. Wich. "Make a date to discuss values and other hard issues so that you know what your elder would want in the event she is unable to speak for herself," she advises. "Discuss the what-ifs of illness, incapacity, and death. Have your elder make her wishes clear. Suggest that she prepare an advance directive, either a medical power of attorney or a living will, to

WHEN TO SEE THE DOCTOR

Being a caregiver could lead to depression. If you have trouble sleeping or your eating habits change or you develop a lack of interest in life, you could be headed for a more serious problem, says Mary Amanda Dew, Ph.D., professor of psychiatry at the University of Pittsburgh. If these symptoms continue for 2 weeks or longer, seek out professional help.

outline her wishes legally. These forms can be obtained from your medical doctor and can be implemented through your attorney."

Make changes now. If an elder is becoming frail but is still capable of caring for herself, consider modifying her living situation now, even if it seems premature, suggests Dr. Wich. "Suggest a move from a too large home to something more manageable. Think about putting her name on an assisted-care housing list. It can take years for a name to get to the top of some housing lists, and there is no harm in saying no if your name comes up before you are ready."

Accident-proof the home. "Don't wait till your elder becomes frail to install safety devices in her home," cautions Dr. Wich. "Install grab bars in the bathroom and handrails in the stairwells. Make sure that lighting is bright and adequate, especially in the kitchen, bathroom, stairwells, and outside of the home. Remove slippery throw rugs and install nonskid carpet on hard floors. Eliminate clutter and uneven surfaces so that walking paths are clear. Set the hot water heater at 120°F or less. Install smoke alarms and make sure that they are operational."

Keep up social activities. "Encourage your elder to maintain her support systems, such as the bridge club, church activities, or whatever she likes doing," says Dr. Wich. "Scout out recreational activities that your community has for seniors and encourage her to attend. Check with your local agency on aging for information and referrals. Also, newspapers, senior centers, and churches may have information on resources in your area that provide social support and enjoyable activities geared toward older persons."

Think it through. If your older loved one has violent outbursts, has substance abuse problems, smokes in bed, or is given to wandering or other dangerous behavior, then she requires continuous supervision, says Dr. Wich. "Taking such an individual into your home may create divided and stressful demands. You'll crash very quickly, and you stand the chance of destroying your relationship with yourself, your elder, your children, and your spouse." The same applies if your elder has round-the-clock nursing needs or is uncontrollably incontinent, says Dr. Wich.

Consider options that are acceptable to both you and her. Such care services are expensive, so you will need to plan ahead to finance them. Inquire about community resources, Medicare funding, medical assistance, sliding-scale payment options, and Veterans Administration assistance, if eligible.

Seek out support. For help with any caregiving need, contact Children of Aging Parents at 1609 Woodbourne Road, Suite 302A, Levittown, PA 19057. If your elder lives far away, contact the National Association of Professional Geriatric Care Managers at 1604 North Country Club Road, Tucson, AZ 85716. Two other organizations that can offer assistance are the Alzheimer's Association (also known as the Alzheimer's Disease and Related Disorders Association), 919 North Michigan Avenue, Suite 1100, Chicago, IL 60611, and the National Stroke Association, 9707 East Easter Lane, Englewood, CO 80112.

Energy Conservers

As a caregiver, you need 10 times more energy than most women. Here is a life plan designed to boost your energy, increase endurance, and enhance your vitality, specifically designed for caregivers by Michael Janson, M.D., director of the Center for Preventive Medicine in Barnstable, Massachusetts.

Skip the coffee. "For some women, even one cup of coffee in the morning can disturb their sleep at night," says Dr. Janson.

Moderate your alcohol intake. "A glass of wine (5 ounces) or a beer (12 ounces) at dinner, one to three times a week, may have healthful benefits. But more than that can affect your performance—even the next day," says Dr. Janson.

Avoid soda altogether. "The sugar, phosphoric acid, and caffeine in soda leach calcium from your system," Dr. Janson says.

Lighten up on sweets. "Too much sugar can be devastating to a woman who is stressed-out," says Dr. Janson. "It causes blood sugar fluctuations, which in turn can cause mood swings." Sugar that occurs naturally in fruits is fine, but avoid candy, cookies, cakes, and ice cream. "And be careful about 'naturally sweetened' foods," he says. "They often use highly concentrated fruit juice or other sweeteners that have similar effects to refined sugar. Even natural sweets like honey and maple syrup are easy to overdo, so be sure to read food labels and avoid products with ingredients like fructose and glucose."

Take a divided-dose multivitamin/mineral supplement. "I tell caregivers to take a good high-potency multivitamin every day," says Dr.

Dispense a 30-Minute Vacation

A half-hour break. It's the impossible dream when you care for someone with Alzheimer's disease. "What caregivers need most is just a little time to themselves," says Dale A. Lund, Ph.D., professor of gerontology at the University of Utah College of Nursing in Salt Lake City. So Dr. Lund helped develop "Video Respite," a series of videotapes that simulates a visit by a warm, caring person. Each tape offers simple, interactive experiences like familiar old songs or holiday memories. Some even feature friendly dogs and gentle hand exercises. "The videos can calm people who are in the moderate or advanced stages of Alzheimer's disease," he says.

"If someone can watch TV, they are likely to enjoy these tapes—over and over again," Dr. Lund says. That can give you, the caregiver, the chance to slip into a hot bath, read a book, or do absolutely nothing. The tapes range in length from about 25 to 55 minutes, and cost from $35 to $58 each.

For more information, write to Innovative Caregiving Resources at PO Box 17809, Salt Lake City, UT 84117.

Janson. "Look for the kind found in health food stores that are divided into four to six pills daily."

Take 400 to 500 milligrams of magnesium a day. "It's an important supplement for women who are under stress because it helps mitigate nervousness and irritability," says Dr. Janson.

The recommended dosage of 500 milligrams exceeds the Daily Value for magnesium, which is 400 milligrams. If you decide to give supplements a try, and particularly if you have heart or kidney problems, you should be working with a doctor who is willing to monitor your progress. Also, if you experience diarrhea when taking these supplements, cut back your dosage until your symptoms subside.

Eliminate stress with exercise. The stress of caregiving can obviously wear you out. Ironically, exercise can help counteract stress. How? Exercise makes your body produce endorphins, brain chemicals that promote a feeling of well-being.

Many kinds of exercise can be stress solutions, like biking, jogging, or brisk walking. Even housework and gardening may qualify, as does any activity that gets your heart pumping and makes you sweat.

In general, you should exercise four or five times a week and work up at least a mild sweat for ½ hour or so. "The sweatier you get, the better," says Dr. Janson, "but don't get too out of breath." And if you can, try to exercise outside of the house. "Though you could use an at-home exercise bike, it's important that caregivers take breaks away from the home. If you can't get out on the bicycle or track, make a commitment to join a gym and to use it regularly," advises Dr. Janson.

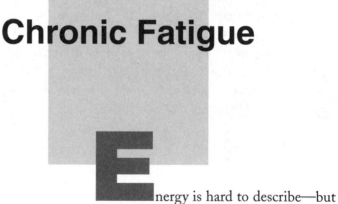

Chronic Fatigue

Energy is hard to describe—but easy to achieve—for most people. Step into a shower in the morning, and your whole body wakes up. Grab a cup of coffee in the middle of the afternoon, and you get a second wind. Get a good night's sleep after a trying day, and you're ready to get back into the fray.

Now, imagine never getting a good night's sleep. Never feeling fully awake and energized, no matter how many showers you take or cups of java you drink. You have entered the Chronic Fatigue Zone.

Four out of five people in the United States who enter the Chronic Fatigue Zone are women who are exhausted almost all the time, often for no apparent reason. No one knows what causes chronic fatigue, though experts say that it probably stems from any number of factors, including poor diet, viral illnesses, weak immune systems, stress, or even sinus problems.

For years, doctors distinguished between simple chronic fatigue and outright chronic fatigue syndrome. Now, it seems, you qualify as chronically fatigued with or without some or all of the classic symptoms of chronic fatigue syndrome: faulty memory and poor concentration, constant sore throat, joint and muscle pain, headaches, and poor sleep.

So far, no one has a cure for chronic fatigue. Doctors say that most people recover eventually, but it may take as long as 5 years. The encouraging news is that by making some changes in your routine—what you eat and when, for example, or timing forays outdoors just right—you can regain some of your lost energy.

Working Out Seems to Work

Sounds crazy, but the experts say that exercise is a major force in launching someone out of the Chronic Fatigue Zone. You might feel as though you can't lift a finger, let alone a dumbbell. But, in fact, moving your body—and establishing an exercise routine—can help you regain physical and mental pizzazz. Women with chronic fatigue be-

WHEN TO SEE THE DOCTOR

If you have unexplained severe fatigue for a month, see your doctor. Also, consult your doctor if you are still tired no matter what strategies you try to regain energy, says Alexander C. Chester, M.D., professor of medicine at the Georgetown University Medical Center in Washington, D.C.

come deconditioned when they don't do any exercise and they spend a lot of time lying down, explains Daniel Hamner, M.D., a psychiatrist in New York City.

The same thing happens to astronauts, says Nelson Gantz, M.D., chief of the department of medicine at Pinnacle Health System in Harrisburg, Pennsylvania.

Remember astronaut Shannon Lucid? After 188 continuous days in space, she could barely walk away from the space shuttle under her own power. Many astronauts are so deconditioned after even a few days in space that they have to be carried off, Dr. Gantz explains.

The key to exercise is to think small, experts say. Here are some ways to get started.

Start step by step. Dr. Hamner suggests doing this literally by walking 5 minutes at a moderate pace every other day. As you grow comfortable with that amount of exercise, try to increase your walking time by 2 to 3 minutes a week. Or if you don't feel like walking, you can ride a stationary bicycle for 5 minutes or go swimming.

Do it early. Most people with chronic fatigue find that exercise is best done first thing in the morning, says Dr. Hamner. And don't be afraid that you will use up the energy that you need to do housework or other activities. "Exercise really gives more energy in the long run," he says.

Take advantage of sunny days. Lack of sunlight seems to lead to more fatigue, especially during the winter months when there are fewer hours of daylight, says Allan Magaziner, D.O., president of Magaziner Medical Center in Cherry Hill, New Jersey. Your pineal gland, a pea-size organ in your brain, needs natural light to secrete melatonin, a hormone that helps you sleep and makes you feel better. So, try to take your 5-minute walk first thing in the morning to take advantage of the sun's rays when you can.

Keep an exercise diary. Write down how you feel right after exercise, later that morning or afternoon, that evening, and the next day. Over the weeks, refer to your notes. In time, you should note an improvement in your energy levels.

Some fatigue is normal for the first couple of weeks. If you experience unrelenting or recurring joint pain, though, see a doctor before continuing, says Dr. Gantz.

Expect some limitations. A lot of people with chronic fatigue were once very active, says Dr. Hamner. "If they don't exercise the way they used to, they feel that they're not really exercising, so they get discouraged and think, 'Why do it?' Don't defeat yourself before you start," he says. Even a few minutes of exercise will lessen fatigue.

Other Fatigue Fighters

Not surprisingly, women with chronic fatigue can no sooner prepare full-course meals from scratch than they can fly to Mars under their own power. The natural tendency is to rely on frozen pizza, canned spaghetti, and other processed foods, says Dr. Magaziner. The problem is that a diet built on convenience foods skimps on beans, fruits, vegetables, whole grains, and other foods rich in vitamins and minerals. Without energy-building nutrients, he says, you will be tired all the time. Here's his nutritional prescription for beating chronic fatigue.

Start your day with fruits and grains. A healthy breakfast is crucial for anyone, and that goes triple if you have chronic fatigue, says Dr. Magaziner. You don't have to make pancakes from scratch; quick-cooking or microwaveable oatmeal and a sliced apple will do the trick. Oatmeal is a good source of magnesium, which the body needs to get energy from food. One sign of magnesium deficiency is muscle weakness.

Have a cup of soup for lunch. Everyone knows that homemade soup is best, but when you're pinched for time, look for instant soups featuring beans or grains (like split pea or barley soup) in supermarkets and health food stores. Beans and grains provide B vitamins that shore up your immune system, says Dr. Magaziner. Just add boiling water to the ingredients and let the mix sit for a few minutes, according to the package directions.

Serve beans and grains with dinner, too. You can choose any kind of beans or grains you like, says Dr. Magaziner. Lima beans or chickpeas, for example, or rice or couscous will do.

Eat some seeds. Pumpkin and sunflower seeds provide zinc, a mineral that can help restore energy by boosting the immune system and reducing the risk of infection, says Dr. Magaziner. And seeds take no time to prepare. The same goes for nuts, another reliable source of zinc.

(continued on page 406)

Clear Your Sinuses, Escape Fatigue

Who would have thought that there might be a link between sinus trouble and chronic fatigue? Yet an enormous number of people who have chronic fatigue also have chronic sinus problems, says Alexander C. Chester, M.D., professor of medicine at the Georgetown University Medical Center in Washington, D.C.

"A lot of chronic fatigue relates to sinusitis," Dr. Chester says. Sinusitis is often a systemic illness, one that affects the entire body. People with sinusitis can feel sick all over, and extreme fatigue or malaise may be the chief complaint.

When your head is stuffed up and heavy with congestion all the time, and you have a pounding headache that won't go away, it's no surprise that you feel exhausted, says Dr. Chester. People who have mild sinusitis symptoms can also feel quite tired. A study that looked at patients in two Boston otolaryngologists' offices compared the general health of people with chronic sinusitis with that of the general population. Researchers found chronic sinusitis to be much more debilitating than angina, congestive heart failure, chronic obstructive pulmonary disease, chronic back pain, or sciatica. The people with chronic sinusitis described having intense body pain, physical limitations, and decreased energy that affected their everyday activities, and at surprisingly high levels. If you have chronic fatigue *and* sinusitis, here's some advice on how to keep your sinuses clear—and maybe lessen your chronic fatigue in the bargain.

- Avoid alcohol. Beer and wine in particular contain sulfites and other substances that may aggravate your sinuses by provoking an allergic reaction. Alcohol in general may dehydrate you and clog your sinuses, says Dr. Chester.

- Avoid milk and wheat, too. Milk and, less often, wheat products often provoke allergic responses in women with chronic fatigue and sinus conditions, says Dr. Chester.

- Steam out your sinuses. Breathing dry air clogs your sinuses in the worst way. Old-fashioned nasal treatments four times a day—like breathing in the steam from a steaming pot of hot water for 5 to 10 minutes—will shrink and moisturize your nasal membranes, Dr. Chester says. Be careful not to burn yourself; you should keep your face at a comfortable distance from the hot steam.

- Stay wet. Nasal saline sprays are often helpful in moistening dry, inflamed nasal membranes, and they sometimes can also have a decongestant effect. Spray your nose four times a day, says Dr. Chester. If your nose feels swollen, you may want to try a decongestant spray, he suggests.

Caution: Decongestant sprays should be taken no more often than three times a day for 3 days, or you may actually end up feeling more congested than before, says Dr. Chester.

Nasal steroid sprays or nasal antihistamine sprays can also be helpful, but you will need to see your doctor first, because they are available by prescription only.

Charge up with Q₁₀. Coenzyme Q_{10} is a natural compound that's available in supplement form in health food stores. Taking 30 milligrams a day improves the body's ability to use oxygen efficiently and ultimately gives you more energy, says Dr. Magaziner.

Consider an apple acid. Taking 300 milligrams of malic acid a day in pill form helps feed the energy-producing cycles of the body, says Dr. Magaziner. Malic acid is available in health food stores.

Get some vigor from vitamins. Take a daily multivitamin/mineral supplement that includes 400 milligrams of magnesium and up to 25 milligrams of each B vitamin, says Dr. Magaziner. Your body needs magnesium in order to get energy from food. Deficiencies of B vitamins—especially B_{12}—have been linked to fatigue and memory loss, among other symptoms.

If you have heart or kidney problems, check with your doctor before taking supplemental magnesium. Supplemental magnesium may cause diarrhea in some people. Also, doses of folic acid exceeding 400 micrograms per day should be taken only under the supervision of a doctor. In large amounts, the nutrient can mask signs of a vitamin B_{12} deficiency.

Inhibit fatigue Indian-style. Gotu kola is an Indian herb that contains no caffeine but has other stimulant properties that make it an effective treatment for fatigue, says Stephen T. Sinatra, M.D., director of the New England Heart Center in Manchester, Connecticut. Take 60 to 100 milligrams in capsule form each day. In addition to simply providing an energy boost, gotu kola may help lift your spirits, since fatigue can lead to depression.

See if this natural "hormone" helps. Many people with fatigue don't produce enough adrenal hormone, and licorice root is the closest herbal equivalent to that hormone that you can get, says Steven Margolis, M.D., an alternative family physician in Sterling Heights, Michigan. He recommends taking 150 to 200 milligrams a day in capsule form. Look for a product that is standardized to contain 12 percent licorice root to ensure that you're taking a safe dose. Licorice root can raise blood pressure, which is why you shouldn't take it in large doses. That said, though, a slight boost in blood pressure might be just what you need if you're fatigued.

Pick another energizing plant. Take 400 milligrams of a blend of

American, Asian, and Siberian ginseng daily. "Ginseng has helped quite a few of my older patients with fatigue," says Dr. Sinatra.

According to Dr. Margolis, these different types of ginseng attack stress fatigue at different levels while also providing a nice circulatory boost, so the sum is greater than the individual parts. This blend is available at health food stores.

Respiratory Remedies

In some people, chronic fatigue has been tied to allergies, especially to the dust, molds, and mold spores that develop in unused heating ducts and unventilated homes. The problem is most likely to occur during the winter months, when you keep your windows shut all the time, says Dr. Magaziner. His advice follows.

- If possible, have good ventilation and air filters installed in your home.

- Have the heating and ventilation system cleaned every 1 to 2 years. And don't forget to change the furnace air filters every month or so.

- If possible, and even in the wintertime, open your windows an inch if you are going out for an hour or so to allow some fresh air exchange.

Wake up. Sleeping too much can make you feel more, rather than less, fatigued, says Alexander C. Chester, M.D., professor of medicine at the Georgetown University Medical Center in Washington, D.C. Most people need 7 to 8 hours of sleep a night, no more.

If you feel tired when you get up, try a hot bath. It might refresh you in ways that a shower can't, says Dr. Chester.

Colds and Flu

Considering the hundreds of different cold and flu viruses out there and everywhere, it's amazing that we aren't all constantly hacking and heaving. Luckily, a healthy immune system stops most of these microscopic invaders before they can reproduce by the billions in our noses, throats, and lungs. Doing your best to strengthen immunity and avoid germs are the top two ways to prevent a cold, with its stuffy nose, sneezing, sore throat, and slight fever. These tactics will also reduce your chances of getting the flu, with its higher fever, muscle aches and pains, and tail-dragging fatigue.

Colds and flu really do have a season, and it's winter, says Keiji Fukuda, M.D., chief of the epidemiology section at the Centers for Disease Control and Prevention in Atlanta. "During the cold-weather months, people are confined to tight quarters, so an ill child in day care or a sneezing adult at work has the opportunity to infect many others," he explains.

In fact, you don't even need to be in the direct line of a sneeze or cough to contract a cold or the flu, notes Michael Fleming, M.D., a family doctor in Shreveport, Louisiana. You don't even need to be in the vicinity at the same time. "All you need to do is to touch something—a doorknob, a telephone, a hand—that someone sick touched or coughed or sneezed on, even up to 24 hours later, then touch your face, nose, or mouth," he explains. Most cold and flu viruses are spread that way.

Antibiotics can't help when you have a mild cold or the flu. They work only against bacteria, not viruses. "That's why a strong immune system is so important," says Anne Davis, M.D., professor of clinical medicine at New York University in New York City. "If you're healthy, you might harbor a cold or flu virus without coming down with symptoms. But when your resistance is low, you are more likely to get sick."

Here's how to minimize the discomfort of a cold or the flu and to make yourself less inviting to viral invaders.

If you're tired, go to bed. "Flu viruses often have a whole-body effect. Maintaining normal activities, including intense exercising, when you have the flu can make your symptoms worse, set the stage for secondary bacterial infections such as pneumonia, and lead to fatigue that lingers for weeks," says David C. Nieman, D.P.H., professor of health and exercise at Appalachian State University in Boone, North Carolina.

"Two full days in bed is not excessive for a full-blown case of flu," says Dr. Fleming. If that's impossible, at least get 8 hours of sleep at night and put off whatever can wait. Give yourself up to 2 weeks to ease back into your normal routine. You will bounce back faster.

You may not feel the need to rest if you simply have a head cold, Dr. Nieman says. In fact, mild exercise may help resolve head cold symptoms by boosting the number of virus-fighting white blood cells circulating throughout your body.

Drink tea, chicken soup, hot lemonade, or other hot fluids. "Whether you're fighting a cold or flu virus, fluids help to keep mucus thin enough to cough up or blow out. Trapped thick mucus promotes secondary bacterial infections such as pneumonia," says Dr. Davis. And feverish sweating can dry you out, which can lead to dehydration and may drive your fever up, she adds. So the advice is to drown a cold *and* a fever. And hot liquids relieve congestion better than cold drinks.

WHEN TO SEE THE DOCTOR

See your doctor if your cold or flu hasn't gotten better after a week or so, especially if it is accompanied by yellow, green, or bloody nasal discharge; a persistent severe headache; or a fever of 101°F or higher. Also go to the doctor if your breathing becomes difficult or painful or you experience sharp pains when you cough, pain around your eyes or cheekbones, or an earache.

Spice yourself up. Ginger is well-known and widely used for its stomach-soothing and ache-relieving properties, so it's just the ticket for colds and flu accompanied by nausea, says Nan Kathryn Fuchs, Ph.D., a nutritionist in Sebastopol, California. To make the tea, simmer 1 teaspoon grated fresh ginger and 1 cup water in a covered pot for 10 minutes. Then strain the tea and drink it. You can drink ginger tea up to four times a day.

Add some astragalus or echinacea. Astragalus—a popular Chinese herb—and echinacea have proven antiviral, immunity-boosting properties, says Dr. Fuchs. At the first sign of illness, take a dose of astragalus or echinacea tincture. Repeat every hour or two for the first day, then three times a day for about 3 days longer than it takes for your symptoms to resolve, she says. You can buy both of these herbs in health food stores. For dosages, follow label instructions.

Note: A tincture is a highly concentrated herbal liquid. It's made by soaking leaves in alcohol or glycerin—which extracts the herb's medicinal properties—for at least 6 weeks. Tinctures are sold in health food stores in small bottles with eyedroppers to give doses. Be sure to always store them out of the reach of children.

Try this cold-killing combo. Combining echinacea with goldenseal may get you good results. Echinacea stimulates the production of natural killer cells, which are a type of white blood cells that fight off viral infections. Goldenseal stimulates white blood cell activity and contains antiviral and antibacterial compounds, chiefly berberine. It works well with echinacea because it has properties that enable it to reduce inflammation and mucus production.

So when symptoms strike, take 300 milligrams of each of these herbs every 2 to 4 hours for the first 2 to 3 days, says Kristy Fassler, N.D., a naturopathic physician in Portsmouth, New Hampshire. Continue with the same dosage of each three times a day until symptoms disappear.

Consider sage. A few years ago, several leading herbalists were sitting around talking shop when the subject of cold remedies came up. Interestingly, neither echinacea nor goldenseal won by consensus. The winner? Sage.

"Sage is antiseptic and astringent," says Cascade Anderson Geller, an herbal educator and consulting herbal practitioner in Portland, Oregon. That means that it helps fight infections while drying up problems like postnasal drip. Steep 1 teaspoon of dried medicinal sage leaves in ½ cup of water and drink it slowly because it's strong and bitter. The recommended dose is ½ cup of tea twice a day between meals. The tea will make you feel better, but sage's drying effects are not something that you want to expose yourself to for more than a day or two, according to Geller.

Take frequent, comfortably hot showers or baths. Humidity fights congestion, says Dr. Fleming. Or keep a humidifier running at 60 percent humidity or more in your bedroom for the duration of your illness. "You'll feel more comfortable and breathe easier," he says.

Prop up your head when you sleep. Sneezing, coughing, and congestion are often worse at night, Dr. Davis says. Particularly if you have postnasal drip, sleep sitting up or prop your head up with extra pillows to make it easier to breathe.

recipe

GINGER-GARLIC SUPER SOUP

You think chicken soup is the sure kitchen cure for a cold? Then you haven't tried this doctor's ginger and garlic soup. "Both ginger and garlic are very boosting to the immune system," says Mary Bove, N.D., a naturopathic physician at the Brattleboro Naturopathic Clinic in Vermont. "And garlic is just great for colds," she adds. The mung bean sprouts are added for extra doses of folate, potassium, and magnesium for overall good health. Here's Dr. Bove's recipe for cold relief.

4	cups chicken broth
½	cup finely chopped fresh garlic
½	cup finely sliced fresh ginger
½	cup mung bean sprouts

Place the broth in a large saucepan and warm over medium-high heat.

In a medium saucepan, sauté the garlic and ginger for 3 to 4 minutes, or until soft. Add to the broth. Stir in the sprouts and simmer for 2 to 3 minutes, or until heated through. Keep any leftover soup in the refrigerator for later "treatments."

Double up on your vitamin C as soon as symptoms appear. In one study, people taking 1,000 milligrams of vitamin C twice a day had less nasal discharge and sneezing and colds of shorter duration than people not taking extra vitamin C.

If you are taking 500 to 1,000 milligrams of vitamin C a day, try increasing that amount to no more than 2,000 milligrams at the first sign of illness. Continue with your larger dose for a few days after you feel better, Dr. Fuchs recommends.

If you experience diarrhea with large doses of vitamin C (as some people do), cut back to 1,200 milligrams or less a day.

Take aim with A. Vitamin A is known as the anti-infection vitamin. It battles viruses and bacteria by keeping the cells healthy all along your respiratory tract and providing antibodies and lymphocytes to destroy the malevolent microorganisms that cause colds.

As soon as you notice cold or flu symptoms, take 100,000 IU of vitamin A daily for 3 days, says Dr. Fassler, then reduce the dosage to 25,000 IU for 1 week or until symptoms disappear. She cautions, however, that these are very high doses, and you need to check with your doctor before taking this much.

Zinc up. Researchers at the Cleveland Clinic Foundation in Cleveland found that people who started taking zinc gluconate lozenges within 24 hours of noticing cold symptoms had colds lasting only 4.4 days, about 3 days fewer than usual. They also had less coughing, headaches, hoarseness, nasal congestion, and drainage than usual.

"Scientists think that zinc helps prevent viral replication or that it may keep viruses from entering cells," says Michael Macknin, M.D., the study's main researcher. The lozenges studied contained zinc gluconate. Theoretically, other forms of zinc can bind with sweeteners in lozenges and become inactive.

You'll find zinc gluconate lozenges in health food stores and some drugstores. Follow the dosage recommendations on the label.

Antigerm Actions

To cut down on the number of cold and flu episodes you experience, you need to avoid germs when possible and fight them off when you are exposed.

Wash your hands frequently throughout the day. This is very important, especially if you are around kids who are sick, directs Dr. Davis. It's just too easy to transfer cold or flu viruses from your hands to your face, eyes, mouth, or nose.

Disinfect your house. This will prevent the spread of infection. Spray doorknobs, phones, and faucets with a disinfectant such as Lysol, making sure that you leave it on as long as the directions call for, Dr. Davis says.

Cover your mouth and nose when you sneeze. It's not just polite; a high-intensity sneeze can propel viruses a distance of up to 10 feet.

Stay away from smoke. Don't smoke and stay away from smoke-filled cars, restaurants, and the like. Cigarette smoke impairs many of your body's respiratory defenses against cold and flu viruses, says Dr. Davis.

Constipation

With so many laxatives on the market today—and with each one promising to work faster, gentler, and better than the rest—which product do doctors recommend?

Truth be told, none. Relying on laxatives to get things moving, so to speak, can eventually lead to what doctors call a lazy bowel. In effect, you lose your ability to void naturally. Only in rare instances—for relief during travel, to treat side effects from medications you may be taking temporarily, or for any other short-term circumstance—do doctors advise using laxatives to relieve constipation, says Anne Simons, M.D., professor of family and community medicine at the University of California, San Francisco, Medical Center.

In fact, if you move your bowels at least once every 3 days, you don't even have constipation, according to Dr. Simons. Only if you void less than that, or if you suddenly go from one bowel movement a day to one a week, do you have a problem.

Constipation usually results from poor nutrition—that is, eating too many processed foods such as potato chips, cookies, and other snacks and too few fiber-rich foods such as grains, fruits, and vegetables. Lack of exercise plays a role, too, as does rushing your toilet time so that you can't void completely.

Women sometimes become constipated during their periods—whether because of hormonal fluctuations (the change in estrogen and progesterone balance decreases bowel motility) or because of cravings for fatty, sugary foods, says Dr. Simons. Constipation is also a frequent vis-

WHEN TO SEE THE DOCTOR

See your doctor if you suddenly develop constant pain or cramping that does not resolve when the constipation is relieved, says Anne Simons, M.D., professor of family and community medicine at the University of California, San Francisco, Medical Center.

Also see your doctor if you experience any persistent and substantial change in your bowel movements, such as a drastic decrease in frequency—for example, from two a day to one every 4 days. This is especially important after age 40, when your risk for colon cancer increases, says Joel Mason, M.D., professor of gastroenterology at Tufts University in Boston.

Finally, if constipation lingers for more than 2 weeks, with less than one bowel movement every 3 days, and is accompanied by abdominal pain or blood in the stool, have it checked out. While it's probably easily remedied, it may be a symptom of something more serious, such as inflammatory bowel disease or another bowel disorder.

itor during the first trimester of pregnancy, when the uterus expands and puts pressure on the abdomen and pelvis.

Regularity Restorers

If constipation has your gut in its grip, you can restore regularity naturally with any of the following remedies.

Eat more fruits and vegetables. Try to have at least one serving of fruit and one serving of vegetables at every meal. Produce has plenty of fiber, and fiber increases the bulk and water content of your stool, says Dr. Simons. That makes the stool easier to pass. Good fruit sources of fiber include raspberries (8 grams of fiber per ½ cup) and prunes (6 grams per ½ cup). Among vegetables, choose sweet potatoes (3 grams per potato) and brussels sprouts (2 grams per ½ cup).

Bulk up with flaxseed. Take a teaspoon of whole flaxseed, mixed in an 8-ounce glass of water or juice, with each meal for 2 to 3 days, or until your symptoms improve. Though flaxseed won't dissolve completely, it does wash down easily. And it's rich in fiber, so it helps increase the bulk and water content of your stools. You will find whole flaxseed in health food stores, says Mitchell Fleisher, M.D., professor of family medicine at the University of Virginia Health Sciences Center in Charlottesville.

Consider psyllium. Take a rounded teaspoon of powdered psyllium seed, mixed in an 8-ounce glass of water or juice, with each meal until your symptoms subside. Follow this with a second glass of water or juice, says Joel Mason, M.D., professor of gastroenterology at Tufts University in Boston.

Try the sacred shell. The herb cascara sagrada (Spanish for "sacred shell") may be the world's most popular laxative, says Theresa MacLean, R.Ph., N.D., a naturopathic physician and pharmacist based in Berwick in Nova Scotia, Canada. It's even an ingredient in several over-the-counter laxatives.

Cascara contains compounds known as anthraquinones, which stimulate the intestinal contractions that we recognize as the urge to go. Take 15 to 20 drops of tincture once daily. You shouldn't use cascara sagrada for long periods of time, however, warns Dr. MacLean. Two weeks is the maximum.

Note: A tincture is a highly concentrated herbal liquid. It's made by soaking leaves in alcohol or glycerin—which extracts the herb's medicinal properties—for at least 6 weeks. Tinctures are sold in health food stores in small bottles with eyedroppers to give doses. Be sure to always store them out of the reach of children.

Get some "lemon aid." Lemon juice is a gentle laxative that is best used for prevention, says Dr. MacLean. And it's cheap. If you find yourself in need and unable to get to an herb store, simply go to any grocery store or produce stand and pick up a handful of lemons. Squeeze half a fresh lemon into a glass of water 15 minutes before meals and drink up.

Oil your intestines. Castor oil is pressed from the seeds of the *Ricinus communis* plant and is slightly yellow or sometimes colorless. Its lingering aftertaste leaves something to be desired, but it works, says Varro E. Tyler, Ph.D., Sc.D., distinguished professor of pharmacognosy at Purdue University in West Lafayette, Indiana. That's because a component in the oil breaks down into a substance that goes to work on both the small and large intestines.

Take 1 to 2 teaspoons on an empty stomach. You can expect results in about 8 hours.

An Herbal Prescription to Soothe a Balky Bowel

Certain herbal teas can help gently coax your bowel back into action. One such tea, called Smooth Move, contains a blend of herbs (senna leaf, licorice root, ginger, cinnamon, and fennel) that gets your stool moving without side effects, explains Mitchell Fleisher, M.D., professor of family medicine at the University of Virginia Health Sciences Center in Charlottesville. He suggests sipping one to two cups of the tea each day for 3 to 4 days. You can buy Smooth Move in health food stores and some drugstores.

See if this weed works. The bitterness of dandelion can stimulate contractions of the colon and move stools along, says Patricia Howell, an herbalist from Atlanta. Use between 1 and 3 dropperfuls of dandelion root tincture in ¼ cup of water. (A dropperful is roughly 15 drops.) Then drink it slowly by holding each mouthful for about a minute. The bitter taste will stimulate bile flow. Drink it three times a day, says Howell.

If all else fails, try licorice. "Licorice root tea will loosen the bowels in obstinate constipation," says Douglas Schar, an herbalist from London. "If you consume licorice tea and prunes before going to bed, you will have no problem moving your bowels in the morning." To make the tea, boil a tablespoon of licorice root for 30 minutes in a cup of water. Strain the tea and let it cool slightly before drinking.

Preventive Prescriptions

The good news about constipation is that it is easy to avoid. These strategies can help.

Get your gut going with fiber. Get at least 25 grams of fiber a day (the Daily Value) by eating at least five servings of fruits and vegetables and two servings of whole grains. In addition to the foods mentioned earlier, try a ½-cup serving of kiwifruit (3 grams of fiber), barley (2.9 grams), or broccoli (2.3 grams).

Drink up. Drink at least ½ ounce of water for each pound of body weight every day. For a 140-pound woman, that works out to 70 ounces—a little less than nine 8-ounce glasses. Water keeps your stool soft so that it's easier to pass, explains Dr. Fleisher.

Walk for 15 to 20 minutes every day. Scientists can't explain why, but walking stimulates bowel function, so you stay regular, explains Dr. Simons.

Train yourself. Sitting on the toilet for about 10 minutes after each meal trains your body to void at the same time every day. And after you have eaten, your digestive system is on standby, ready to process food and empty waste. Stick with this schedule, says Dr. Simons, and within a few weeks, the urge to void after a meal will come naturally. But if you can't go within 10 minutes, don't force it, as straining creates problems of its own.

Depression

The World Health Organization predicts that by the year 2020, depression will rank right behind heart disease as the world's second most disabling illness. And if the current trend continues, most of its victims will be female. Right now, women are three times more likely than men to develop depression.

"Women do have times in their lives when they seem especially vulnerable to depression," says Laura Epstein Rosen, Ph.D., supervisor of family therapy training for the Special Needs Clinic at Columbia-Presbyterian Medical Center in New York City. Sometimes the risk is biologically driven, as when hormone levels fluctuate just after childbirth and just before menopause. Other times it is externally driven—perhaps by the death of a parent, divorce, job loss, or some other major life event.

Even everyday conflict can brew into mild depression, says Susan Heitler, Ph.D., a clinical psychologist in Denver. "When you want X and your partner wants Y, you have a problem," she explains. If you repeatedly give up what you want so that your partner gets what he wants, without seeking a mutually satisfying compromise, you may pay an emotional price in the long run.

Mild depression often manifests itself as deeply negative feelings of sorrow, guilt, discouragement, and powerlessness. More severe cases may be accompanied by symptoms such as loss of appetite, lack of sleep, and difficulty concentrating.

The good news about depression is that once you recognize that you have it, you can easily treat it. "By knowing when you are vulnerable to depression and by recognizing its signs and symptoms, you can get the help you need," says Dr. Rosen.

What's more, depression may draw your attention to some aspect of your life that needs evaluation and change, says Margaret Jensvold, M.D., director of the Institute for Research on Women's Health in

Rockville, Maryland. "If you find yourself repeatedly getting upset or sad about the same situation, you need to come to terms with that situation, one way or another," she advises.

Mood Medicine for Mom

For severe depression, you will need to see a doctor, who may recommend a combination of talk therapy and antidepressant drugs. Mild depression responds well to self-care measures like these.

WHEN TO SEE THE DOCTOR

Read and respond to the following two questions.

1. Have you had a distinct period during which you felt down and unhappy or you lost your pleasure and interest in life?

2. Have you suffered from at least five of these eight symptoms for 2 weeks or longer?
   - Appetite or weight changes
   - Sleep problems
   - Excessive fatigue
   - Excessive agitation or lethargy
   - Loss of interest or pleasure in usual activities
   - Guilty feelings
   - Slow thinking or indecisiveness
   - Suicidal thoughts

If you answered yes to both questions—and especially if you have had suicidal thoughts—see your doctor. You may have severe depression, which requires professional care, says Gary Emery, Ph.D., director of the Los Angeles Center for Cognitive Therapy.

Try a tea. Research suggests that St. John's wort is just as effective as commonly prescribed antidepressant drugs, but with fewer side effects. Compounds in the yellow-flowered herb appear to stimulate brain cells.

To make the tea, pour 1 cup boiling water over 1 to 2 heaping teaspoons dried herb (available in health food stores). Allow the herb to steep for 10 minutes. Then strain the tea and set it aside to cool a bit before drinking it. Drink one to two cups every day.

Because of its stimulant properties, St. John's wort should not be taken at bedtime, advises Varro Tyler, Ph.D., Sc.D., distinguished pro-

A Visualization Prescription for Confronting Conflict

Depression often stems from an unresolved problem with another person—be it a spouse, a sibling, or a coworker. The following exercise, recommended by Susan Heitler, Ph.D., a clinical psychologist in Denver, can help you work through the situation so that both of you come out ahead—and happy.

- Recognize your negative feelings as depression.

- Look for the cause of your depression. Ask yourself what conflict or frustrating situation lies behind your sad feelings.

- Visualize your way out of the conflict with these simple steps.

    1. Close your eyes. Ask yourself, "If I were mad at someone, who would it be?"

    2. Allow the image of the person you feel mad at to appear on your mental screen.

fessor of pharmacognosy at Purdue University in West Lafayette, Indiana. The herb also increases your sensitivity to sunlight, making you burn more easily. So while you are using St. John's wort, limit the time you spend in the sun and use a sunscreen on all exposed areas.

Get your vitamins. The most common deficiencies in people who are depressed are the B-complex vitamins and vitamin C, says C. Norman Shealy, M.D., Ph.D., director of the Shealy Institute, a holistic medicine clinic in Springfield, Missouri.

The B vitamins help energize brain cells and manufacture important chemicals to keep your moods high. Vitamin B_6, for example, plays a

3. Pretend that you're Alice in Wonderland. You have just sipped the growth drops. See yourself grow bigger and bigger until you tower over the person with whom you are in conflict.

4. From your new, powerful vantage point, reassess the other person and what each of you wants.

5. Use what you can now see about that person to discover new possibilities for resolving your conflict in a mutually beneficial way.

To understand how this exercise supports conflict resolution, think of a woman who views herself as small and powerless in her relationship with her husband. Because of her self-image, she may be unable to assert herself effectively when a problem arises. Leaving the problem unresolved could cause her to become depressed.

If she visualizes herself as bigger and more powerful than her husband, she may notice things about him that she never did before. "For example, her husband's body language might tell her that he is actually scared or insecure," says Dr. Heitler. "Understanding him more fully can help her devise solutions to the problem that will benefit both of them."

role in the production of serotonin, a brain chemical that has a direct impact on your moods and emotions.

Another B vitamin that has been linked to depression is folate, the naturally occurring form of folic acid. In fact, depression is considered the most common symptom of a folate deficiency. Harvard Medical School researchers found that as many as 38 percent of adults diagnosed with depression had low levels of folate in their blood. Another vitamin that's just as important in maintaining high spirits is vitamin C. Low levels can leave you feeling gloomy, says Ray Sahelian, M.D., a physician in Marina del Rey, California. Vitamin C helps manufacture serotonin and two other essential brain-related chemicals, dopamine and norepinephrine, which lift your mood, keep you alert, and sustain your sex drive.

For mild to moderate depression, you may want to take a high-potency multivitamin/mineral supplement daily after talking to your doctor, says Dr. Shealy. He also suggests 100 milligrams each of thiamin, riboflavin, niacin, and B_6, along with 400 micrograms of folic acid, 100 micrograms of B_{12}, and 2,000 milligrams of vitamin C in divided doses daily.

Try a natural pick-me-up. 5-HTP is a natural compound produced by the body from tryptophan, an amino acid found in many foods. It's also a precursor of serotonin, which means that more serotonin is produced when 5-HTP is present. Serotonin is a brain chemical that produces a feeling of well-being.

When you take 5-HTP in supplement form, it's absorbed in your gastrointestinal tract and then journeys to your brain, where it's converted into serotonin, says Dr. Sahelian.

If you've been diagnosed with depression and you have a doctor's approval, you can take 50 milligrams of 5-HTP late in the evening, says Dr. Sahelian. But he doesn't advise taking larger amounts. Any dosage over 50 milligrams can cause vivid dreams, nightmares, and nausea.

Eat a lot. Six small meals, spaced 3 hours apart over the course of the day, can help keep your blood sugar on a more even keel. "For some people, low blood sugar can trigger depression," says Dr. Jensvold. Of course, you should make sure that each of the six meals is well-balanced. Cheetos or chocolate don't count. Choose whole grains, fruits, vegetables, and fat-free or low-fat dairy products.

Avoid this depression duo. "The more severe your depression, the more you will benefit from purging your diet of caffeine and sugar, though we're not sure why," says Larry Christensen, Ph.D., professor of psychology at the University of South Alabama in Mobile.

You probably already know the caffeine culprits: coffee, tea, cola, and chocolate. As for sugar, avoid candy, baked goods, and other treats. The sugars that naturally occur in fruits and other foods are okay, according to Dr. Christensen.

If your symptoms do improve during 2 weeks of abstention, you could try reintroducing caffeine and sugar one at a time. You may find that you can tolerate one but not the other.

Move to improve. Do some aerobic exercise (the kind that pumps up your heart and respiration rates) for 20 to 30 minutes at least 3 days a week. "Any depressed woman who makes herself work out will experience a definite improvement in the way she feels about herself," says Robert S. Brown Sr., M.D., Ph.D., professor of psychiatric medicine at the University of Virginia in Charlottesville. "The effort and vigor with which you work out is proportional to the physical and emotional benefits that you receive." In other words, the more you sweat, the better you'll feel.

Write down how you feel. "Keeping a diary can help you work through your depression," notes Dr. Jensvold. It allows you to articulate, vent, and come to terms with your unhappiness.

Turn to your friends for support. "You need to have a friend or two to call upon when you are sad, someone who can give you the gift of listening," says Dr. Jensvold. But, she adds, make sure that you share good times with that person, too.

Inactivity

Some women view exercise the same way that they view sex. They think it is important and would like to do it more often, but they just can't seem to find time—or to make time.

That's too bad, because exercise has a lot to offer healthwise. It helps you maintain a healthy weight. It lowers your cholesterol and blood pressure, which in turn slashes your risk for heart disease. It even bolsters your resistance to certain types of cancer.

"Exercise literally gives you more time," says Ralph Paffenbarger, M.D., professor emeritus at Stanford University School of Medicine. In his own studies, Dr. Paffenbarger has found that for every hour you work out, you gain an additional hour of life.

But if you are accustomed to an inactive lifestyle, even the promise of living healthier longer may not motivate you enough to get a move on. Here is what you can do to leave the sedentary lifestyle behind.

Make exercise a priority. "Tell yourself that exercise is important," says Ross Andersen, Ph.D., director of exercise science at the Johns Hopkins Weight Management Center in Baltimore. "Remind yourself every day, especially on those days when the rest of your life seems to be conspiring to keep you from your workout."

As important as exercise is, it almost never has a deadline attached to it, explains Dr. Andersen. So it is easily bumped to the back burner . . . unless you make a mental commitment to it.

Focus on how you feel rather than how you look. If you dream of achieving a supermodel physique, you will probably be disappointed. "Most women simply can't look like Cher or Jamie Lee Curtis. It's not in their genetic makeup," notes Dr. Andersen. But you can feel good about yourself and your body. "Women tell me that exercise makes them stronger, helps them sleep better, gives them energy as well as a sense of accomplishment," he observes. "That's what I want them to home in on." These positive changes arrive within a few weeks after beginning an exercise program. They help keep people going.

Substitute positive affirmations for negative self-talk. "People come up with horrible ways of describing themselves, like 'fat' or 'gross,'" says Michael Scholtz, director of fitness at the Duke University Diet and Fitness Center in Durham, North Carolina. "All they are doing is beating up on themselves." When one of these critical messages floats through your brain, he suggests countering it with a positive statement, such as "I am a capable person who exercises every day and enjoys it." While this won't instantly change your self-image, it will make you aware of all the negative self-talk going on in your head and encourage you to think more positively.

Sign up for beginner-level exercise classes. You will get the instruction you need to avoid injury, along with the support and encouragement you need to keep going. "Classes are especially helpful for women who have never exercised, who don't think they can exercise, or who feel embarrassed and self-conscious," says Christina Frederick, Ph.D., professor of psychology at Southern Utah University in Cedar City. "For them, the right class and the right instructor can make all the difference in the world."

Recruit an exercise partner. That way, on those days when you will use any excuse not to work out, knowing that someone is expecting you just may compel you to slip into your sweats and sneakers after all, according to Dr. Frederick.

Consider hiring a personal trainer if you can afford one. Particularly if you have a health problem that makes exercise difficult, a personal trainer can provide individualized guidance. "Find someone whose personality complements yours but who challenges you to improve," advises Dr. Frederick.

Create a Routine That Works for You

When it comes to customizing your exercise routine, keep in mind that you want to make your exercise sessions relatively hassle-free and as non–time-consuming as possible. Follow these guidelines to shape a routine that you can live with.

Set aside at least 30 minutes every day for your workout. Mark it in your daily planner, just as you would any other appointment. This affirms the importance of exercise, explains Dr. Andersen. "You can say to yourself, 'I don't need to feel guilty. I'm doing exactly what I planned to be doing right now.'"

Your body actually appreciates this regularity, adds Scholtz. "Over time, your biological clock sets itself according to your workout schedule, so your body expects and wants an exercise fix at a certain time of day," he says. "If it doesn't get a workout, you end up feeling less energetic."

Get your family's support. Make sure that family members, especially children, understand that you are not available during your scheduled workouts. You may want to write your workout times on a calendar and post the calendar in your kitchen. This can help you avoid last-minute requests for rides to soccer games and dance lessons.

Select a gym wisely. If you join a gym, choose one that is close to home or work. You are more likely to stop by the facility if you pass it on your daily commute, observes Scholtz.

Create a home gym. If you exercise at home, invest in some basic equipment. This means things such as a foam floor mat, a jump rope, an aerobic step, exercise tubing (for easy resistance training), and a pair of dumbbells.

Be prepared at all times. Keep workout clothes and a pair of sneakers in your car. That way, you can exercise whenever the opportunity presents itself.

Exercise first thing in the morning. You are least likely to get outside interference at this time of day. "In my experience, even people who say that they are not morning exercisers adapt in a few weeks' time," notes Scholtz.

Focus on consistency rather than intensity. When you are first starting out, your goal is to make exercising a habit, says Dr. Andersen. So don't worry too much about how fast or how far you walk, for example, as long as you are doing something for the amount of time you have allotted. You can worry about speed and distance later on if you want.

Divide and conquer. Break a 30-minute workout into 5- to 10-minute chunks. "Time is such a huge barrier to exercise that being active for a few minutes here and there throughout the day really excites people," explains Dr. Andersen. "They say, 'I can do that.'"

Look for opportunities to be active. Despite your best efforts, things will occasionally intrude on your workout time. Rather than bag your workout altogether, do as much as you can wherever you can, even if it is only for 5 minutes. "Take the stairs rather than the elevator at work, or park farther away from the building rather than in the closest spot you can find," recommends Scholtz.

Work through normal muscle soreness. What's normal? Well, you should expect a little tightness and discomfort in your muscles after you exercise, according to Scholtz. This type of soreness usually subsides over time, as your muscles adapt to your workout routine. If, on the other hand, you have pain that causes you to limp or leaves you unable to get out of bed in the morning, that's a sign that you are overdoing it and need to cut back.

Do Something You Enjoy

You have penned your workouts into your daily planner. Now the big question: How, exactly, should you spend that time? The answer is entirely up to you—but just remember that the activity you choose can make or break your motivation. To keep exercise accessible and fun, heed this advice from the experts.

Adjust your personal definition of exercise. "You can probably come up with at least one physical activity that you enjoy," says Scholtz. "You may not think of that activity as exercise, but it actually is."

Try various activities until you find one that appeals to you. "Doing something pleasurable gives you the motivation to stick with it," according to Dr. Frederick. "Even though you may not engage in the activity every day, you will likely put in more hours per week than people who don't enjoy their workouts."

To find an activity you like, ask yourself these questions: What did you enjoy doing when you were younger? What sports were you good at? What activities have you always wanted to try? Perhaps ballroom dancing? Or inline skating? Or scuba diving?

Plan an active vacation. Take a walking tour of Paris or Rome, do a bed-and-breakfast bicycle tour of Vermont, or volunteer for a week with an environmental or community service organization.

Infertility

I t's something that most women take for granted. Some even spend most of their reproductive years trying to avoid it. So imagine the irony and despair, the frustration and sense of loss that comes when a woman finally decides to have kids—and then just can't make it happen.

Technically, a couple is considered infertile when they have tried for a year or more to produce a baby, without success. This happens to about one in six couples. And the problem seems to be equally divided between men and women, says Marc Goldstein, M.D., director of the Center for Male Reproductive Medicine at New York Hospital–Cornell Medical Center in New York City.

Often the problem can be figured out and fixed. A woman's fallopian tubes may be blocked with scar tissue, for instance. Or a man may have a varicose vein (called a varicocele) in his scrotum that slows bloodflow and raises the temperature too high for sperm production. Surgery can correct such problems.

But sometimes the cause of infertility is not so obvious and seems to be related to hormonal or metabolic imbalances. True, just getting older slows the productivity of a woman's ovaries. (Men, by comparison, can go strong into their midsixties with little effect on their fertility, says Dr. Goldstein.)

The stressful part of infertility is the uncertainty of it all. Is it me? Is it him? Is it just bad timing? Do we try harder? Do we try less? Stop trying to guess the answers. Science has gotten a whole lot smarter about this stuff. If you sense there is a problem, both you and your partner should get your reproductive gear checked out. That said, there is much that you—and your husband—can do on your own to increase the chances of conceiving. First, here are some options that you can try.

Take a folic acid supplement each day. A study by researchers in Budapest, Hungary, found that women who took daily prenatal supplements containing 800 micrograms of folic acid (the synthetic form of folate) got pregnant slightly faster than women who were not taking prenatal supplements.

Doses of folic acid exceeding 400 micrograms per day should be taken only under the supervision of a doctor. In large amounts, the nutrient can mask signs of a vitamin B_{12} deficiency.

Try using some unicorn. Although this herb has yet to be researched scientifically, many herbalists consider it to be *the* herbal antidote for infertility. False unicorn root, which was included in many traditional fertility formulas, is believed to contain compounds called steroidal saponins that herbalists suspect may be responsible for its normalizing effect on female hormones. Use 5 to 15 drops of the tincture or take up to ½ cup of an infusion daily, sipped slowly throughout the day. Herbalists suggest using false unicorn root in fertility formulas for at least 3 to 6 months.

Herbalists say that wild false unicorn root is becoming rare and endangered in nature. Help protect this wild plant by buying products that use the cultivated herb. You can find these products in health food stores.

Note: A tincture is a highly concentrated herbal liquid. It's made by soaking leaves in alcohol or glycerin—which extracts the herb's medicinal properties—for at least 6 weeks. Tinctures are sold in health food

WHEN TO SEE THE DOCTOR

If you are under age 35 and you and your partner have not been able to conceive during a year of unprotected sex, see your gynecologist, says Jacqueline Gutman, M.D., professor of reproductive endocrinology at the University of Pennsylvania in Philadelphia. If you are age 35 or over, see your doctor after waiting 6 months.

stores in small bottles with eyedroppers to give doses. Be sure to always store them out of the reach of children.

Brew this traditional tonic. Combine 1 ounce each of dried partridgeberry, false unicorn root, cramp bark, and blue cohosh. Add 1 tablespoon of the herb blend to 1 cup of water and simmer over low heat for about 15 minutes. Drink one cup a day, suggests Cascade Anderson Geller, an herbal educator and consulting herbal practitioner in Portland, Oregon.

Yet to be heavily studied by researchers, partridgeberry is reported to contain saponins that herbalists believe are responsible for the herb's hormone-balancing effects. It has a long history of use among women preparing for pregnancy. Research has shown that cramp bark contains antispasmodic substances that herbalists believe make it effective in preventing miscarriage.

Consider another useful herb. The herb chasteberry acts like a mild progesterone, says Liz Collins, N.D., a naturopathic physician in Portland, Oregon. When you take it, you're lending support to progesterone and estrogen, the two hormones that are essential to reproduction. If infertility is the result of the estrogen-to-progesterone ratio being out of balance, chasteberry might tip the scales just enough to improve your chances of success.

She recommends the standard dosage, which is 175 to 225 milligrams a day.

Control your caffeine consumption. You may not have to give up caffeine for good. But one study conducted by researchers from the Johns Hopkins University School of Hygiene and Public Health in Baltimore found that women who got more than 300 milligrams of caffeine a day from coffee, cola, or tea were 26 percent less likely to get pregnant over the course of a year than women who avoided the stuff, says Chris Meletis, N.D., a naturopathic physician at the National College of Naturopathic Medicine in Portland, Oregon. If you are monitoring your caffeine consumption, keep in mind that 6 ounces of coffee supplies 103 milligrams; 12 ounces of cola, 37 milligrams; and 6 ounces of tea, 36 milligrams.

Take your time . . . and enjoy yourself. The vaginal lubrication that occurs with sexual arousal is slightly more alkaline than normal vaginal secretions. This creates a more hospitable environment for sperm during the short time that they may be in the vagina.

Also, while orgasm is not necessary for conception, it does help semen move upward in the female reproductive tract, says Jacqueline Gutman, M.D., professor of reproductive endocrinology at the University of Pennsylvania in Philadelphia.

Help for Your Husband

It takes only one sperm to do the job. But nature demands that millions be deployed and that the majority be good candidates for fatherhood. "It's a team effort," Dr. Goldstein explains. "Sperm actually travel in packs and help each other create a pathway through the cervical mucus to penetrate the egg."

To determine a man's fertility, his sperm are examined under a microscope for quantity, motility (their ability to wriggle and thrash through the female reproductive tract en route to the egg), and form. Most cases of male infertility reflect a low sperm count—less than 20 million sperm per milliliter, which is about ⅛ teaspoon. (The average count is 66 million per milliliter or, on average, 200 million per ejaculation.) Poor-quality sperm can also cause problems, Dr. Goldstein says. For a man to be considered fertile, more than 50 percent of his sperm must be swimming vigorously, in a straight line, and have good form. They can't be sticking together, for instance, or have crooked tails.

Sometimes sperm problems are linked to a hidden infection such as chlamydia, a treatable sexually transmitted disease. (Both you and your partner need to be treated, however.) Prescription drugs and thyroid problems can also cause difficulties. Here are some things that your mate can do to boost your chances of conceiving.

Ask him to wear boxer shorts and baggy pants as much as possible. Tight underwear and pants tuck the testicles too close to the body, causing their temperature to rise. And anything that cooks a man's testicles can lower his sperm count, says Dr. Meletis. Research has shown that sperm production drops sharply at temperatures above 96°F.

Make sure his sperm stay in shape. Encourage him to take 1,000 to 2,000 milligrams of vitamin C, 400 IU of vitamin E, and 100 micrograms of selenium each day. These nutrients help keep sperm from becoming misshapen, sticking together when they shouldn't, and dying, says Dr. Meletis.

Some people develop diarrhea when they take more than 1,200 milligrams of vitamin C a day. If he is one of them, he should simply cut back the dose to a more tolerable level.

Think zinc. Encourage him to take 30 to 50 milligrams of this mineral each day. Zinc is essential for male reproduction. A low level of the mineral can diminish production of the male hormone testosterone, which in turn can lead to a reduced sperm count, says Dr. Meletis.

Your partner should take this much zinc only with medical supervision. A too high intake of the mineral can cause problems of its own.

Better the odds with pygeum. This African tree bark extract is a common treatment for enlarged prostate, as it's known to help relieve some urinary symptoms. Pygeum also causes an increase in prostate secretions, however, improving the composition of semen and the odds for conception, says Steven Rissman, N.D., a naturopathic physician at American WholeHealth in Littleton, Colorado. The recommended dose is a capsule containing 100 to 200 milligrams each day.

Get him some Asian assistance. Asian ginseng, also called panax, Chinese, or Korean ginseng, is a traditional Chinese virility tonic. In a number of animal studies, it has been shown to increase testosterone, testicle size, and sperm formation. It's commonly available. "Check the label so you know the amount of ginsenosides in each capsule," says Dr. Rissman. He should take 100- to 200-milligram capsules that provide a total of 15 milligrams of ginsenosides daily.

General Fertility Tips for Both of You

Here is what men and women can do to achieve optimum fertility.

Give up smoking. It's just plain bad news if you or your partner continues smoking while you are trying to conceive, says Dr. Gutman. In women, smoking has been found to reduce blood levels of estrogen as well as the motion of the fallopian tubes, which encourages the union of egg and sperm. Nicotine, which is toxic to sperm, is found in the cervical mucus of female smokers.

In men, cigarette smoking in particular is associated with decreased sperm counts and sperm motility as well as an increased frequency of abnormal sperm, Dr. Meletis says.

Try to limit toasting. Limit alcohol consumption to three drinks per week, with a drink equaling one 12-ounce beer, one 5-ounce glass of wine, or a mixed drink made with 1½ ounces of liquor. This goes for you and your partner. Experts agree that alcohol is a reproductive-tract toxin for both men and women. The more you consume, the more you jeopardize your chances of parenthood.

Maintain a healthy weight. Body fat plays an important role in hormone levels, especially for women but also for men, experts say. "Thin women may have too little estrogen, and overweight women too much, to become pregnant," Dr. Gutman says. "Thin women need to gain enough weight to ovulate regularly. "They may not need to gain a lot, just 5 pounds or so," she says. And overweight women don't need to become svelte, but they do need to lose enough to get within 30 percent of their ideal body weight.

Thin men, especially those on no-fat, no-cholesterol diets, may have low sperm counts. "You actually need some cholesterol every day to produce hormones, including testosterone," Dr. Goldstein says. "And extremely overweight men have high estrogen levels and, frequently, overheated testes, which impede sperm production." Losing some weight can set things right. Staying within 30 percent of their optimum body weight is a good guideline for men to follow, too, he says.

Create a schedule. Plan to attempt conception either 2 days before ovulation or the day of ovulation. These are the best times of the month to make babies, says Allen Wilcox, M.D., Ph.D., a researcher at the National Institute of Environmental Health Sciences in Research Triangle Park, North Carolina. In fact, your odds of conceiving remain decent for up to 6 days before ovulation, but they drop dramatically within 24 hours after ovulation. "One possibility is that changes occur in the cervical mucus after ovulation, blocking sperm from entering the uterus," he explains. "In any event, it's better not to wait until ovulation and possibly miss your chance."

To determine when you are ovulating, use a urine test that measures luteinizing hormone, advises Dr. Gutman. This test turns positive about 24 hours before ovulation occurs. Women with regular, 28-day menstrual cycles tend to ovulate 10 to 14 days prior to menstruation. Ovulation test kits are available in drugstores.

Don't do it. You read right. If your partner has a low sperm count, abstain from sex for 48 to 72 hours before attempting to conceive. Waiting will encourage a higher concentration of sperm in the semen, and you'll have a better chance of succeeding, says Dr. Goldstein.

Menopause

No, menopause isn't a disease, although it is sometimes treated as such. Like puberty, it is a time of transition that all women go through sooner or later, like it or not. Most women actually reach menopause (officially defined as 1 year without periods) somewhere between the ages of 48 and 52. Many women, though, have at least a few years of so-called perimenopausal symptoms before this, as hormonal fluctuations cause symptoms such as hot flashes, irregular periods sometimes accompanied by heavy bleeding, and mood swings.

Surveys show that some women have a particularly tough time during menopause, while others breeze right through it. The majority are somewhere in between, with bothersome but tolerable symptoms. "Women who have had their ovaries surgically removed or who have gone through early menopause (before age 50) are especially likely to have more severe symptoms," says June LaValleur, M.D., professor of obstetrics and gynecology at the University of Minnesota Medical School in Minneapolis.

There is no preventing menopause. Even replacement hormones can't fully mimic your body's natural cycle. But whether you decide on hormone-replacement therapy or choose to sweat it out, you have plenty of ways to minimize menopause's impact on your mind and body.

Natural Hormone Helpers

Dietary and lifestyle changes, along with certain herbs, can protect your health as you go through menopause. Here is what the experts recommend.

Consume 30 to 50 milligrams of isoflavones each day. Isoflavones are weak, plant-derived forms of the hormone estrogen that are found in soy foods such as tofu, tempeh, and soy milk. Studies have shown that women who eat about 4 ounces of soy foods a day—which supplies 30 to 50 milligrams of isoflavones—are less likely to have bothersome menopausal symptoms such as hot flashes and vaginal dryness, says James E. Williams, O.M.D., a doctor of Oriental medicine with the Center for Women's Medicine in San Diego.

Consider flaxseed. "Flaxseed contains lignans, plant compounds that, like isoflavones, have some weak estrogen-like activity in the body," notes Dr. Williams. In studies, lignans also seem to confer some protection against breast cancer and other hormone-dependent cancers, adds Dr. Williams. Eat about 1 tablespoon of ground flaxseed each day. You can bake with it, or try sprinkling flaxseed on cooked foods, cereals, and salads.

It's best to buy fresh flaxseed and grind it yourself (you can find it at health food stores). And keep it refrigerated when you are not using it, since it tends to go rancid rapidly.

WHEN TO SEE THE DOCTOR

Many women have irregular periods as they approach menopause. In most cases, there is no need for concern, says June LaValleur, M.D., professor of obstetrics and gynecology at the University of Minnesota Medical School in Minneapolis. Do see a doctor, though, if your periods are fewer than 21 days apart, if you bleed between periods, or if your periods become much heavier. See a doctor, too, if you become unusually tired. Thyroid problems are more common at this stage of life.

Even if your menopausal years go smoothly, you should see your gynecologist for preventive care, advises Dr. LaValleur. This includes regular Pap tests, mammograms, and cholesterol, blood pressure, and bone-density screenings.

Plant yourself. The plants from the *Umbelliferae* family—which includes fennel, parsley, and celery—contain compounds with estrogen-like activity. "Fennel is particularly rich in phytoestrogens," says Michael Murray, N.D., a naturopathic physician in Bellevue, Washington. Fennel root, a large bulb that has a delicate, licorice-like flavor, can be sliced into a salad or stir-fry or used to season soups.

Vitamize. Take 1,000 milligrams of vitamin C and 50 milligrams of B-complex vitamins twice each day. (Make sure that your B-complex supplement contains pantothenic acid.) These vitamins support your adrenal glands, tiny powerhouses on top of your kidneys that continue

Hormone Replacement: Menopausal Help or Hindrance?

Conventional medicine treats menopause as a deficiency disease of estrogen in much the same way that diabetes is considered a deficiency disease of insulin," says naturopathic physician Tori Hudson, N.D., professor at the National College of Naturopathic Medicine in Portland, Oregon. So just as physicians are quick to prescribe insulin for diabetes treatment, many are equally quick to prescribe estrogen and other hormones, called hormone-replacement therapy (HRT), for heart and bone protection. HRT can also relieve hot flashes and other menopausal symptoms, notes Dr. Hudson.

"But menopause, unlike diabetes, isn't a disease process, and it's not something to be halted or reversed," says Dr. Hudson. "It's a perfectly normal part of life. All women stop menstruating. It's a part of normal aging. True, some women have problems associated with menopause, but we have to be realistic about treating those problems in a way that best suits the individual woman."

to produce small amounts of estrogen, says Helen Healy, N.D., a naturopathic physician in St. Paul, Minnesota. "I especially recommend this to women who are leading stressful lives or who in the past tended to burn the candle at both ends," she says. "Their adrenals have less reserve power."

Some people experience diarrhea when they take more than 1,200 milligrams of vitamin C a day. If this happens to you, simply reduce your intake of the vitamin until the diarrhea subsides.

Also, take 400 IU of vitamin E each day. Scientists have yet to determine exactly how vitamin E helps to ease menopausal symptoms. But

HRT uses either synthetic or natural female hormones, like estrogen (collected from the urine of pregnant mares or plant sources), to compensate for the normal decline in production experienced by women at midlife. Some herbalists and many M.D.'s agree that HRT may be an appropriate choice for certain women with severe menopausal symptoms or for those at high risk for heart disease and osteoporosis.

Using HRT does not necessarily guarantee a problem-free passage, however. Among women who choose HRT, roughly one out of three will stop using it before a year is up because of uncomfortable side effects. Fully 50 percent of all women who take HRT will experience one or more problems, including menstrual bleeding, bloating, premenstrual irritability, cramps, and breast tenderness. There can be other problems, too, like headaches, weight gain, depression, abnormal uterine bleeding, and changes in hair and skin. Using estrogen can double your chances of developing gallbladder disease. And many doctors tell women to shun HRT if they've had breast cancer or have a family history of the disease.

In other words, some women feel better and may be better off with the side effects of menopause than with the side effects of menopause medicine, says Dr. Hudson.

To determine if HRT is right for you, see your doctor.

the nutrient seems to alleviate hot flashes and vaginal dryness for some women, says Dr. Murray.

Many experts believe that you can take this much vitamin E without side effects. But if you have had a bleeding disorder or a stroke, if you are taking anticoagulants, or if your family has a history of stroke, you should use vitamin E supplements only under medical supervision. It is possible that large amounts of vitamin E interfere with the absorption and action of vitamin K, which is involved in blood coagulation.

Eat small meals 2 to 3 hours apart. To make this easy, you can divide your breakfast and lunch in half, then make your dinner roughly the same size. All-day-long grazing maintains a normal blood sugar level in your body and may even help you eat less because you never become ravenously hungry, explains Elaine Moquette-Magee, R.D., an expert in menopausal nutrition. Both of these factors may help you avoid menopausal weight gain.

Get comfortable with this herb. Black cohosh has a long history of use for menopausal discomfort, says Willow Moore, D.C., N.D., a chiropractor and naturopathic physician in Owings Mills, Maryland. A good dose to take is 40 milligrams twice a day, she says. You probably won't feel relief until 2 to 4 weeks after you start taking it. Also, you should continue taking black cohosh even after menopause ends, says Dr. Moore. She recommends taking it for 6-month periods, with a month off in between.

Recruit an Asian ally. Dong quai is yet another great all-around supplement to take for menopausal problems. "Many women in China and Japan who take a dose of dong quai every day, from the time they start menstruating all the way through menopause, have a reduced incidence of menstrual problems," says Dr. Moore.

Dong quai is thought to be good for relieving all kinds of female troubles, from premenstrual syndrome to heavy periods to menopausal problems, says Dr. Moore. For best results during menopause, follow the dosage directions on the package you buy, she says. The instructions for a product from Gaia Herbs, for example, are to put 30 to 40 drops in a small amount of warm water and take it three or four times a day between meals.

If you have hot flashes, try this herbal trio. "My own standard recommendation for hot flashes and other symptoms of menopause is a trio of traditional herbs," says Andrew Weil, M.D., director of the Program in Integrative Medicine at the University of Arizona in Tucson.

Dr. Weil recommends taking one dropperful each of tinctures of dong quai, chasteberry, and damiana once a day at midday. Continue taking the herbs until your hot flashes cease, then taper off gradually.

Damiana is a nervous-system tonic, said to ease depression and anxiety. Chasteberry may counteract the effectiveness of birth control pills. Don't use dong quai while menstruating, spotting, or bleeding heavily, because it can increase blood loss.

Note: A tincture is a highly concentrated herbal liquid. It's made by soaking leaves in alcohol or glycerin—which extracts the herb's medicinal properties—for at least 6 weeks. Tinctures are sold in health food stores in small bottles with eyedroppers to give doses. Be sure to always store them out of the reach of children.

Suspend the sweats with sage. Hot flashes that strike while you're asleep are called night sweats, and sometimes feelings of terror or anxiety will precede them. Garden sage is famed for the way it reduces or even eliminates night sweats. It acts fast, within a few hours, and a single cup of infusion can stave off the sweats for up to 2 days, says Susun S. Weed, an herbalist from Woodstock, New York. What's more, you probably have a bottle of sage sitting on your spice rack. Just make sure it's still nice and aromatic before you use it medicinally.

To make a sage infusion, put 4 heaping tablespoons of dried sage in a cup of hot water. Cover tightly and steep for 4 hours or more.

Activate yourself aerobically. How long and how often you should get a move on depends on your current level of fitness. If you have been inactive, for instance, start by walking at a comfortable pace for 15 minutes, 3 days a week. Gradually increase your time, frequency, and intensity until you are going for 20 to 60 minutes every day. If you like, you can switch from walking to bicycling, swimming, rowing, or aerobic dance—that is, any activity that elevates your heart rate.

Research has proved that regular exercise helps combat weight gain, heart disease, and osteoporosis—conditions for which a woman's risk increases following menopause, says Mona Shangold, M.D., director of the Center for Women's Health and Sports Gynecology in Philadelphia. It may also improve your mood and the quality of your sleep.

Lift weights two or three times a week. Strength training helps to prevent the muscle loss and weakness that are inevitable in older, sedentary women after menopause, explains Dr. Shangold. You can use dumbbells, a barbell, or strength-training machines. It all depends on what you're most comfortable with.

If you haven't tried lifting weights before, contact your YM/YWCA or local health club for a reference to an experienced, knowledgeable instructor. An instructor can show you proper form and technique, then supervise you until you have it down pat.

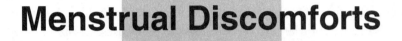

Menstrual Discomforts

Figure 1 or 2 days a month, 12 months a year, from age 14 to age 50 or so. Subtract some time off for pregnancy, and that's about 2 years' worth of menstrual cramps by the time a woman reaches the end of her reproductive years. Add in tagalong symptoms—backaches, bloating, nausea, diarrhea, fatigue, and headaches—and that's a heck of a lot of time spent feeling not-so-great.

Most women have some menstrual discomfort at some point in their lives. Older teenagers and women in their thirties typically experience the most pain.

Cramps, headaches, diarrhea, and fatigue are caused by chemicals called prostaglandins that are released into the body during menstruation. Certain prostaglandins cause blood vessels in the uterus to constrict, for example, decreasing bloodflow to the area. The uterine muscle then goes into spasm, tensing up like a tight fist. Older women sometimes have so-called congestive menstrual pain, thought to be due to poor fluid flow in the pelvis and usually preceded by premenstrual bloating, headaches, and breast pain, explains Mary Bove, N.D., a naturopathic physician at the Brattleboro Naturopathic Clinic in Vermont.

Ibuprofen—the standard drug approach for relieving menstrual discomfort—targets prostaglandins. "This drug inhibits the body's production of cramp-causing prostaglandins, and it works best if you start taking it before the specific prostaglandin that causes the uterine spasms is released into the bloodstream," says Robin Phillips, M.D., a doctor in the department of gynecology at Mount Sinai Medical Center in New York City. If you go this route, she suggests taking 400 milligrams of ibuprofen just prior to or at the onset of pain and then every 6 to 8 hours, with food, for the first day or two of your period. (*Note:* If you have a history of ulcers, Dr. Phillips cautions against using ibuprofen.)

Ibuprofen isn't your only option, however. Here's what else you can do for menstrual problems.

Try cramp-easing herbs. Two in particular, black haw and cramp bark, have a long history of use to relax the muscles of the uterus and relieve menstrual cramps, says Dr. Bove. In fact, black haw works so well

WHEN TO SEE THE DOCTOR

If you have severe cramps and heavy bleeding (defined as bleeding through a pad and or tampon every hour), try lying down, suggests Mary Lake Polan, M.D., Ph.D., professor of gynecology at Stanford University School of Medicine. If the bleeding continues at that rate for 12 to 24 hours, call your doctor.

You should also call your doctor in the following circumstances, says Dr. Polan: if you have heavy bleeding and lower abdominal pain and cramping and believe that you could be pregnant; if you have heavy bleeding and feel weak and light-headed; if you have severe menstrual cramps for the first time or start passing clots for the first time; if you are on birth control pills and have severe cramps; if you have nausea, headaches, fever, diarrhea, and vomiting as well as cramps; or if your cramps interfere with normal activity and aren't relieved by self-care, including normal doses of aspirin or ibuprofen.

that it is sometimes used to help prevent miscarriage. "I tend to use both, interchangeably or in combination," she says.

If your cramps are mild, make a tea: Add 2 teaspoons dried black haw or cramp bark per cup of water. Boil 10 minutes, cool, strain, and drink up to three cups a day. Severe cramps may require stronger medicine: a teaspoon dose of herbal tincture every ½ hour for 2 to 3 hours, Dr. Bove says. It is best not to wait until your pain peaks to start dosing, she adds. "Women who regularly have cramps may want to start taking this a few days before they expect their periods." Since these herbs (which can be purchased at health food stores) contain an aspirin-like compound, they should not be used by women who are sensitive to aspirin.

Note: A tincture is a highly concentrated herbal liquid. It's made by soaking leaves in alcohol or glycerin—which extracts the herb's medicinal properties—for at least 6 weeks. Tinctures are sold in health food stores in small bottles with eyedroppers to give doses. Be sure to store them out of the reach of children.

Sip ginger tea. This pungent spice has several properties that make it a good choice for menstrual cramps: It reduces inflammation and muscle spasms; it dilates blood vessels and so increases bloodflow; and it has warming, energizing character that helps dispel sluggishness, Dr. Bove says. Add six to eight thin slices or a couple of teaspoons grated fresh or ground ginger to 2 cups freshly boiled water and simmer 15 to 20 minutes. Strain before drinking. "You can add ginger to cramp bark tea to augment the effects of cramp bark," she adds.

Get in the tub. Fill your tub with comfortably warm water, then add 5 drops each of bergamot, chamomile, and rosemary essential oils, along with 10 drops of evening primrose oil. Then soak in the tub, adding hot water as necessary to keep the water warm, suggests Dr. Bove. "These essential oils have tension-relieving and muscle-relaxing qualities."

Pressure yourself. The traditional Chinese acupressure points for relieving menstrual cramps are found in the middle of the crease where the leg joins the trunk of the body, explains Michael Reed Gach, Ph.D., director and founder of the Acupressure Institute in Berkeley, California. You can press here with your fingertips, or you can stimulate these points one at a time by positioning your left fist over the points on your left side and your right fist over the right side, then, lying on your stomach with your fists in place, using the weight of your body to apply pressure. Find a comfortable position to relax in for at least 2 minutes, Dr. Gach says.

Walk pelvic problems off. Walking stimulates the pelvic region and gets fluids moving through the area, so it reduces pelvic congestion, says Dr. Bove. "I tell women to work on opening their pelvis, letting their hips lead their stroke as they walk, letting their hips and arms swing freely so that their whole body has a chance to stretch out." A daily 20-minute-or-so walk will decrease the likelihood of cramps, reduce them if you have them, and brighten your mood, she says.

Drink lots of water. No one knows why, but "it's been shown scientifically that increased hydration relieves menstrual cramps," says Dr. Phillips. "If a woman happens to be in the hospital when she has her period and the flow of fluid through her IV is increased, the cramps get better. I tell women to drink as much water as they can until their cramps go away, then cut back." This is particularly helpful in the summer, she says, when women are more likely to be slightly dehydrated.

Friendly Foods

For long-term prevention of menstrual discomfort, you need to make some dietary changes. Doctors offer these recommendations.

Lighten up. Reduce your consumption of meats; dairy products such as butter, full-fat cheese, and whole milk; and egg yolks. The saturated fat in these foods contains a type of prostaglandins that triggers muscle contractions. So you will want to cut back on fat from these sources.

Eat more fish and raw nuts and seeds. Flax, sunflower, sesame, and pumpkin seeds and certain fish, such as trout, mackerel, and salmon, contain two kinds of fatty acids—linoleic and linolenic. These fatty acids help relax muscles, says Dr. Bove.

You can also try capsule supplements of evening primrose or black currant oil, which also contain linoleic and linolenic acids, says Dr. Bove. She prescribes 1,000 to 3,000 milligrams a day, depending on the severity of the symptoms. Be sure to take the supplements daily with meals for 3 to 6 months. Both supplements can be purchased at health food stores.

Mineralize. Magnesium and calcium play an important role in maintaining normal muscle tone. Take 500 to 600 milligrams of each. Getting enough of both can help your muscles relax, reducing the severity of menstrual cramps, says Dr. Bove. "I like to use equal amounts of both, as liquid or buffered supplements, which seem to get into the muscles faster than tablets," she says. "I tell women to try these daily supplements and other dietary changes for at least 3 months because it often takes some time to see an improvement."

But taking magnesium and calcium only when you have cramps isn't likely to be helpful, adds Adriane Fugh-Berman, M.D., chairperson of the National Women's Health Network. "You need to take them during the entire month."

If you have heart or kidney problems, talk to your doctor before taking supplemental magnesium. Also, if you experience diarrhea when taking these supplements, cut back your dosage until your symptoms subside.

Get your Bs and E. The B vitamins are important—especially vitamin B_6—because they help your body metabolize hormones. Dr. Fugh-Berman recommends taking a daily 50-milligram supplement of a B-complex vitamin formula all month long.

Also add vitamin E. In clinical studies, 150 IU of vitamin E—administered daily for 10 days premenstrually and during the first 4 days of the menstrual cycle—helped relieve menstrual discomfort within two menstrual cycles in approximately 70 percent of the women who tried it.

Vitamin E also seems to relieve heavy bleeding, Dr. Bove says. "I'll start someone on 800 IU daily, and then increase to 1,200 IU in the days before menses begins. I might have them use 1,200 to 1,600 IU during days of heavy bleeding, and then, as their bleeding decreases, decrease the dosage." Usually, by the second or third cycle, they no longer have heavy days, she says. Before taking amounts above 600 IU, you should check with your doctor, she adds.

Consider vitamin A. Some doctors have women with heavy menstrual bleeding take extra vitamin A for several months to see if it lightens their bleeding. "I wouldn't recommend vitamin A alone but might give an amount higher than the Daily Value of 5,000 IU in a good multivitamin or even a prenatal vitamin," Dr. Bove says. In one study, 71 women with heavy bleeding had significantly lower blood levels of vitamin A than women with normal periods. And when these women were given 25,000 IU of vitamin A twice a day for 15 days, blood loss normalized or was reduced in more than 90 percent of the women. "I'd stick with no more than 25,000 IU a day," she adds.

Any vitamin A supplement of more than 15,000 IU a day should be taken only with medical supervision. Women who are pregnant should rely on their doctor-prescribed prenatal vitamins and avoid taking vitamin A supplements altogether.

Overweight

Every year, more than half of all Americans are either dieting or trying to keep off pounds that they have already lost. For too many of us, weight wars wage on and on. Why do we have so little success when it comes to weight loss?

"I think it's because we want a quick fix rather than a long-term cure," says Cheryl Norton, Ed.D., professor of human performance, sport, and leisure studies at the Metropolitan State College of Denver. "Once typical Americans pass age 20, they gain about a pound a year because they live sedentary lifestyles. So they try all sorts of diets and even starve themselves to take off the weight fast." Sure, the extra pounds disappear . . . for a while. But inevitably, they creep back on.

Make no mistake: If you are overweight, you will do yourself a world of good by aiming for a healthier weight—one that's right for your age and your size, says G. Michael Steelman, M.D., a physician in Oklahoma City. To figure out your healthy weight, you can use the following guideline recommended by Dr. Steelman: Start at around 100 pounds if you are 5 feet or taller. Then add 5 pounds for every inch that you are over 5 feet. To that number, add 10 percent if you have a large frame, or subtract 10 percent if you have a small frame.

If you want to slim down sensibly and permanently, there is only one "secret formula" that works: You must burn more calories than you consume. You can do that by eating healthfully and exercising regularly.

Before you start, try to be realistic about your goals. *Baywatch* bodies don't come overnight, and drastic measures can hinder more than they help. A reasonable goal is losing no more than 2 pounds per week. Take off more than that, and your metabolism (your body's calorie-burning mechanism) will slow down in an effort to conserve energy. "It's your body's way of protecting you from starvation," explains Dr. Norton. Your weight loss will taper off, and you'll regain those pounds quite easily.

Also, it's better to start your weight-loss program in the spring or summer. You naturally tend to eat more during the fall and winter months, when the weather turns cold. That undermines your chances for success from the get-go. Warm weather, on the other hand, encourages you to head outdoors and get active. Finally, if you use a scale to monitor your progress, weigh yourself at the same time every day. Your weight fluctuates over the course of 24 hours. Stepping on the scale in the morning one day and at bedtime the next can leave you with an inaccurate (and discouraging) picture of how you are doing.

Start with the Obvious

This is pretty simple: Watch what you eat. Well, you might say, I've already done that, and it didn't work. That's because what you probably did was diet. Diet books come and go because diets don't work in the long run. If they did, millions of people would be skinny, and these so-called diet experts would have to do something else—probably something less lucrative—to earn a living. Still, eating right isn't exactly easy either, or else overweight wouldn't be as big a problem as it is in this country. The following basics will help you get the hang of eating like a loser—a weight loser, that is.

Measure serving sizes. "Many women have cut way back on dietary fat but overcompensate with too large portions of fat-free or low-fat foods," says Dr. Steelman. "These foods can be quite high in calories."

WHEN TO SEE THE DOCTOR

If you exceed your healthy weight by 20 percent or more, you have a higher-than-average risk for developing health problems such as heart disease, diabetes, and some forms of cancer. You should see your doctor for a checkup and for assistance in developing a weight management program that works for you.

Favor fiber. Most weight-loss experts agree: If you want to lose weight, eat more foods high in fiber, such as fruits, vegetables, beans, potatoes, and whole grains. High-fiber foods take up more space in your stomach than fat-laden fare, and they tend to be low in fat and calories.

But fiber-rich foods do more than shush a growling tummy. Fiber may slightly reduce the number of calories your body absorbs from food each day.

Fiber also stabilizes levels of glucose, or blood sugar, your body's main source of fuel, says Dana Myatt, N.D., a naturopathic physician in Phoenix. Some people produce higher-than-normal amounts of insulin, the hormone that controls the rate at which blood sugar is absorbed by cells. In response to this abnormally high insulin level, the body manufactures more fat cells than normal. The more fat cells you have, the slower your metabolism is likely to become, and the more likely you are to gain weight. Fiber-rich foods don't appear to stimulate the production of insulin as much as foods made with white flour, such as white bread and baked goods, do.

Divide and conquer. Break your usual three meals a day into five or six mini-meals. By eating smaller meals more often, you stave off hunger and prevent yourself from overeating when you finally do sit down at the table, says Dr. Steelman.

Eat breakfast every morning. Breakfast jump-starts your metabolism and keeps calories burning efficiently throughout the day, says Dr. Steelman. Plus, by filling up first thing in the A.M., you are less likely to overindulge at lunch or dinner.

For breakfast, choose healthful foods such as toast with all-fruit preserves, fat-free or low-fat yogurt, or fat-free or low-fat cottage cheese with fruit. Fatty, sugary foods such as doughnuts and Danish send your blood sugar for a roller-coaster ride. That pumps up your appetite and sparks sugar cravings, according to Dr. Steelman.

Build up your stash. Keep healthful snacks such as dried fruit, single-serving cans of vegetable juice, and low-fat granola bars in your purse, briefcase, or car. These foods make great antidotes for between-meal munchies. They satisfy your hunger without a lot of calories or fat, notes Ingrid Lofgren, R.D., of the University of Massachusetts Medical Center in Worcester.

Eat dinner at least 3 hours before going to bed. Based on his patients' experience, Dr. Steelman has concluded that people who eat the majority of their calories close to bedtime have a harder time losing weight. Blame it on your body's metabolism: It slows down at night, so your body stores fat more easily.

If you must eat less than 3 hours before hitting the sack, choose fruits, vegetables, whole grains, and lean proteins such as fat-free or low-fat dairy products. These foods supply the most vitamins and minerals in exchange for a modest number of calories, explains Dr. Steelman.

Pepper your food with cayenne. Add a dash of cayenne pepper (also known as red pepper) or hot-pepper sauce (like Tabasco) to your food several times a day, suggests Dr. Myatt. The active ingredient in cayenne pepper, capsaicin, is a stimulant of saliva, salivary amylase (an enzyme involved in the digestion of starch), and hydrochloric acid, which improve the digestive process, she says. "People with sluggish digestion tend to gain weight. Those with efficient digestion tend to maintain a normal weight."

Capsaicin may also accelerate metabolism. In research conducted at Oxford Polytechnic Institute in England, dieters who added 1 teaspoon of red-pepper sauce and 1 teaspoon of mustard to every meal raised their metabolic rates by as much as 25 percent.

Treat yourself to tea. Drink one cup of green tea with a meal two or three times a day, suggests Dr. Myatt. Green tea contains caffeine, a stimulant that revs up metabolism, as well as theobromine, a compound similar to caffeine. Depending on how long it's steeped, one cup of green tea contains from 40 to 100 milligrams of caffeine—up to the amount in one cup of coffee. So if you're cutting back on caffeine for other reasons, don't drink more than two or three cups.

Green tea has something that coffee doesn't, however: It's rich in vitamin C and flavonoids, compounds that are potent antioxidants. These protective nutrients help reduce the risk of illnesses such as heart disease and cancer, especially of the colon. And it promotes weight loss due to its thermogenic effect, which improves metabolism, Dr. Myatt says.

Green tea is sold in health food stores and some supermarkets. It is sold as loose, dried tea leaves and in tea bags, which is an easier form to use for some people, she says. It also comes in capsule form. The recommended dosage is usually two capsules three times a day, says Dr. Myatt, but she prefers the tea because you get a lot more of the antioxidants in a cup than you will in a pill.

Measure out a mix to get your metabolism going. Schisandra berry (which means "five-flavor seed" in Chinese) grows in the most remote parts of the world. Gum guggul is extracted from a plant related to myrrh, and bladderwrack is a type of brown seaweed. Team these exotic ingredients with some basic herbs, and the result is a remedy that very gently helps weight loss along by improving metabolism, says David Winston, an herbalist in Washington, New Jersey. Blend the following tinctures (also called extracts) in an 8-ounce or larger bottle: 1 ounce of nettle, 1 ounce of dandelion leaf, 1 ounce of bladderwrack, 2 ounces of guggul, and 2 ounces of Chinese schisandra berry (all are available at health food stores). Take ½ to 1 teaspoon three times a day. (Hold your nose, though: This concoction isn't the most pleasant-tasting around, says Winston.)

Bladderwrack is a folk remedy for overweight. Schizandrin, the active ingredient in schisandra berry, gently stimulates metabolism. Dandelion is used by herbalists to boost the liver's secretion of bile, which helps break down the fats in food. Nettle is rich in minerals, which help maintain overall health during weight loss, Winston says. And guggul helps normalize thyroid function, which is sometimes disturbed in overweight people.

Note: A tincture is a highly concentrated herbal liquid. It's made by soaking leaves in alcohol or glycerin—which extracts the herb's medicinal properties—for at least 6 weeks. Tinctures are sold in health food stores in small bottles with eyedroppers to give doses. Be sure to always store them out of the reach of children.

Burn Off That Weight

Exercise is an essential component of the weight-loss equation. Remember that to slim down, you need to burn more calories than you consume. And the best way to burn more calories is to work out regularly. To develop a more physically active lifestyle, give these tips a try.

Aerobicize. Do at least 30 minutes of aerobic exercise 5 to 7 days a week, suggests Dr. Steelman. *Aerobic* doesn't necessarily mean desperately trying to keep up in a killer kickboxing class. While that will burn off those excess calories, there are plenty of other less intense options out there. Aerobic exercise can be any activity that makes you breathe harder and your heart beat faster, like walking, running, or bicycling.

It's very important to choose an aerobic activity that you enjoy. The more you like what you're doing, the more you will want to stick with it, notes Dr. Steelman.

Grab some iron. You don't need to be a female bodybuilder to benefit from weights. Lifting weights helps you lose weight because it increases muscle tone in your body. Since muscle burns more calories than fat, your metabolism speeds up. And it stays up, whether you are active or at rest. And don't worry about looking like a refugee from the World Wrestling Federation. Male hormones like testosterone are what build Schwarzenegger-style bodies, and you have very little of that. To get those kinds of muscles, you'll probably need a little illegal pharmaceutical assistance. Without that, you'll just have a toned, feminine body that gobbles up calories even as you sleep.

You can do a combination of strength training and aerobic exercise on the days you work out or alternate between aerobic exercise one day and strength training the next. Just be sure to substitute strength training for aerobic exercise on no more than three of your workout days, Dr. Steelman adds.

Find moments to move. Use little ways to increase your physical activity throughout the day. If you walk to work, for example, tack an extra block onto your route. You will burn 10 more calories per day, or roughly 3,500 more calories per year, the number of calories in one pound of fat, says Dr. Norton. Some other strategies are to take the stairs instead of the elevator, go for a brisk walk at lunch, and park your car at the far end of the parking lot when you go to the supermarket.

Tension Headaches and Migraines

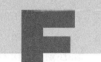

From bad-hair days to bounced checks, life sometimes seems like one headache after another. But truth be told, most of us would prefer these minor annoyances to the real McCoy—the persistent, pounding pain that grips our heads from time to time and then stubbornly refuses to let go.

Headaches occur for any number of reasons. They can be driven by emotional factors, such as depression or anxiety, or by high blood pressure, says Seymour Diamond, M.D., director of the Diamond Headache Clinic in Chicago. Blocked or inflamed sinuses can trigger headache pain. Even changes in your sleeping or eating pattern can make your head hurt because they disrupt your body's internal clock, explains Joseph P. Primavera III, Ph.D., a psychologist at Thomas Jefferson University Hospital in Philadelphia.

But the most common by far are tension headaches. Almost everyone—about 90 percent of the population—has experienced a tension headache at some point, says Fred D. Sheftell, M.D., founder and codirector of the New England Center for Headache in Stamford, Connecticut. The pain typically starts in the muscles at the back of your head and neck and works its way to your forehead. You may feel mild throbbing in your temples or just behind your eyes.

Tension headaches are usually a by-product of stress, but even sitting in a cramped position or straining your eyes at a computer screen can provoke pain. Fortunately, these headaches generally last no more than a few hours, and they often respond to over-the-counter pain relievers or just quiet relaxation, Dr. Sheftell says.

A migraine, on the other hand, can last from 4 hours to 3 days, says Dr. Diamond. And the pain's duration only magnifies its intensity. Typically, a migraine begins as a dull ache that progresses to an overwhelming, throbbing agony. Sometimes the pain is preceded by an aura, a visual disturbance characterized by brightly colored lines, flashes of light, dots, or spots. The pain itself usually affects only one side of the head. But you may feel ill all over with nausea, numbness, weakness, and extreme sensitivity to light and noise.

Approximately 65 percent of women who experience migraines get their headaches around the time of their periods, a fact that Dr. Diamond attributes to changing levels of the hormone estrogen throughout the menstrual cycle. Scientists can't yet explain the mechanics of it, but somehow these hormonal fluctuations make women more susceptible to the chemical chain reaction that causes blood vessels feeding the brain to rapidly constrict and then expand, producing pain. For similar reasons, some women who take hormone-replacement therapy during or after menopause also experience migraines during the interval when they are not taking estrogen. For example, if a woman takes hormone replacement for 21 days and then is off for 7 days, she may experience a headache during the 7-day drug-free period.

Headache Help

Tension headaches respond well to certain herbs. When pain sets in, turn to one of these herbal remedies for relief. (All of these herbs are available in health food stores and some drugstores.)

WHEN TO SEE THE DOCTOR

If your headache is accompanied by any of the following symptoms, have someone take you to an emergency room right away, advises Seymour Diamond, M.D., director of the Diamond Headache Clinic in Chicago: fainting; seizures; clear fluid or blood coming from your nose or ears; vomiting; a stiff neck, along with nausea and fever; problems with speech, coordination, or vision; weakness or numbness on one side of your body; fever of 101°F or higher; or lethargy immediately after a head injury.

Make a mix. Make yourself a soothing herbal tea of equal parts wood betony, chamomile, vervain, and lavender. These herbs are tonics that relieve pain, gently relax your body, and help release tension. They can improve the way your body handles stress and, if used regularly, can help reduce the frequency of tension headaches, explains Elizabeth Wotton, N.D., a naturopathic physician in Plymouth, Massachusetts.

To make the tea, simply steep 1 heaping teaspoon of the herb blend in 1 quart freshly boiled water for 10 minutes, says Dr. Wotton. Strain the herbs and allow the tea to cool before sipping it. If you have a tension headache, drink one to two cups. If you are prone to tension headaches, drink up to four cups a day.

Soak in a lukewarm herbal bath for 20 minutes. Steep 2 tablespoons lavender and 2 tablespoons lemon balm in 1 cup hot water for 10 minutes, then pour the tea into your bathwater, says Dr. Wotton.

Rub out the pain. Choose peppermint essential oil if you have a headache in the front of your head, because the scent's stimulating effects help improve circulation and draw energy away from the pain. Choose lavender essential oil if you have pain in the back of your head, because the scent's relaxing properties help soothe muscle spasms.

To use either oil, moisten your fingertip with less than a drop. Then rub the oil on your temples, across your forehead, and on the back of your neck, suggests Michael Scholes, director of the Michael Scholes School of Aromatic Studies in Los Angeles. If the oil is working, you should feel a slight tingling sensation. Repeat again within the hour if necessary. You can buy essential oils in health food stores.

Migraine Minimizers

Among headaches, migraine is exceptionally excruciating—and stubborn, too. But you don't have to just live with the pain. The following remedies can help rein in migraine and its symptoms.

Try feverfew. If your migraines are the type that feel as if the top of your head is about to explode, the herb feverfew may help, say David Winston, an herbalist in Washington, New Jersey. Research demonstrates that small amounts of feverfew can prevent migraines, according to Winston. The herb contains parthenolide, a substance that, along with other constituents of the plant, may maintain levels of serotonin, a nerve messenger, within blood platelets. Serotonin helps to reduce pain.

Nutrition Prescriptions for Menstrual Migraines

Are your migraines as predictable as your periods? That's no coincidence. For many women, monthly hormonal fluctuations set the stage for migraines both before and during menstruation. You can reduce your chances of developing a migraine at "that time of the month" with the following vitamin and mineral supplements, recommended by Fred D. Sheftell, M.D., founder and codirector of the New England Center for Headache in Stamford, Connecticut.

- Take 200 to 400 milligrams of riboflavin every day. Riboflavin might play a role in the way your brain's energy system works, improving its ability to short-circuit migraine pain.

- Take 50 milligrams a day of vitamin B$_6$ the week before your period. Then increase your dosage to 100 milligrams a day and continue the supplements right

"I recommend taking ½ teaspoon daily of feverfew tincture (also called an extract) made from the whole leaf (the bottle usually indicates if it is from whole leaves) or 500 milligrams in capsule form once a day," says Lisa Alschuler, N.D., a naturopathic physician and chairperson of the department of botanical medicine at Bastyr University in Bothell, Washington.

Note: A tincture is a highly concentrated herbal liquid. It's made by soaking leaves in alcohol or glycerin—which extracts the herb's medicinal properties—for at least 6 weeks. Tinctures are sold in health food stores in small bottles with eyedroppers to give doses. Be sure to always store them out of the reach of children.

through your period. Vitamin B$_6$ stimulates production of serotonin, a brain chemical that constricts blood vessels and so staves off migraine. Don't rely on the benefits of B$_6$ on a daily basis, however. Unstable gait and numb feet may occur with doses of vitamin B$_6$ at 50 milligrams to 2 grams daily over a prolonged time.

- Take 400 IU of vitamin E every day. Vitamin E helps to stabilize your body's level of the hormone estrogen. The vitamin's antioxidant properties may have some benefit as well.

- Take 200 to 400 milligrams of magnesium a day. Research has shown that women who get migraines during their periods tend to have low levels of this mineral in their brain cells.

  If you have heart or kidney problems, check with your doctor before taking magnesium supplements. Some people who take 350 milligrams or more of supplemental magnesium a day may experience diarrhea.

- Take a daily multivitamin in addition to the supplements above. That way, you can be sure that all your nutritional bases are covered.

Get some ginkgo. Ginkgo improves blood supply to the brain, helps maintain vascular tone, and keeps the blood vessels from leaking inflammatory chemicals. Therefore, it helps prevent the initial vasoconstriction and ischemia (blood deficiency) that can occur in classic migraines, says Tieraona Low Dog, M.D., a family practice physician at the University of New Mexico Hospital in Albuquerque.

For migraine prevention, Dr. Alschuler recommends taking ginkgo in standardized extract capsules, 40 milligrams per capsule two or three times a day.

Ginkgo has been shown to have potentially harmful interactions with some pharmaceutical drugs (MAO inhibitors) and should never be used with aspirin or other nonsteroidal anti-inflammatory medicines.

Freeze your head. Apply ice for 10 minutes to the part of your head that hurts. Some women find that cold works better than heat in relieving their migraines. Cold helps constrict expanded blood vessels and block pain messages to your brain. If you get headaches a lot, fill a paper cup with water and put it in your freezer, suggests Robert Kunkel, M.D., of the headache section for the Cleveland Clinic Foundation in Cleveland. Then when you need a cold compress, just tear off the top inch of the cup and rub the ice against your head. You can also buy a gel pack and keep it on the ready in your freezer.

Have some coffee. The caffeine that coffee contains helps constrict dilated blood vessels in the brain, says Patricia Solbach, Ph.D., director of the Center for Clinical Research at the Menninger Center for Clinical Research in Topeka, Kansas. Be careful, though: Too much coffee can make your pain even worse. Limit your daily intake to one 5-ounce cup, which contains about 100 milligrams of caffeine.

Preventive Points

If you are prone to headaches, you can take steps to reduce their frequency and intensity with the following strategies.

Keep a headache diary to track down what triggers your pain. When you get a headache, make note of what you have eaten in the previous 24 hours, what you are doing when the pain sets in, whether you are under stress, whether your period is approaching, or any other factors that you think may be connected to your headache, Dr. Primavera says. Then after 2 weeks, see if you notice any pattern to your pain so that you can start to eliminate or regulate those triggers in your life.

Bypass cured meats such as frankfurters, bologna, and salami. These foods contain nitrites, which trigger migraines in some people. Other common offenders include monosodium glutamate (found in Chinese food as well as lunchmeats and frozen dinners), aspartame (an artificial sweetener that goes by the brand name NutraSweet), and tyramine (an amino acid found in aged cheeses, pickled herring, and the pods of lima beans and snow peas). In general, if you end up with a migraine more than half the time after you eat a particular food, then you should not be eating it, advises Dr. Sheftell.

Limit yourself to one drink a day. Alcoholic beverages—particularly red wine and beer—are notorious for triggering migraines, because the alcohol makes blood vessels dilate. In fact, if you consistently get a migraine after imbibing, you should cut out the booze entirely, advises Dr. Diamond. A drink, incidentally, is defined as one 12-ounce beer, one 5-ounce glass of wine, or a mixed drink made with 1½ ounces of liquor.

Urinary Tract Infections

"Every year around the third week in September—just as predictably as the leaves turn color—teachers in the state of Maine show up in my office with urinary tract infections," says Brenda Sexton, M.D., director of Internal Medicine for Women in Yarmouth, Maine.

The cause, says Dr. Sexton, can be traced to a typical schoolteacher morning: a cup of coffee at home, a quick restroom break before classes begin, then no opportunities to void until lunchtime. And after lunch, no toilet breaks occur again for several hours, until the children go home. To avoid the discomfort of a full bladder, schoolteachers avoid drinking water.

"Even 8 ounces of water means disaster," says Dr. Sexton.

Within a few weeks of limited water intake and infrequent voiding, a teacher will wake up in the night with the urge to urinate. Yet when she goes to the bathroom, she feels burning, stinging pain, accompanied by the feeling that she hasn't completely voided—signs of a urinary tract infection, or UTI, says Dr. Sexton.

The constant need to urinate and feeling pain along with a stinging sensation when urinating are the classic characteristics of UTIs, says

Paul Nyirjesy, M.D., associate professor of obstetrics and gynecology at Temple University School of Medicine in Philadelphia.

Schoolteachers aren't the only ones who get them. One out of five women will get a UTI at some time in her life . . . eight times as often as men do. And if a woman gets one infection, she has a good chance of getting more. UTIs account for nearly 7 million doctors' visits a year, more than any other disorder besides colds and flu. And treatment costs are estimated at $1 billion a year, according to the American Medical Women's Association.

Dr. Sexton's experience—treating women for UTIs at the same time every year—demonstrates just one of the many classic conditions that foster this infection.

UTIs occur when bacteria make their way up the urethra, the little pipe through which your urine exits, says Richard J. Macchia, M.D., professor of urology at the State University of New York Health Science Center at Brooklyn. Bacteria often get pushed up the urethra during in-

WHEN TO SEE THE DOCTOR

Before treating symptoms of what may be a urinary tract infection (UTI), make an appointment with your doctor to rule out vaginitis or a sexually transmitted disease such as chlamydia. You want to be sure that you're about to treat the right condition.

If your symptoms are accompanied by fever, chills, nausea, vomiting, upper back pain, or blood in the urine, call your doctor immediately. This could be a sign of a more serious problem. And always see a doctor if you have any symptoms of a UTI and you are pregnant, have diabetes, or have any other serious illness.

Also, if you have more than two UTIs (or what you think are UTIs) within 6 months or more than three episodes in a year, see a doctor.

tercourse, and condoms and diaphragms also have been associated with an increase in the number of infections.

Other peak times for UTIs are right before menstruation, when hormonal changes are thought to have an effect, and at menopause, when the vaginal walls thin out and become more susceptible to bacteria, says Helene Leonetti, M.D., an obstetrician/gynecologist in Bethlehem, Pennsylvania. UTIs also often occur within the first few weeks of having a new sex partner, though no one knows exactly why (although it probably has something to do with the frequency of sex).

These year-round conditions set the stage. Cut back on your water intake and voiding habits—as did the schoolteachers Dr. Sexton observed—and you eliminate one of nature's means of flushing the system of bacteria.

Nature's UTI Neutralizers

If you are otherwise healthy, urinary tract infections will usually clear up themselves within 3 to 7 days, says Dr. Macchia. But most women don't want to live with the pain that long, so doctors generally prescribe a 3- to 5-day regimen of antibiotics. If you can't get to a doctor for some reason or you want some relief in addition to medication, try these natural prescriptions.

Drink one glass of water every hour for 8 hours. Drinking a lot of water increases urine flow, explains Kristene E. Whitmore, M.D., chief of urology and director of the Incontinence Center at Graduate Hospital in Philadelphia. This washes out the bacteria that are attempting to adhere to the cells lining your urethra.

Stunt bacteria growth with some C. Taking 2,000 milligrams of vitamin C every day for up to 3 days inhibits the growth of bacteria, says Dr. Macchia.

Taking more than 1,200 milligrams of vitamin C a day may cause diarrhea in some people. If this happens to you, switch to a buffered supplement.

Stop the sticking with cranberry. Drink three 8-ounce glasses of cranberry juice cocktail every day until you urinate normally again, says Dr. Macchia. For decades, women and their doctors have been using cranberry juice as a treatment for UTIs. This modern folk remedy was once thought to stunt bacterial growth by acidifying urine. But several studies now suggest that cranberry juice contains a substance that prevents bacteria from sticking to the walls of the urethra, thus helping to control infection.

As an alternative to drinking cranberry juice, take three cranberry capsules a day, suggests Dr. Leonetti. Available in health food stores, cranberry capsules provide the healing effect of cranberry juice cocktail without all the sugar.

Avoid coffee, tea, colas, alcohol, and citrus fruits and juices. The acids in these foods and beverages act as stimulants, increasing the frequency and urgency of urination, says Gretchen Lentz, M.D., professor of obstetrics/gynecology at the University of Washington in Seattle.

Have a seat. Sitting in an herbal sitz bath can help relieve the external burning of a UTI and hasten healing, says Feather Jones, an herbalist in Boulder, Colorado. She recommends using uva-ursi and marshmallow root powder. To make this soothing soak, boil 1 gallon of water and add a handful of powdered uva-ursi leaves (approximately 1 ounce by weight). Steep for 20 minutes, then strain. Add 1 ounce of marshmallow powder. Transfer the brew to a large pan, be sure the water is comfortably warm, and soak for 20 minutes. Jones suggests doing this once or twice a day for several days or as long as it's needed.

"Uva-ursi is an astringent, so it will help reduce swelling, and the marshmallow root soothes irritated tissues," says Jones.

Pick up this perennial herb. "Goldenrod is the number one urinary herb in Europe," says Ed Smith, an herbalist in Williams, Oregon. A tea made from the yellow flowering tops of this perennial herb is an ultra-safe, mildly astringent antiseptic that promotes healing of inflammation in the urinary tract. Steep 1 well-rounded teaspoon in 1 cup of hot water for 5 to 10 minutes, then strain. Drink three to four cups a day of this gentle, diuretic tea until your symptoms are gone.

Try this tongue twister to terminate a UTI. The herb pipsissewa will increase urine flow and stimulate the removal of waste products from the body. The herb contains substances called hydroquinones, which have a disinfectant effect on the urinary tract. So this should help wash away bacteria and relieve pain and itching.

Steep 1 teaspoon of dried leaves in 1 cup of hot water for 10 to 15 minutes, then strain. Drink this tea three times a day until your infection is gone.

Ease irritation with marshmallow. Marshmallow makes a thick, rather slimy tea that works as a demulcent to soothe irritation in the urinary tract, says Lynn Newman, a medical herbalist in Glen Head, New York. Both the leaves and root contain mucilagen, the substance in the plant that makes it slimy. The root, which contains about 35 percent mucilagen, is generally available in the United States. Marshmallow is particularly useful for older adults who have chronic inflammation of the urinary tract. Make a solution of 1 teaspoon of root powder soaked in 1 cup of cold water overnight. Drink it one to three times a day for as long as you have the infection.

Wear cotton underwear. Bacteria grow in warm, moist environments. Cool, absorbent cotton won't allow bacteria to thrive. Cotton underwear is especially helpful if you are experiencing external discomfort such as swelling, rawness, or dryness, says Betsy Foxman, Ph.D., associate professor of epidemiology at the University of Michigan School of Public Health in Ann Arbor.

Keeping UTIs from Coming Back

Once your urinary tract is free and clear of infection, experts offer these prescriptions for keeping it so.

Keep on with the cranberry. You should continue drinking three 8-ounce glasses of cranberry juice cocktail every day, especially if you are prone to UTIs. You will know that you are sufficiently hydrated when your urine appears clear like water rather than deep yellow, says Dr. Macchia.

Just go. Go whenever you need to because the more you urinate, the less chance bacteria have to grow and thrive, says Dr. Lentz. Try to urinate every 3 to 4 hours daily.

Void before and after sex. Urinating before intercourse means that bacteria won't have a place to breed; urinating afterward will flush out any bacteria that might have been pushed up the urethra during intercourse, says Dr. Lentz.

Skip the panty hose for a month. You may be getting UTIs because you wear nylon panty hose, says Dr. Foxman. So in addition to switching to cotton underwear, switch to stockings to discourage colonization of bacteria. If you still end up with an infection, at least you know that your undergarments aren't causing the problem.

Check your birth control method. The use of the diaphragm as a birth control method, with and without spermicidal jelly, has been linked to UTIs. So if you are prone to bladder infections, consider another form of birth control, such as a cervical cap, an intrauterine device, or oral contraceptives, says Dr. Lentz.

Condoms have been associated with UTIs, too, says Dr. Foxman. By all means, don't stop using condoms when you have sex. But if you are getting UTIs, try switching to a different type of condom. For example, if you use a spermicidally treated condom, try a lubricated condom instead, she says. If you have been using a lubricated condom, try a condom with a different type of lubricant.

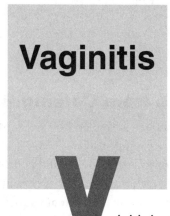

Vaginitis

aginitis is a catchall term for any inflammation of the vagina. Generally, the itching, burning, and discharge that typify vaginitis can be traced to one of three causes: infection, irritation, or hormones.

Yeast infections are one form of vaginitis. (For more information on yeast infections, see page 473.) Another is trichomoniasis, which is an inflammation triggered by a protozoan that invades the genitourinary tracts of men and women alike. Trichomoniasis is transmitted sexually and causes itching, burning, and an abnormal, fishy-smelling discharge.

The most common form of vaginitis is bacterial vaginosis, an infection often associated with, but not caused by, sex. Like trichomoniasis, bacterial vaginosis is characterized by an abnormal, often yellowish, fishy-smelling discharge that often becomes worse after intercourse. Much less commonly, the infection can cause itching and burning pain, says Paul Nyirjesy, M.D., associate professor of obstetrics and gynecology at Temple University School of Medicine in Philadelphia.

As for irritants, reactions to chemicals or other substances in douches, bubble baths, soaps, or even sperm can disturb the vagina, leaving you vulnerable to vaginitis, says Helene Leonetti, M.D., an obstetrician/gynecologist in Bethlehem, Pennsylvania.

Vaginitis can plague a woman any day of the year. But because of changes in hormone levels, women tend to experience symptoms more often before menstruation, during pregnancy, or after menopause, when the vaginal walls become thinner and more susceptible to infection as women lose estrogen, Dr. Leonetti says.

If you think you might have vaginitis, see your doctor without delay, especially if you are sexually active. Though trichomoniasis rarely leads to more serious illness, it may put women at risk for other sexually transmitted diseases. If it goes untreated, bacterial vaginosis may lead to an upper urinary tract infection, pelvic inflammatory disease, premature labor in pregnant women, and post-hysterectomy infection in other women, says Dr. Nyirjesy. For vaginitis, doctors generally prescribe antibiotics or vaginal creams, which can soothe the irritation in 2 to 3 days and prevent complications.

After you have seen a doctor and have your medical prescriptions in hand, try these remedies. They may help speed relief of itching and discomfort.

WHEN TO SEE THE DOCTOR

If you have vaginitis and your symptoms don't start to subside after 2 or 3 days of treatment, consult your health care provider, who can rule out more serious medical conditions such as pelvic inflammatory disease, says Paul Nyirjesy, M.D., associate professor of obstetrics and gynecology at Temple University School of Medicine in Philadelphia.

Get plenty of neutralizing nutrients. Whether your bout with vaginitis is caused by bacteria, yeast, or hormonal changes, supplementing with a powerful arsenal of vitamins and minerals may help shorten the duration and lessen the severity of the infection, says Pamela Sky Jeanne, R.N., N.D., a naturopathic family physician in Gresham, Oregon.

Among these stars are vitamins A, C, and E; beta-carotene; and zinc. Taken together, they can help reduce the pain and inflammation associated with vaginitis, says Dr. Jeanne.

Vitamin A is a renowned infection fighter that will keep vaginal tissues healthy. It cranks up your immune system, stimulates growth of healthy vaginal tissues, strengthens cell membranes, and protects the vagina from further infection. But it does have some drawbacks, she notes. If you take too much, it could affect your liver, and if pregnant

Homeopathic Prescriptions for Vaginitis

Homeopathic remedies can effectively relieve vaginal infections, says Judyth Reichenberg-Ullman, N.D., a naturopathic physician with the Northwest Center for Homeopathic Medicine in Edmonds, Washington, and coauthor of *Homeopathic Self-Care*.

Widely available in most health food stores as tablets, pilules, or granules, homeopathic remedies are extremely diluted doses of substances that would otherwise cause the symptoms that you are experiencing. According to homeopathic practice, the correct remedy depends on your particular constellation of symptoms. Dr. Reichenberg-Ullman suggests trying these remedies.

- Caladium for vaginal infections in which itching is the primary symptom

women take high doses for long periods of time, there's a chance that their babies may have birth defects.

As an alternative, you can take beta-carotene. It helps to produce more vitamin A in your body, but unlike vitamin A, beta-carotene can be taken in large doses without the worry of side effects.

If you have a vaginitis infection, you can take 5,000 to 10,000 IU of vitamin A daily if you're not pregnant, not trying to conceive, and are using a reliable method of birth control, Dr. Jeanne advises. Alternatively, you can take 100,000 IU of beta-carotene daily, she says. But you need to talk to your doctor if you're taking this much beta-carotene.

Similar to vitamin A, vitamin C kicks your immune system into high gear, strengthening your body's ability to fight off the infection. Vitamin C helps reduce the inflammation and strengthens capillary walls and mucous membranes lining your vagina so they can ward off infec-

- Mercurius solubilis or Mercurius vivus for infections with an offensive discharge accompanied by rawness and soreness

- Apis (or honeybee) for vaginal infections accompanied primarily by swelling, but also by redness and soreness, in the genital area

- Kreosotum for vaginitis with extreme burning, rawness, and abrasions in the genital area

Take a 6X dose of the remedy that most closely matches your symptoms up to three times a day, says Dr. Reichenberg-Ullman. (The notation 6X is a standard measurement in homeopathy and refers to a remedy's potency, which is listed on the label.)

Start the remedy at the first sign of symptoms—vaginal discharge, pain, itching, and swelling—and stop as soon as your symptoms improve. "If they are no better after three doses, change to another remedy," advises Dr. Reichenberg-Ullman.

tion. "Make sure the vitamin C you take contains bioflavonoids or rose hips," says Dr. Jeanne. "Bioflavonoids prevent the infected vaginal cells from releasing immune system chemicals called histamines, which cause the inflammation."

Take 2,000 milligrams of vitamin C daily to maintain a healthy vagina, Dr. Jeanne suggests. If you suffer from chronic vaginal infections, take 3,000 to 4,000 milligrams a day over a 2-week period until symptoms improve.

Vitamin E should be the number one nutrient for women during and after menopause, says Dr. Jeanne. Estrogen levels drop and remain low once menopause is under way, leading to the irritation, inflammation, and other vaginal problems related to low estrogen. Dr. Jeanne believes that vitamin E can lower this risk by strengthening the cell membranes lining your vagina. The stronger the membranes, the less likely it is that bacteria will invade them and wreak havoc.

With your doctor's consent, you can take 400 to 800 IU of vitamin E daily, says Dr. Jeanne. Sometimes, higher dosages are recommended, depending on your condition.

The trace mineral zinc is another powerful healer and protector against vaginal infections. It will support your immune system so you can battle infections. It's vital for the production of collagen, the connective tissue that helps wounds heal, and it can create new skin.

During an infection, take 30 to 60 milligrams of zinc daily in divided doses, says Dr. Jeanne. Since zinc can cause stomach upset, you might want to take a partial dose with each of your meals. You shouldn't take zinc if you have certain health conditions, however, so talk to your doctor before starting these dosages.

Comfort yourself with comfrey. An active bout of vaginitis—no matter what the cause—brings burning and stinging. This is especially apparent during trips to the bathroom, when urine makes contact with raw skin. While you are using other treatments or medications to directly address the cause of the problem, the herb called comfrey can be a symptom-relieving comfort, says Virginia Frazer, N.D., a naturopathic physician and licensed midwife in Kennewick, Washington.

Comfrey leaf has anti-inflammatory properties. While it won't cure an infection, rinsing your vaginal area with a tea made from comfrey will soothe inflamed tissues. Make a double-strength tea using 2 heaping tablespoons of dried comfrey leaf to 1 cup of boiling water. Steep, covered, for 10 minutes, then strain the cooled tea into a plastic spray bottle.

Keep the bottle handy when you visit the bathroom, recommends Dr. Frazer. Spray your nether parts liberally as needed to ease the burning. Use it topically as needed for 3 to 5 days.

Avoid bubble baths. Soaps often contain harsh chemicals, which can provoke an allergic reaction leading to vaginitis, says Dr. Leonetti. For similar reasons, don't use commercial douches, feminine hygiene sprays, or scented panty liners while you have vaginitis. Let your insides clean themselves, she advises.

Take time for yourself. Repeated rounds of vaginitis seem to be related to stress, according to Dr. Leonetti. Stress seems to depress immune defenses. And it often triggers cravings for sugary, processed foods, which some experts believe may lead to bacterial imbalances that cause vaginitis.

"Check that you're sleeping enough and not eating junk food," says Dr. Leonetti. "Focus on eating lots of fruits and veggies. Stay away from colas and other caffeinated beverages, which act as stimulants. And most of all, try to relax." She suggests that you choose whatever technique works best for you—deep breathing, listening to music, or just "taking five" for yourself.

Varicose Veins

Ah, summertime. The flowers are in bloom, the skies are blue, and the beach beckons. Meanwhile, you're rifling through your closet, desperately trying to find something to wear that will keep your legs covered and hide those unsightly blue veins that you'd rather not share with the world at large.

If this tactic sounds familiar, you're one of the millions of women who are bothered by varicose veins. More than twice as common in women as in men, varicose veins can be brought on by pregnancy, obesity, prolonged standing, or unlucky genes. Whatever the catalyst, the root cause is the same: misbehaving veins and the valves in them.

A varicose vein happens when valves in a leg vein malfunction or the vein wall becomes weak and can't support the blood as it's pumped back to the heart. When the valves don't close as they should, some of the blood pools in the veins and flows backward due to gravity. Pressure builds up, and the veins begin to stretch and twist. The result? Those knotted, purple veins that make summer—with its almost compulsory uniform of shorts and swimsuits—the least favorite season for many women.

Varicose veins rarely indicate a serious problem, says Howard C. Baron, M.D., associate professor of surgery at the New York University School of Medicine in New York City. Although your legs may ache by the end of the day, symptoms are often mild or even nonexistent. The veins do tend to become more prominent over time,

WHEN TO SEE THE DOCTOR

If you have varicose veins and experience shortness of breath or chest pain, see your doctor at once. In severe cases, blood clots form in the vein and can end up lodged in the lung. If your leg is painful, red, swollen, or warm, you should see a doctor; these are symptoms of inflammation in a vein. You could also have a blood clot, which is a complication of varicose veins.

Also, consult your doctor if the skin around a varicose vein, especially on your ankle, is turning purplish brown and is itchy or flaky; these symptoms could indicate that a varicose ulcer is developing. And if you accidentally cut the skin over a varicose vein, see a physician.

though, so the sooner you start taking steps to hinder their progress, the better.

An Antivein Arsenal

If you already have varicose veins, the following remedies can help minimize symptoms and improve the veins' appearance.

Tighten them up. The herb horse chestnut contains aescin, which tightens the veins. "We call it a venotonic," says Mark Stengler, N.D., a naturopathic physician in Oceanside, California. "That's an herbal substance that increases the contraction of the elastic fibers in the vein wall. Usually, varicose veins have lost their elasticity and are sagging, so it tones them up." Take 45 drops of tincture of this herb, available in health food stores, three times a day. Mix the tincture with 2 tablespoons of hot water to help it taste better.

Note: A tincture is a highly concentrated herbal liquid. It's made by soaking leaves in alcohol or glycerin—which extracts the herb's medicinal properties—for at least 6 weeks. Tinctures are sold in health food stores in small bottles with eyedroppers to give doses. Be sure to always store them out of the reach of children.

Assist your veins with an astringent. Witch hazel is an astringent herb that helps tighten vein walls. It's available in liquid form in almost any supermarket or drugstore. Soak a cotton swab in witch hazel water and rub it over varicose veins twice a day, says Dr. Stengler.

Sweep them with the broom. Butcher's broom is used extensively in Europe for varicose veins and hemorrhoids. The active ingredient in butcher's broom is ruscogenin, which, says Dr. Stengler, has an anti-inflammatory, vasoconstricting (vein-tightening) effect. Take 300 milligrams of extract standardized to 10 percent ruscogenin with breakfast, lunch, and dinner. You can take this dosage for about 3 months or indefinitely, if you wish.

Get this fruit into the fight. Bilberry, which is a European cousin of the blueberry, "helps to stabilize the connective tissue around a vein so it's not so lax," says Dr. Stengler. That may help prevent blood from pooling in the vein. Take an 80-milligram capsule of extract standardized to 25 percent anthocyanosides three times a day. Bilberry is safe to take long-term.

Strengthen your veins. You can do this by taking bioflavonoids, which are the compounds in fruits and vegetables that give them their color. According to Stephen T. Sinatra, M.D., director of the New England Heart Center in Manchester, Connecticut, bioflavonoids can help protect the vascular walls. Two bioflavonoids that seem to promote vascular health are grape seed and pycnogenol. If you have varicose veins, you should take about 200 to 300 milligrams of grape seed extract or pycnogenol a day with meals for at least 6 months, says Dr. Sinatra. If your discomfort improves, you can continue taking the supplement indefinitely.

Lift up your legs. Elevate your legs at or above the level of your heart for at least 20 minutes, three or four times a day. You can use pillows to raise your legs to the proper height. This helps drain your veins of pooled blood, explains advises J. A. Olivencia, M.D., a vascular surgeon and medical director of the Iowa Vein Center in West Des Moines.

If your job has you on your feet all day long, elevate your legs for at least 30 minutes as soon as you get home, suggests Dr. Olivencia.

When you don't have your legs elevated, sit with your feet flat on the floor. Crossing your legs puts pressure on your veins and ultimately blocks the flow of blood in your legs. While 5 minutes of leg crossing probably won't do any long-term damage, 25 minutes or more can cause problems.

Avoid wearing knee-high nylons and socks. These garments usually have tight elastic bands that grip just below the knees and leave long-lasting indentations in the skin. "If you have varicose veins, tight-banded knee-highs are going to cause the veins to swell and stretch even more," says John Mauriello, M.D., medical director of the Vein Clinic of Charlotte in North Carolina.

Wear sneakers or low-heeled shoes as often as possible. High heels can aggravate varicose veins. "When you step into a high-heeled shoe, you are no longer using your calf muscle," notes Dr. Mauriello. "And your calf muscle is what pushes blood up into the central part of your body."

Keep your showers brief and lukewarm or cool in temperature. Starting your day with a hot half-hour shower will only exacerbate already dilated veins. Because your veins are below the level of your heart while showering, the blood will pool, and the hot water will dilate the vein, explains Dr. Olivencia.

Stop Varicose Veins in Their Tracks

Whether or not any of these risk factors apply to you, you can take steps now to stop varicose veins from developing. Doctors recommend the following preventive measures.

Maintain a healthy weight. Carrying around extra pounds stresses your veins, causing them to stretch and even collapse, explains Dee Anna Glaser, M.D., assistant professor of dermatology and internal medicine at St. Louis University School of Medicine.

While there are a number of complex formulas for calculating your ideal weight, one simple formula used by some experts can let you know if you're close: If you're 5 feet tall, you should weigh 100 pounds. If you're taller, add 5 pounds for each additional inch of height. Then to that number, add 10 percent if you have a large frame, or subtract 10 percent if you have a small frame. (For more information on losing weight, see the Overweight chapter on page 445.)

Exercise for at least 30 minutes every day. Physical activities such as walking, bicycling, and jogging strengthen your calf muscles and push pooled blood back into circulation, says Dr. Glaser.

Stretch your calf muscles when you sit for long periods of time. You can do this simple exercise just about anywhere: Push your foot down for 1 to 2 seconds, as though you were stepping on the gas pedal in your car, then pull it up. Do this for a few minutes each hour. This movement contracts your calf muscle. "Every time you contract your calf muscle, it pushes the blood from your leg toward the central part of your body," explains Dr. Glaser.

Use compression hose. If your family has a history of varicose veins, wear compression hose from the beginning of your pregnancy up until your ninth month or until your obstetrician instructs otherwise. Compression hose put pressure on leg veins to keep them from dilating. This keeps the veins' valves working more efficiently. Put the hose on first thing in the morning and don't take them off until you go to bed, advises Dr. Olivencia. You can find nonprescription compression hose in drugstores and medical supply stores. Some are designed specifically for use during pregnancy.

Ideally, you should put them on before you get out of bed. (For this to work, you'll need to shower at night rather than in the morning.) Once you stand up, gravity pulls blood backward through the vein valves in your legs, explains Dr. Mauriello. The blood then pools in your veins, causing them to swell.

On long car trips, move your legs around as much as you can. Try wiggling your toes, flexing your feet, rotating your ankles, or bending and straightening your knees. Motions like these help keep your blood circulating, says Dr. Glaser.

Eat at least 25 grams (the Daily Value) of fiber every day. A fiber-rich diet, featuring whole grains, fruits, and vegetables, helps prevent constipation by making stool easier to pass. If you must strain to move your bowels, you create pressure in your abdomen that can block the flow of blood to your legs. Over time, the increased pressure may weaken the walls of the veins in your legs, says Dr. Mauriello.

One-half cup of great Northern beans supplies more than 6 grams of fiber. Certain breakfast cereals can be good sources of fiber as well. For example, 100% Bran contains more than 8 grams and All-Bran contains 10 grams, each per 1-ounce serving.

Take 500 milligrams of vitamin C twice a day. Your body uses vitamin C to build collagen and elastin, connective tissues that help strengthen vein walls, says Dr. Mauriello. And because it's an antioxidant, vitamin C also protects your veins from free radicals, unstable molecules that occur naturally in your body and that damage cells and tissues.

Take gotu kola. This herb seems to be able to strengthen the sheath of tissue that wraps around veins, reduce formation of clogging scar tissue, and improve bloodflow through affected limbs. Therefore, it may be useful as a preventive measure. Roberta Bourgon, N.D., a naturopathic physician in Billings, Montana, recommends taking 60 to 120 milligrams a day in capsules.

Yeast Infections

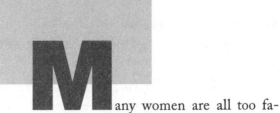

Many women are all too familiar with the intense itching, burning, and cottage-cheese–like white discharge that epitomize a yeast infection. In fact, it's estimated that 75 percent of women get at least one yeast infection during their lives.

While yeast infections can—and do—occur anytime, many episodes fall just before menstruation, when the normal balance of "good" and "bad" organisms in the vagina is disrupted. The bacterial balance can also be upset by hormonal shifts that occur during pregnancy or menopause, use of oral contraceptives or antibiotics, or flagging immunity from fighting a cold or another viral infection. Under these circumstances, a yeast called *Candida albicans*, a type of fungus, runs rampant in the vagina.

Yeast infections also have been linked to wearing nylon underwear and wet bathing suits. Wet or tight, sticky clothes trap heat and moisture, providing a wonderful arena for fungal growth, says Mary Lake Polan, M.D., Ph.D., professor of gynecology at Stanford University School of Medicine.

Yeast infections are only one form of vaginitis and can also mimic urinary tract infections or sexually transmitted diseases. In fact, women misdiagnose themselves at least half the time, says Betsy Foxman, Ph.D., associate professor of epidemiology at the University of Michigan School of Public Health in Ann Arbor.

"The data suggest that most women who think that they have a yeast infection actually have something else or nothing at all," adds Paul Nyirjesy, M.D., associate professor of obstetrics and gynecology at Temple University School of Medicine in Philadelphia. "Getting an accurate diagnosis is very important before beginning treatment."

So if this is your first experience with symptoms of a yeast infection or if you are pregnant or have an underlying condition such as diabetes, head to your doctor. He can take a laboratory specimen and determine whether or not you have a yeast infection or another type of vaginal infection.

Anti-Itch Allies

If, in fact, yeast is what's vexing you, your doctor will almost certainly prescribe an antibiotic or suggest an over-the-counter anti-yeast medication. (The best known are Gyne-Lotrimin and Monistat-7.) But over-the-counter antifungals have been found to work only a little more than half the time, says Helene Leonetti, M.D., an obstetrician/gynecologist in Bethlehem, Pennsylvania.

If your system needs extra help fending off yeast infections, try these natural prescriptions.

For external itching, apply a yogurt compress. Place ½ cup of plain yogurt on a clean cloth or towel and place it on the outside of your vagina for 15 minutes. Rinse off the yogurt with warm water, then use

WHEN TO SEE THE DOCTOR

If you've never been diagnosed with a yeast infection before, if you're pregnant, or if you have diabetes, you should see your doctor to determine the exact cause of your symptoms. You could have another type of infection that requires different treatment. If itching and soreness don't subside after 2 or 3 days of using antibiotics and these natural prescriptions, consult your doctor. And if lower abdominal pain, fever, or painful urination accompany your symptoms, see a doctor immediately, says Margaret Polaneczky, M.D., professor of gynecology at New York Hospital–Cornell Medical Center in New York City. You should also turn to your doctor if you see no improvement after using home remedies for a maximum of 2 weeks.

A Homeopathic Prescription for Yeast Attacks

T o help relieve the discomfort of yeast infections marked by a burning sensation; lots of white, curdy discharge; and violent itching, you might consider trying Kreosotum, a homeopathic remedy, says Judyth Reichenberg-Ullman, N.D., a naturopathic physician with the Northwest Center for Homeopathic Medicine in Edmonds, Washington, and coauthor of *Homeopathic Self-Care*.

Homeopathic remedies like Kreosotum work by using very diluted doses of the same substance that causes symptoms to cure them, according to practitioners. The minuscule doses used in homeopathy can't hurt and often help, says Dr. Reichenberg-Ullman. She suggests taking a 6X dose of Kreosotum up to three times a day, stopping as soon as your symptoms subside. (The notation 6X is a standard measurement in homeopathy and refers to a remedy's potency, which is listed on the label.) The remedies are usually sold in most health food stores as tablets, pilules, or granules.

If you see no improvement after three doses, try another remedy.

a blow-dryer on the warm setting to make sure that you are totally dry, says Dr. Leonetti.

Go for a sea-salt soak. Sea salt actually has the ability to kill candida, says Virginia Frazer, N.D., a naturopathic physician and licensed midwife in Kennewick, Washington. Once a day, dissolve 1 cup of sea salt in warm bathwater, swish it around, then ease yourself in for a soak. Repeat until symptoms subside.

Try douching. This plant-based home remedy for yeast infections involves white vinegar, which is really just the fermented juice of white grapes. Douching is never recommended for healthy women because it can throw a perfectly normal vaginal environment off-balance. During a yeast infection, though, the vagina's pH balance is already off-kilter. That's when an internal cleansing with the mild acidity of a vinegar solution can really help, says Mercedes Cameron, M.D., a family practitioner at St. Mary's Hospital in Grand Junction, Colorado.

Twice a day for 2 days, use a standard douche bag to douche with 2 tablespoons of white vinegar added to 1 quart of water. If you are clearly getting better, continue this treatment until symptoms subside, but for no longer than 1 week. If you don't see any improvement in 2 days, you may have a problem other than a yeast infection, so it's time to visit your doctor, says Dr. Cameron.

Change condoms. Buy your guy some polyurethane condoms. Allergies to latex condoms may be associated with increased susceptibility to yeast infections, says Margaret Polaneczky, M.D., professor of gynecology at New York Hospital–Cornell Medical Center in New York City. So, if you use condoms for protection and get frequent yeast infections, consider switching to a nonlatex brand.

Remedies to Avoid Repeat Episodes

If only yeast infections were like mumps—once you have had it, you're immune. Unfortunately, that's not how it works. In fact, if you have had one yeast infection, chances are that you will get another, doctors say. Try these natural prescriptions, however, to fend off repeat or resistant episodes.

Arm yourself with acid. Boric acid suppositories are an effective way to treat yeast infections and may be particularly effective against resistant ones, says Dr. Nyirjesy.

Buy a bag or box of boric acid and a package of gelatin capsules (size "1") at your drugstore or health food store, then fill the capsules with boric acid. Insert one suppository in the vagina in the morning and another before bedtime for 2 weeks, says Dr. Nyirjesy.

Caution: Boric acid is poisonous, so never take it orally or leave the capsules around where children could get at them, Dr. Nyirjesy says.

Alternate boric acid with acidophilus. Some doctors believe that combining boric acid suppositories with acidophilus suppositories works best to maintain the delicate bacterial balance in a woman's vagina. Alternate one boric acid suppository in the morning with one acidophilus suppository (available in health food stores) every night for 5 nights, suggests Judyth Reichenberg-Ullman, N.D., a naturopathic physician with the Northwest Center for Homeopathic Medicine in Edmonds, Washington. Don't use these suppositories while you menstruate, or you may actually upset the bacterial balance rather than prevent infection.

Grab some garlic. "Garlic is one of the best things to take for yeast infections," says Tori Hudson, N.D., a naturopathic physician and professor at the National College of Naturopathic Medicine in Portland, Oregon. It is both antifungal and immunity-boosting, she says.

Two garlic capsules a day are enough to protect against yeast, according to Dr. Hudson. It's best to take enteric-coated capsules because the coating prevents the active ingredients in garlic from breaking down in the stomach. Look for garlic capsules with 4,000 milligrams of allicin-alliin, which is the antifungal agent found in garlic.

Employ echinacea and goldenseal. A German study found that women taking antifungal medicine plus echinacea extract had only a 10 percent recurrence of yeast infections. In the study, this group was compared to women who took only antifungal medicine. Nearly 60 percent of that group had recurrent infections.

Another great anti-yeast herb is goldenseal, says Lorilee Schoenbeck, N.D., a naturopathic physician in Middlebury, Vermont. Goldenseal contains berberine, a chemical that has antibiotic properties and works particularly well against yeast. You can buy echinacea and goldenseal separately or in combination capsules. Whichever you choose, take them daily as directed on the product you buy. If the capsules are 450 milligrams of an echinacea and goldenseal combination, a typical dose would be two or three capsules daily with water. Do not use goldenseal if you are pregnant, however.

Never wash inside the vagina with soap. This may give you an allergic reaction that leads to a yeast infection, says Dr. Leonetti. And don't worry that your vagina won't get clean. The vagina has a self-cleaning mechanism that does not need soaps or lotions.

Use cotton panties. Yeast thrive in the dark, moist, dank environment that nylon underwear and panty hose provide. Cotton underwear will reduce yeast's ability to thrive, says Dr. Leonetti.

Loosen up. You can be fashionable in looser-fitting clothes and keep out the yeast-infection–creating fungi that thrive in the environments created by tight, constricting outfits, says Dr. Leonetti.

Sleep naked. Sleeping nude, or at least without underwear, will air out your vagina and keep the yeast-infection–causing bacteria from having a place to thrive, says Dr. Leonetti. Another benefit of this strategy is that it may spice up your love life a bit.

Cool it with the candy. It doesn't have to be forever, thank goodness, but you should probably avoid sweets for a month. No one is sure if eating too much sugar really leads to yeast infections. If, however, you know that you get a yeast infection whenever you have gone overboard on chocolates, try avoiding sugary confections for a month and see if your yeast infections disappear, doctors say.

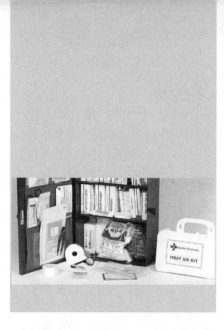

First Aid

Basic Lifesaving Techniques

+

When it comes to emergencies, all too often people think that the person next to them will be able to help or that somehow there will be a doctor in the house. Don't take that chance. You want to be prepared—make that very prepared—when the life of a friend, a relative, a child, or even a total stranger is at stake.

One of the most important things that you should know is how to get in touch with your local emergency medical services, says Jedd Roe, M.D., professor of emergency medicine at the University of Colorado School of Medicine in Denver. In most but not all communities, the emergency number is 911. If this isn't true in your community, check the inside cover of your telephone directory for the emergency number. In a serious situation, calling your local emergency services is your best first step, advises Dr. Roe.

First, Read This

Below, you'll learn five lifesaving techniques that every person should know how to perform properly. But first, there are two important points you need to remember.

The first one is that it's not enough just to know what to do. You must know how to do it properly. Skills such as rescue breathing and cardiopulmonary resuscitation (CPR) can't be learned from a book alone. Take a first-aid and CPR class at your local hospital or community center, advises Paul Matera, M.D., an emergency medical technician-paramedic and vice chairman and professor of emergency services at Providence Hospital in Washington, D.C. They'll teach you the right way to do these lifesaving techniques, which will come up repeatedly in this emergency first-aid section. What's offered here is just a short refresher for those of you who have already learned these skills. The information given is only for adults; children and infants require different procedures.

The second important point to consider while giving first aid is avoiding disease transmission. While chances are that you will be helping a family member or friend, you may be helping a stranger. There are simple ways to reduce the risk of disease. Try not to come in contact with the victim's body fluids, such as blood or saliva. Wear disposable latex gloves, or place layers of clean cloth between you and body fluids. Have the victim use his own hands to stop bleeding. You should have a face mask or face shield for doing rescue breathing and CPR. Protect your eyes as well. If you have glasses or sunglasses, wear them, or borrow a pair from a friend. Wash your hands thoroughly after giving first aid, even if you wore gloves. If you did come in contact with body fluids, tell your doctor. You can get disposable gloves at drugstores and face masks at medical supply stores.

If there is an emergency in a public place like a restaurant or sports arena and you decide to assist, ask the manager or security officer for a first-aid kit. Public places are usually required to have first-aid kits that should contain universal precaution kits with gloves, eye protection, and face masks, says Dr. Matera.

Five Critical First-Aid Tactics

The following techniques may help save the life of someone you love. Just remember: Whenever possible, call 911 before taking any of these steps.

Rescue Breathing

In rescue breathing, you supply the breath for someone who has stopped breathing. You usually need to use it after some type of trauma—a bad fall, a seizure, an accident—when the heart is still beating. "Most times, after a few breaths, they'll wake right up and breathe on their own. You only need to breathe for them until spontaneous respiration is reestablished," says Dr. Matera.

If the victim isn't breathing, roll him gently on his back, keeping his head and back in a straight line. Sometimes all it takes to restore someone's breathing is to reopen his airway with the head-tilt/chin-lift technique. Kneel beside the patient and place the palm of your hand on his forehead and push backward to tilt the head back. Take the fingers of your other hand and hook them under the bony point of the chin and lift the chin upward.

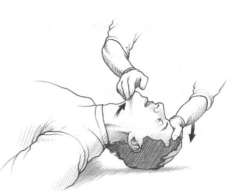

If you suspect a neck or spine injury, use this technique instead. Place your hands on the side of the victim's head, behind the angles of his lower jaw, and move the jaw forward without tilting the head backward.

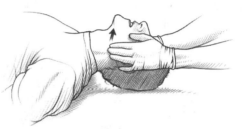

Take 3 to 5 seconds to check for breathing. Place your ear over the victim's mouth and nose and listen and feel for breathing. Look at his chest to see if it is rising and falling. If he is breathing, and there are no spinal injuries, place him in the recovery position.

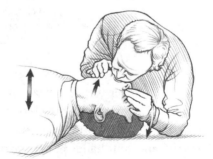

If he is not breathing, start rescue breathing. Keep his head tilted back and pinch his nose shut. Seal your lips tightly around his mouth. (If you are using a mask or shield, be familiar with how to use them.) Give two slow, deep breaths, each lasting 1 to 2 seconds. Check that the chest rises with each breath. If the first breath does not go in, retilt the head and try again.

Checking for a Carotid Pulse

To see if you have to move on to CPR, check for a pulse. Many people can easily find the carotid arteries, making it a good place to look for a pulse. But the carotids are also the closest major arteries to the heart muscle. "If you find a carotid pulse, you can be pretty sure that the heart is pumping out some blood," Dr. Matera says. If you locate a pulse, then continue with rescue breathing until the person starts breathing on his own.

If you don't find a pulse, it means that the heart isn't doing its job of pumping blood. Move on to CPR, Dr. Matera says. Don't make the fatal mistake of just listening for a heartbeat in the chest, he warns. You can have a heartbeat yet not have a pulse. "In certain shock situations, the heart can be beating, but nothing is being pumped out. The heart can be technically beating and even contracting, but there may be no blood available to pump," he says. Check for a pulse to make sure that blood is pumping through the person's system.

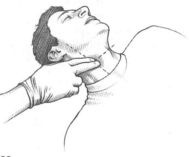

After two deep breaths, check to see if there is a pulse. Find the victim's Adam's apple and slide your fingers down the side of the neck nearest you. You should find the pulse as you approach the level of the angle of the jaw. Use your fingers, not your thumb, to check the carotid artery for a pulse. This should take 5 to 10 seconds.

If there is a pulse but no breathing, give one slow breath every 5 to 6 seconds. Every 10 to 12 breaths, check for a pulse. If there is a pulse, continue the cycle of breathing and checking for a pulse until help arrives, the victim breathes on his own, or there is no pulse.

CPR

For whatever reason—heart attack, an accident, loss of blood—the person's heart stops pumping blood and the person stops breathing. CPR gets the heart pumping and lungs working manually. You supply the breaths, and your hands pump the heart. Without this, the major organs, including the heart and brain, will die within minutes because they aren't getting oxygenated, nutritious blood, Dr. Matera says. "When you are giving breaths, you must see the chest rise. When you are giving compressions, a pulse must be detected. Then you know that you are doing your job," he adds.

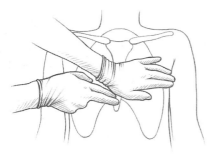

If there is no pulse, start CPR. Your hands must be positioned properly. Slide the fingers of your hand nearest the victim's feet up his rib cage and find the notch at the bottom of the sternum. Put your middle finger on the notch, and place your index finger next to it. Place the heel of your other hand next to the index finger.

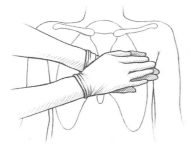

Remove the hand at the notch and place it on top of the hand on the chest. Keep your fingers off the chest. Use the heel of the bottom hand to apply pressure to the chest.

Pivot at hips

Straight arms

Use heel of hand

Your shoulders should be directly over your hands. Keep your arms straight and your elbows locked. Push down with your upper body, pivoting from your hips. Don't rock from your knees; instead move straight up and down like a piston. With each compression, the victim's chest should be pushed straight down about 2 inches. Keep up a steady rhythm and don't stop between compressions. Compress the chest 15 times. Then give the victim two deep breaths. Make sure you do the compressions quickly so that in about a minute you've done 80 compressions.

Do three more cycles of 15 compressions and two breaths. Then check the pulse. If there is no pulse, continue doing four cycles of 15 compressions, two breaths, and a pulse check until help arrives, the victim revives, or you are too exhausted to continue. If there is a pulse, return to rescue breathing.

Shock Position

After a severe emotional or physical trauma, a person may slip into a state of shock. He may be awake but appear confused, lethargic, or shaky, and he may have pale, cool, moist skin. This happens because the circulatory system is failing to provide enough oxygen-rich blood to the body. Putting the person in the shock position helps restore circulation, says Dr. Roe.

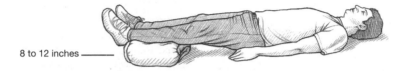

8 to 12 inches ———

Lay the victim on his back. If you are absolutely certain that there are no head, neck, or spine injuries or broken bones in the legs or hips, raise his feet 8 to 12 inches. If you are not sure if there are head, neck, spine, or leg injuries, keep the victim lying flat. In either case, if he is feeling cool, cover the victim with a blanket.

Recovery Position

If the victim is breathing and has a pulse but is unresponsive or is vomiting, put him into the left-side recovery position, says Dr. Roe. If you suspect a spine injury, do not move the victim. The recovery position will keep him from choking on or inhaling his vomit if it comes up.

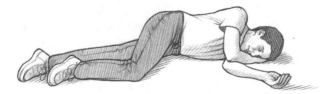

With the victim on his back, kneel at his left side. Bend his left arm at the elbow so his upper arm is next to his head. Place the back of his right hand against his left cheek and hold it there. With your hand behind his right knee, bend the right leg and roll him toward you. In the final position, his right hand supports his head and his bent right leg prevents rolling.

First Aid for Children

Bleeding

If your child has punctured or severed an artery, bright red blood will spurt out with each beat of the heart. Arterial bleeding can be life-threatening.

Severe bleeding from a vein is usually less dangerous and is distinguished by flowing rather than spurting blood.

If your child is bleeding heavily—from either an artery or vein—you should take the following steps as soon as possible.

1. Calm and reassure the victim. The sight of blood can be very frightening.
2. Locate the source of the bleeding.
3. Wash your hands.
4. Put on sterile gloves if you have them. Remove any obvious loose debris from the wound.
5. Using a sterile dressing or clean cloth, apply direct pressure to the wound to stop the bleeding. Direct pressure is almost always appropriate for brisk bleeding; however, do not use direct pressure on an eye injury, on a wound that contains an embedded object, or on a head injury if there is a possibility of skull fracture.
6. Raise the bleeding part above the level of the victim's heart if you don't suspect a broken bone and if elevating the injury doesn't cause the victim more pain.
7. If the bleeding doesn't stop or if you need to free your hands, apply a pressure bandage. This is a roller bandage or long strip of cloth tied firmly over the wound. (The pressure bandage should be tight enough to keep pressure on the wound, but not so tight that it cuts off circulation.)
8. If the bleeding doesn't stop after 15 minutes of direct pressure, or if the wound is too extensive to cover effectively, use pressure-point

bleeding control—applying pressure to a major artery—if you are trained in the procedure.

9. If the bleeding stops with direct pressure but then starts up again, reapply direct pressure.

10. If the bleeding is severe, take steps to prevent shock while you await medical help. Lay the victim flat, raise his feet 8 to 12 inches, and cover him with a coat or blanket. Do not place the victim in the shock position if you suspect any head, neck, back, or leg injury or if the position makes the victim uncomfortable.

11. If bleeding is not severe, wash the wound with soap and water. Rinse well and cover with a sterile dressing or a clean cloth, then apply direct pressure for a few minutes.

Breathing Problems and Suffocation

If your child is having severe breathing problems, they may be caused by a number of conditions, including injury, sudden illness, or an underlying medical problem. Here's what to do.

- Call for emergency medical service.

- Loosen any tight clothing.

- While you wait for help to arrive, do not move your child or put him in any position that he finds uncomfortable.

- Do not put a pillow under your child's head, since this can close his airway.

- Do not give him anything to eat or drink.

- Be as calm and reassuring as you can. Anxiety can worsen the problem.

- If your child becomes drowsy or stops wheezing, do not assume that his condition is improving. His condition may have taken a turn for the worse. But if you've already called the emergency medical service, help should arrive quickly.

Minor Burns

If a burn appears to be superficial (red skin and perhaps a blister) and is smaller than a quarter, you can treat it as minor. Take these steps.

1. Cool the burn immediately by immersing it in cold water (not ice water) or placing it under gently running cold water for at least 10 minutes. A clean, cold, wet towel might also help reduce the pain. If a blister forms, leave it alone.
2. Pat the area dry with a clean (sterile, if possible) cloth and cover it with a nonadhesive sterile dressing. This will help prevent infection.

   Caution: Call for medical attention for any burn that involves your child's airway, eyes, face, hands, or genitals. Additionally, if a minor burn doesn't heal normally, call your doctor. Even with a minor burn, you should make sure your child is up-to-date on his tetanus immunization.

Severe Burns

A severe burn can be caused by any prolonged exposure to intense heat, fire, electricity, chemicals, or scalding liquids. It destroys all skin layers and may affect the underlying fat and muscle. The child needs immediate emergency medical treatment. Call an ambulance and take the following steps while you wait for medical help to arrive.

1. Check your child's ABCs: Make sure the airway is open, and check his breathing and circulation. Start rescue breathing, CPR, or bleeding control as needed.

   Caution: Someone who is certified in CPR and first aid is best suited to do these techniques. You and every member of your family can easily learn them and become certified. First-aid and CPR courses are offered by local chapters of the American Red Cross. The American Heart Association also gives instruction in CPR.
2. Calm and reassure your child.
3. Treat your child for shock. Have the child lie down and elevate his feet 8 to 12 inches. If you think he has a head, neck, back, or leg injury, just keep your child calm and comfortable.
4. Don't take any other steps to treat your child for a severe burn. Also, don't give him anything to eat or drink, and never apply cold compresses, creams, ointments, sprays, or oils. Trying to remove blisters or dead skin may cause severe complications.

Choking

If your child gets food, liquid, or an inedible object in his airway, he will automatically begin coughing to eject the obstruction. The choking sensation can be frightening to a child, but as long as he can speak, breath, or cough forcefully, he will probably be able to expel the object by himself.

But you must intervene if your child seems to be in real trouble. Take action right away if your child has convulsions or loses consciousness. You should also take immediate action if he can't breathe, cry, speak, or cough forcefully, or if his face looks pale and bluish. A correctly performed Heimlich maneuver could save his life.

You or someone else should call for emergency help as soon as possible. But don't wait for the ambulance to arrive before performing the Heimlich maneuver.

Heimlich Maneuver for a Baby

For a baby who is newborn or up to 1 year of age, use this method to restore breathing.

1. Place the baby face-down along your forearm, with his head toward the palm of your hand. Lower your arm slightly, so his head is lower than the rest of his body. Support your baby's head with your hand. Hold the baby's jaw between your thumb and finger (illustration A). Rest your forearm on your thigh.

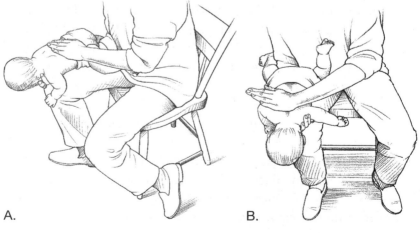

A. B.

2. Deliver four forceful blows with the heel of your hand to the baby's back, between the shoulder blades (illustration B).

3. Then turn the baby over, so he's lying on his back. Place him on your thigh or a firm surface, with his head lower than his chest.

4. Place your index and middle finger on the baby's breastbone just below the nipples and above the notch at the end of the breastplate (illustration C).

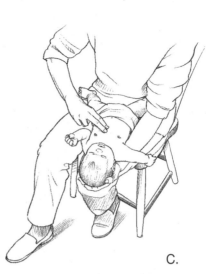

C.

5. Give four quick thrusts down, pressing the breast ½ to 1 inch each time. Each thrust is a separate attempt to clear the airway by forcing air out through the windpipe.

6. Continue the series of four back blows and four chest thrusts—turning the baby from stomach position to back position—until the object is dislodged. If the baby becomes unconscious, however, you should stop this maneuver. (You can provide first aid for an unconscious infant using techniques taught in a first-aid course.)

7. Seek medical attention even if your baby starts to breathe normally.

Heimlich Maneuver for a Child over 1 Year Old

1. Stand or kneel behind your child and wrap your arms around her waist (illustration A).

2. Make a fist with one hand and grab it with the other hand (illustration B). Place the thumb side of your fist in the middle of your child's abdomen. Place

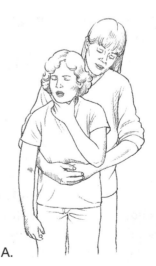

A.

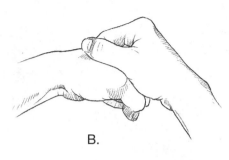

B.

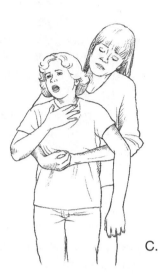

C.

the fist above the navel and well below the breastbone (illustration C).

3. Keeping your elbows out, give four quick, upward thrusts into the child's abdomen (illustration D).

4. Repeat this procedure until the object pops out of her throat and the airway is cleared. But stop the procedure if the child loses consciousness. (You can provide first aid for an unconscious victim using techniques taught in a first-aid course.)

5. Seek medical attention even if your child starts to breathe normally.

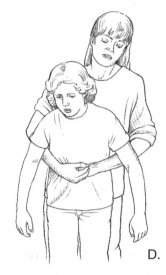

D.

Convulsions without Fever

During a convulsion (also known as a seizure), a child becomes unconscious for a brief period of time. The convulsion may be accompanied by falling; drooling or frothing at the mouth; vigorous, involuntary muscle spasms; loss of bladder or bowel control; and a temporary halt in breathing. In some cases, there are no convulsive movements, but the child becomes pale and limp.

Convulsions are associated with many medical conditions. But if your toddler has no previous history of convulsions and suddenly experiences multiple seizures, he may have swallowed poison. Call the Poison Control Center and get immediate emergency medical aid.

While seizures are frightening to parents, they are usually short-lived, generally lasting from 30 to 45 seconds. Once a seizure has begun, there is no way to stop it. The best thing you can do for your child is to get medical help while you take steps to prevent him from hurting himself. Here's what you should do to protect your child during a seizure.

- Place your child on the ground in a safe area. Clear away any sharp or hard objects.

- Protect his head by placing cushions around it.

- Loosen his collar, pants, belt, or any other tight clothing.

- Roll your child onto his left side to keep his airway clear.

- Do not try to restrain your child during a seizure, and do not try to put anything between his teeth.

- When your child regains consciousness, he may fall into a deep sleep. This is typical: Do not try to wake him.

- Do not give him anything to eat or drink until is he fully awake and alert.

Drowning

If your child has been submerged in the water and is no longer breathing, you may still be able to save his life if you take immediate action. Here's how.

- Call for emergency medical help and rescue the drowning child.

- Check your child's ABCs—airway, breathing, and circulation. If necessary, begin rescue breathing or CPR if you have been trained.

- Remove any cold, wet clothes. Cover your child with a blanket, coat, or any other clothing to prevent hypothermia.

- As your child revives, he may cough and have trouble breathing.

- Try to be calm and reassuring while you wait for medical help to arrive.

- Victims of near-drownings should always be checked by a physician because lung complications may develop as a result of the accident.

Electric Shock Injuries

Electrical injuries can be minor if your child has only brief contact with a low current, but a high-voltage shock from a generated electrical current or a lightning strike can cause devastating injuries: severe burns, internal and external damage, cardiac and respiratory arrest, neurological damage, and sometimes death. If your child has sustained an electrical injury, take the following measures.

- Check to see if your child is still in contact with the electrical current. If he is, don't touch him, even with a wooden branch, pole, or broomstick. A high-voltage current may be able to travel through wood.

- Shut off the power at a wall switch or circuit box.

- Check the ABCs—airway, breathing, and circulation. If necessary, begin CPR if you know how.

- Call for emergency medical service.

Eye Injuries

When your child gets an eyelash or a piece of dirt in her eye, she can probably remove it herself by blinking—or her tears may flush out the small object. But if your child has a more serious eye injury, it could jeopardize her sight.

Be very cautious, however, about touching your child's eye. Even if your child has chemicals or a foreign body in her eye, you may not be able to help her immediately—and if you try, you could make the eye injury worse. Also, your child will undoubtedly resist your attempts to help her.

Because an eye injury requires expert medical care, your main role is to ensure that the eye is protected as much as possible until help arrives. Take these steps.

Foreign Body in the Eye

- If the eye seems seriously injured by the foreign body, call for emergency medical service.

- While you wait for help to arrive, tilt your child's head so that the injured eye is facing downward. Flush the object out of the eye, from the inside corner of the eye outward, using a sterile saline solution if you have it. (If you have none, plain tap water will do.)

- Try to hold your child's eyelid open to make sure the eye is properly flushed. Keep flushing for 15 to 30 minutes, or until you have medical help.

- Do not press or rub the eye.

- Do not try to remove the object with your fingers, a cotton swab, or anything else.

Foreign Body Embedded in the Eye

- Call for emergency medical service even if the object in the eye is small.

- Leave the object alone. Do not touch it or let anything press on it.

- If the object is large, place a cup or cone over the injured eye and tape it into place. Cover the uninjured eye with an eye patch or sterile dressing. If the object is small, cover both eyes with eye patches or a sterile dressing.

- Try to calm and reassure your child.

Chemical Exposure

- Call for emergency medical service, then try to determine the type of chemical. Call the Poison Control Center in your area for specific advice.

- Do not press or rub the eye or allow the child to rub the eye. Tilt your child's head so the injured eye is facing downward. Flush the eye with fresh water, pouring the water from the inside corner of the eye outward. Continue to do this for at least 15 to 30 minutes or until help arrives. (You may have to force the eye open to be effective.)

- If both eyes are affected, do this procedure in the shower.

- Even if only one eye is affected, cover both eyes with sterile dressings after the flushing procedure. Keep the eyes covered until help arrives.

Falls

If an infant or toddler doesn't start to use an injured arm or leg within hours of a fall or he continues to cry when the injured area is touched, assume the child has a broken bone. Take the following measures.

- Call for emergency medical help.

- Don't move the child unless the injured limb is immobilized. If you know first aid, splint the limb in the position you found it.

- Keep your child still while you wait for help to arrive.

- Do not try to straighten or test a misshapen bone or joint.

- Do not give your child anything to eat or drink.

- If the injury involves an open wound, do not blow on it, wash it, or probe it. Cover the wound with sterile dressings.

- Take steps to prevent shock. If you can do so without moving the limb or causing pain, raise the child's feet 8 to 12 inches. Cover him with a blanket.

- Do not attempt to move a child whom you suspect to have a neck injury. Call for help. (You should cover the child with a blanket while you're waiting for help to arrive.)

Finger or Toe Injuries

An injured finger or toe may turn black and blue under the nail. Often there's swelling as well as some bleeding around the cuticle. When there's bleeding underneath the nail, the end of the toe or finger will turn black or dark blue. The pressure underneath the nail will be very painful. If your child has a smashed finger or toe, take the following steps.

- Call your child's physician if there appears to be excessive swelling, a deep cut, blood under the fingernail, bleeding, or if the finger or toe appears broken.

- Don't attempt to straighten the injured part.

- If the swelling and bleeding are less severe, wash the injured area with soap and water and cover with a soft, sterile cloth. Then apply an ice pack or soak it in cold water to relieve pain and minimize swelling.

- Cover with a soft, sterile cloth.

- If you notice increased pain, swelling, redness, pus, or fever within 24 to 72 hours of the injury, notify your child's physician at once. An infection has probably set in.

Frostbite

A frostbite injury, caused when bitter cold and wind freeze body tissue, can be severe enough to penetrate the skin and everything beneath it including blood and bones. Any part of the body can be affected by frostbite, but it commonly strikes the exposed areas of the face, the fingers, toes, earlobes, and nose. Frostbitten skin is frozen, waxy, and numb; when it thaws, the skin may blister, swell, and turn red, blue, or purple.

It is often hard to judge how serious the frostbite damage is, so you should play it safe by beginning first-aid treatment whenever you suspect your child *might* have a case of frostbite. Then get your child to a doctor as soon as possible. Here's what to do.

- Move your child out of the cold.

- Remove any constricting or wet clothing and replace with dry clothing.

- Rewarm the frozen area for at least 30 minutes by using wet heat. Immerse the frozen limb in water that is slightly warmer than body temperature (100° to 105°F). Help the warming process by circulating the water with your hand. For areas that can't be immersed in water, such as the cheeks and nose, apply warm compresses.

- Expect that rewarming may be painful. Your child will experience a burning sensation, swelling, and color changes on the skin. When the skin looks pink and is no longer numb, the area is thawed.

- After the skin has thawed, apply dry, sterile dressing to the area. If fingers have been affected, place the dressing between each finger, too. Use the same procedure if the toes are frostbitten.

- Move the thawed areas as little as possible.

- Prevent refreezing by wrapping the rewarmed areas.

- Don't thaw out a frostbitten area if it's not possible to keep it thawed.

- Do not use direct heat such as a radiator, car heater, campfire, or heating pad to thaw the frostbitten area.

- Do not massage or rub snow on the frostbitten area.

- Do not disturb the blisters on the frozen skin.

Head Injuries

Your active child may receive a good wallop on the head as she runs, climbs, and plays, but as long she is up and running again after the injury, it is not likely that she has sustained serious damage. You should watch her for the next 24 hours, though, since the symptoms of a serious head injury may be delayed. Check with your doctor at least by telephone for any head injury that causes even momentary loss of consciousness. And, for infants, consult the doctor for all but minor head injuries.

Be alert for such symptoms as severe or repeated vomiting, dazed or confused behavior, increased irritability, restlessness, a personality change, or drowsiness during the times when your child would ordinarily be alert. According to doctors, you should also watch out for headache that is not relieved by over-the-counter headache remedies. Other symptoms that indicate problems include slurred speech, a stiff neck, double vision, difficulty seeing, pupils of unequal size, weak limbs, fluid or blood draining from the nose or mouth, or a slowed rate of breathing.

If you see an obvious wound, dent, or fracture in your child's skull—and some bleeding—you should take immediate action. But you should take the following precautions *any* time you suspect that your child has a serious head injury.

- Call for emergency medical help.

- While you wait for the ambulance, do not move your child unless absolutely necessary.

- Do not shake or pick up your child.

- Do not remove any object that is stuck in the wound or protruding from the skull or head area.

- Check the ABCs—airway, breathing, and circulation. And, if necessary, begin rescue breathing, CPR, and bleeding control.

- Try to keep your child calm and still.

- If you suspect your child has a fractured skull, do not apply direct pressure to any bleeding wound in the head area.

- If your child vomits, lean her forward and support her head so she does not choke. Do not sit her up if you think her neck is injured; instead, support her head and neck and roll her to one side.

- Apply ice to areas of swelling.
  Caution: Ice should be wrapped in a cloth or towel—not applied directly to the skin—as it may cause frostbite.

- If your child is dazed or unconscious, assume that she may have a spinal injury. It is essential that her head and neck are kept immobile.
  Place your hands on both sides of her head, and keep the child's head and neck in the position in which you found them. If the child vomits, roll the child as a unit (head and neck immobile) onto one side to prevent choking and to allow breathing. But otherwise, the child should not be moved at all. Wait for medical help.

FIRST AID +

Poisoning

If you suspect that your child has swallowed, inhaled, touched, or injected some kind of poison, it's important to stay calm to avoid alarming your child. Quietly question your child about what he took and how long ago. (You need this history to be able to respond appropriately.)

Keep the child as quiet as possible while you do the following.

- Look in your child's mouth. If he has chewed on pills or bitten a poisonous plant, remove any bits of pills or plant parts that remain in his mouth.

- Your child should stay with you when you go to the phone to call for help.

- If your child has swallowed a poisonous product or medication, also take the container with you when you go to the phone. Call the local Poison Control Center. If there is no Poison Control Center, call your doctor, a hospital emergency department, or Emergency Medical Service (EMS) and follow instructions. The person you speak to will probably ask you to read product information from the container.

- Give specific information about your child's age and weight, and a description of the product or substance that he swallowed. You should also try to estimate the amount swallowed and exactly when it happened.

- When medical instructions are given to you over the phone, follow them exactly. Never give any poison remedy (even ipecac syrup) without getting medical advice.

First Aid for Adults

Broken Bones

First of all, the person with a broken bone should stay still to keep the bone from moving until you get medical help. Moving it around further harms the bone, and it also increases the risk of damaging surrounding blood vessels and nerves. If you suspect a head, neck, or spinal injury, you should absolutely not move the person. Call for an ambulance right away.

Here are some step-by-step tips to follow while waiting for medical help to arrive.

1. Do not attempt to put bones back together. Moving a broken bone will only cause a lot more pain and further damage. Save the repair work for the doctors at the hospital no matter how bad a break looks.
2. Bandage with saline. If the bone breaks through the skin, soak sterile gauze in saline. Regular contact lens solution will do. Place the gauze over the bone and the injured skin. If you don't have saline solution, use dry sterile gauze. Do not use any kind of tape to fasten the gauze to the wound; just lay it on the area. After the wound is covered, sit tight and wait for the ambulance to arrive. Do not move, splint, or elevate a bone that breaks through the skin, adds Jedd Roe, M.D., professor of emergency medicine at the University of Colorado School of Medicine in Denver.
3. If you are out in the woods or are far away from a hospital, you can make a splint to help keep broken bones still until you get medical help. The splint should cover the areas below and above the break. Splint the bone the way you found it, no matter how mangled it may be.

    Plenty of common items make a quality splint: cardboard, a ruler, branches, magazines, a pillow, or a thick blanket. When applying a splint, use your hands to support the injured area. You can use cloth ties, neckties, torn clothing, or belts to tie the splint to the injured area. Make sure that any knots are not pressing against the injury. Tie them securely, but not so tightly that circulation is impaired, says Dr. Roe.

If the area beyond the splint becomes pale, numb, or throbs, loosen the ties. You may also need to loosen the ties if the injured area swells after you've applied the splint.

How to make an ankle splint ▶

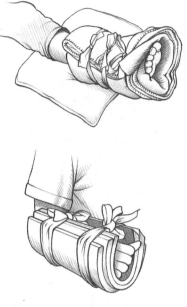

For a broken ankle that has no open wound, place a thick blanket underneath the foot and ankle. Then wrap it lightly with cloth or anything that ties it in place, leaving the toes exposed. After applying the splint, elevate the ankle.

How to make a forearm splint ▶

To splint a broken forearm or wrist, you can place a few fairly thick magazines or newspapers rolled into a "U" shape under the lower arm. Make sure that the splint extends from the elbow to the hand. Tie it snugly in place with cloth ties. Make a sling by tying a jacket, shirt, or some other piece of clothing or cloth around the neck.

If you are alone and have possibly broken your forearm, make a self-splint by holding your broken arm close to your body. Bend the elbow of the broken arm and hold the forearm still against your chest with your opposite hand and arm until you get medical help, says Ian Cummings, M.D., director of emergency services at the Day Kimball Hospital in Putnam, Connecticut.

4. **Put it on ice.** After you make the splint, put an ice pack or a cold compress on the break, Dr. Roe says. Keep the ice on for 20 to 30 minutes at a time, and make sure to wrap it in a towel or cloth to prevent the skin from freezing. Ice the area several times in the first 24 hours. The ice keeps down the swelling and lessens some of the pain.

5. **Raise it.** If the bone that you suspect is broken is in the wrist, hand, finger, toe, foot, or ankle, you should elevate the broken area above

the heart, Dr. Roe says. The person can do this lying down if it makes him more comfortable. This slows the blood from pooling in the fractured area and reduces swelling. Do not elevate larger broken bones, particularly the femur or pelvis.

6. Treat for shock. When a person breaks a major bone like his femur or pelvis, he may go into shock, says Dr. Roe. (For instructions on how to treat for shock, see Basic Lifesaving Techniques on page 486.)

Broken Nose

1. Put ice on the nose. A broken nose will swell up quickly and start to bleed. An ice pack or a cold compress wrapped in a towel to avoid freezing the skin will help reduce the swelling and stop the bleeding.
2. Stop the bleeding. Treat blood from a broken nose the same way you would a nosebleed. Sit up straight and tilt the head slightly forward so the blood flows out of the nose and not down the throat. Then apply pressure by pinching the nostrils closed for a few minutes, says Sanford Archer, M.D., associate professor of otolaryngology at the University of Kentucky A. B. Chandler Medical Center in Lexington.
3. Give the person a painkiller. An everyday over-the-counter pain medicine will help with the pain. But stick with acetaminophen-containing products such as Tylenol, he advises. Nonsteroidal anti-inflammatories such as ibuprofen and aspirin open blood vessels and will actually increase the bleeding.
4. Give him a decongestant. A decongestant nasal spray will help any congestion that may develop after the nose is broken. Pills or nasal sprays work fine, although Dr. Archer advises not to use the sprays for more than a few days because it's possible to become addicted.
5. Later, you can try some natural remedies. Natural remedies can help speed the healing process after the person has been treated for a broken nose. Some herbalists recommend gotu kola as a healer of cartilage, tendons, and connective tissue. You can give the herb as a tea or a tincture. Steep 1 tablespoon of the dried herb in a cup of boiling water. The person with the broken nose can drink two to three cups of gotu kola tea a day for several weeks, says Kathleen Maier, director of the Dreamtime Center for Herbal Studies in Flint Hill, Virginia, and a professional member of the American Herbalists Guild. If you're using the tincture, put 20 to 30 drops in water

and give him this two or three times a day for several weeks. You can find gotu kola in health food stores.

Note: A tincture is a highly concentrated herbal liquid. It's made by soaking leaves in alcohol or glycerin—which extracts the herb's medicinal properties—for at least 6 weeks. Tinctures are sold in health food stores in small bottles with eyedroppers to give doses. Be sure to store them out of the reach of children.

Arnica is another good follow-up option because it reduces swelling, bruising, and pain. You can give him two or three pellets of Arnica 30C internally two times a day for 5 days. If the person doesn't have an open wound, you can also apply arnica cream or gel to the nose area. The cream can also be used as needed for 5 days. Arnica is available at most health food stores and homeopathic stores.

Burns

Although about 2 million Americans are burned every year, only 5 percent of them need hospital treatment. Small heat burns caused by flames or hot items usually don't go beyond first-degree burns (which look red) or mild second-degree burns (which have some minor blistering)—meaning that you can treat them at home.

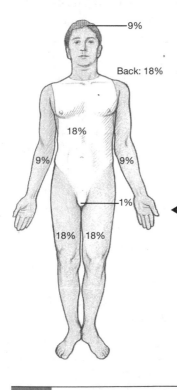

But severe second-degree or third-degree burns—usually indicated by skin that is white with red spots, wet or waxy looking, or severely blistered or charred—should be seen immediately by a doctor.

◀ The Rule of Nines is a way to figure out how much of the body is burned. It divides the body into sections and assigns a percentage value to each section. For example, in an adult, the head and arms each equal 9 percent of the body's total surface area. The front and back of the torso and the legs are each worth 18 percent.

One also should get medical treatment for burns if the burn covers more than 10 to 20 percent of the body; if the face, hands, or genital area has been burned; if the person has suffered chemical or electrical burns; or if the burn becomes infected or the victim starts to develop chills and a fever, says Dr. Roe. Signs of infection usually occur 2 to 3 days later and include increased redness or pain, swelling, pus, and red streaks spreading from the burn up the extremities.

If a person has suffered a severe second- or third-degree burn, you should elevate the burned area and put the victim in the shock position while waiting for medical help to arrive, says Dr. Roe. (For illustrated instructions on how to put someone into this position, see page 486.) Do not disturb any blisters or remove any dead skin, he cautions.

For minor burns, here's what you should do.

1. Place your burn under cool water for at least 15 minutes. Don't use the old standby home remedy of ice. "Ice can cause tissue damage. It essentially freezes the outside layer of the skin," says Dr. Roe.

2. Leave blisters intact. Blisters provide a natural protective layer for the burned tissue, functioning as a nice, sterile dressing. As long as that skin is intact, there's no avenue for bacteria to get in.

3. Change and clean daily. If the burn is blistered or open, you should apply an ointment such as Polysporin and bandage it with dry, sterile gauze. Take off the gauze bandage at least once a day, and gently clean the burn area with antibacterial soap and water. Reapply ointment and cover the wound with fresh gauze. As long as it looks better every day, then you are probably doing all right. You may use the ointment over a small blistered area, but burns with blistering over an area larger than a silver dollar need to be seen by a doctor.

4. Try zinc. The mineral zinc aids wound healing. Give 30 milligrams of zinc supplement twice a day for 10 days to your patient. But you need to check with your doctor first. Doses above 15 milligrams require medical supervision.

Choking

1. Call 911 or your designated emergency number. The choking could be caused by a complete or partial airway obstruction, but since either can be life-threatening, you need to get help right away.

2. Ask him to try to talk. The choking person should try to talk because if he can speak or even make any sound, then his airway is partially obstructed and he is not completely choking yet. He should try to dislodge the piece of food by coughing.

3. Fight the natural urge to thrust your hand into the mouth, whether it's yours or someone else's, to dig out whatever is stuck. One thing that you do not want to do is stick your fingers down the back of a conscious person's throat. You end up pushing whatever's stuck deeper down into the airway, making it even harder to get out.

4. Learn the Heimlich maneuver. Everybody should know how to perform the Heimlich maneuver, both on themselves and on others. For step-by-step instructions on how to do it correctly, see the following illustrations.

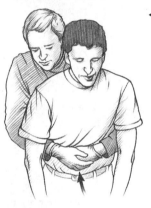

◀ **Performing the Heimlich maneuver on someone else**

If someone else is choking, stand in back of him and wrap your arms around his waist. Then make a fist with one hand and position the thumb side of your fist just above his belly button. Grab hold of your fist with your other hand.

Pull in and then up as hard as you can. You may need to do this four or five times to dislodge the object.

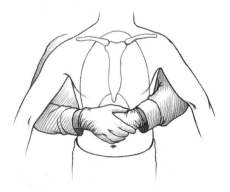

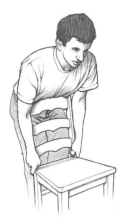

◀ Performing the Heimlich maneuver on yourself

If you're alone and choking, stand at the back of a chair. Lean over the chair so that the top is positioned just above your belly button. Supporting yourself by holding on to the sides with your hands, pull yourself down onto the back of the chair. You may need to do this four or five times until the object comes out.

5. If you can't find a chair to perform the Heimlich maneuver on yourself, throw a large object on the ground. Any object that provides a thrust to the abdominals will do. Just lay something down and flop yourself on top of it.

6. If the person who is choking becomes unconscious, lay him on the floor on his back and check the pulse. If he has a pulse, begin rescue breathing, which is explained and illustrated on pages 482 and 483. Give him two full breaths.

7. If the breaths won't go in, begin abdominal thrusts, which are similar to the Heimlich maneuver. To do this, straddle the unconscious victim with your legs, placing one hand on top of the other with your palms positioned just above the person's belly button. Your fingers should be pointing toward the person's head. Push upward toward the person's face with 6 to 10 good thrusts, says Dr. Roe.

8. Do a finger sweep to see if you have dislodged the object. With your two fingers in a hooked position, place them inside and to one side of the mouth. Using a sweeping motion, move the fingers to the other side. Having your fingers in a hook position pulls the item out toward you instead of pushing it farther down into the airway, Dr. Roe says.

9. If the object has not been dislodged, recheck the victim's pulse and repeat the steps, beginning with two rescue breaths, Dr. Roe says. If the person has no pulse, begin cardiopulmonary resuscitation, which is explained and illustrated on pages 484 and 485. In the event that the person regains consciousness at any time, put him in the recovery position (illustrated on page 486) until medical help arrives.

Drowning

How to Save Yourself

1. Stay calm. Panicking and flailing about in the water will only wear you down, making you more likely to drown. You need to conserve energy. The more energy you use panicking, the more you'll tire yourself and won't be able to help yourself.

2. You should slowly tread water without exerting too much of your energy. Look around and find your bearings—that is, see how far you are from land, how you can possibly get help, and how many people are around. Figure out the best way to get out of this situation.

3. Inflate your clothes. Your clothes make for great flotation devices if you're not wearing a life jacket. While treading water, tuck in your shirt or jacket or you could also tie the shirttail ends together. Unbutton the collar button and take a deep breath. Then bend your head forward into the water, pull the shirt or jacket up to your face, and blow into the shirt. Both your face and your shirt should be in the water when you're blowing the air into your shirt. After inflating your shirt, keep the front of the shirt or jacket underwater and hold the collar closed. The air trapped in the shirt will keep you afloat. With time, the air may seep out of the shirt. If that happens, just repeat the process.

4. Keep winter clothes on. If it's cold out, you shouldn't make the mistake of thinking that heavy winter clothes will weigh you down. Winter clothes may actually help you float and delay hypothermia in cold water. Lie back, spread your arms and legs, and use a winging motion with your arms to move toward safety. The air in the clothes will keep you on top of the water.

5. If you are in cold water, start to swim toward shore. In cold water, there's the added threat of hypothermia. But you should use easy, gentle strokes to get there. Swim forward but conserve your energy by doing a breaststroke or a sidestroke. Once you get tired, float for a while.

6. If caught up in a strong current, go with it. Don't fight it. If the current pushes you farther away from land, swim in a diagonal direction across the current, but not into it.

How to Help Someone Who Is Drowning

1. Find a nearby object—a lightweight pole or long stick—and use it to reach for the victim. If someone else is around, have that person grab your belt or pants and hold you for stability. And make sure that your feet are firmly planted.
2. If you can't find something to reach out with, throw something in the water that floats. An empty picnic jug, life jacket, cushion, piece of wood—anything you can find. If there's a rope handy, tie it to the object so that you can pull it back in or retrieve it to try again.
3. If there's no pole or object to throw, but there's a rowboat, canoe, boogie board, or some other water-worthy craft nearby, then row to the victim. Two cautions if you try this: Wear a life jacket. And to avoid capsizing, pull the victim in over the rear of the boat (the stern), not over the side.
4. Jumping in and swimming to save the victim yourself should be your last option if the other three techniques are impossible. But you should only try this if you are a capable swimmer trained in water lifesaving procedures. If you are untrained in these procedures; have improper equipment to reach, throw, or row to the victim; or would be putting yourself in danger, go get help instead.
5. If you have saved someone from a near drowning, you may need to start emergency measures such as rescue breathing and cardiopulmonary resuscitation. (Look in Basic Lifesaving Techniques on pages 482 to 485 for step-by-step, illustrated instructions.) If the person was rescued from cold water, you should remove their wet clothing and cover them with a dry blanket, adds Michael Espino, senior associate of new products and services development for the American Red Cross in Falls Church, Virginia.

Electric Shock
How to Help Yourself

A jolt of electricity may not always be strong enough to render you unconscious, but it can be strong enough to make your muscles involuntarily contract. If this happens, you may find yourself actually gripping the power source with your hand even though you want to let go.

If you have a free hand, grab a wooden object or a magazine or any nonconductive material and try to pry or slap your other hand from the wire. Or throw your body back so that you pull away from the source, says Paul Matera, M.D., an emergency medical technician-paramedic and vice chairman and professor of emergency services at Providence Hospital in Washington, D.C.

How to Help Someone Else

1. Turn off the power by unplugging the appliance. If that can't be done, then turn off a circuit breaker or a fuse box. If you have difficulty cutting off the source to an outside line, call the power company or 911 to see if they can shut it down.
2. After you have cut off the power, call 911.
3. Before jumping in to save someone who has had an electric shock, make sure that the power is cut off or you could be a victim as well. If someone is trapped in a car with a power line on top of it, tell him to stay put until the power has been shut off. If you feel your legs tingle as you get near a victim, stop. The sensation means that you are on energized ground and that an electrical current is entering your body. Raise one foot off the ground, turn around, and hop on one foot to a safe place.
4. Don't try to move live wires, even with wooden objects such as poles, handles, or tree branches. If the voltage is high enough, even these objects can conduct electricity, and the rescuer will be electrocuted. Definitely don't push wires with metal objects. Wait for properly trained personnel to arrive.
5. As soon as you can safely reach the victim, check his breathing and pulse. If he isn't breathing, start emergency breathing procedures. If he isn't breathing and doesn't have a pulse, start cardiopulmonary resuscitation. (Look in Basic Lifesaving Techniques on pages 484 to 485 for step-by-step, illustrated instructions.)
6. Let him lie. Someone who has experienced an electric shock may also have a spinal injury. Don't move the victim unless absolutely necessary to open his airway or give rescue breathing. Keep him in the position where you found him, and cover him with a jacket or blanket to keep him warm until medical help arrives.
7. Seek medical attention for the victim immediately. Although he may look fine or even say that he's okay, most of the damage from an elec-

tric shock is internal. You can look deceptively normal after a shock but actually have a great deal of nerve, vascular, and muscular damage.

Falling

1. Tell the person who fell not to move. After a hard fall, he should resist the temptation to jump up and deny that the accident occurred. Temporary numbness or pain can mask or exaggerate the severity of an injury.

   It is usually safe to wait a few moments to see if pain persists or dies down unless it is clear that the person is severely hurt—which means that the pain is intense, he is unable to move, or some part of his body is immovable. Only after a little time passes can you and the person accurately gauge the severity of the injury.

   Note: If the person who fell has significant pain in the neck or back; if he experiences weakness, numbness, tingling, or paralysis of an arm or leg; if he can't use an arm or leg; or if he has a deformity of an arm or leg, let the paramedics be the ones to move him. The only exceptions to this are if you're alone in a remote area with no chance of getting help or if the person is in danger.

2. Determine how badly he is hurt. Ask the person the following questions after a fall:

   - Is your pain moderate or severe?

   - Are you bleeding?

   - Can you move the area below the pain, meaning can you wiggle your toes and fingers?

   - Do you have normal sensation below the injured area?

   - Is there any deformity? Compare the injured area with the opposite area if necessary (for example, compare an injured arm to your uninjured arm).

   - Did you lose consciousness, even for only a moment?

   - Did you or are you experiencing any of the following: confusion, dizziness, severe headache, vomiting, weakness, or visual changes such as double vision?

3. Choose a course of action. From the answers to the above questions should come the answer to the next question: Does this person need to see a doctor, or can I handle this myself? Bloody scrapes you can handle. But if the person can't move the area or there's numbness, he may have a broken bone, a dislocation, or a nerve injury. Likewise, if his ankle slumps to one side or a finger points the wrong way, he will definitely need a doctor. And if he has smacked a vital area, like his head, you'd better be safe and have him see a doctor, says Warren Bowman, M.D., a doctor in Cooke City, Montana, and medical director of the National Ski Patrol. If you believe that the person is seriously injured, call 911, he says.

4. If you see an elderly person fall, you should assess the person carefully since fractures (especially of the spine and hip) are more common in seniors. Consult a doctor or take the person to the emergency room if there is any deformity, loss of use, marked swelling, or bruising, or if there is not significant recovery within 24 hours, Dr. Bowman says.

Open Wounds

1. First, put on a pair of latex gloves. Then place sterile gauze or, in a pinch, a piece of the cleanest cloth you have available over the wound and press down firmly to try to stop the bleeding. For a shallow cut, hold for 5 minutes; for a deep wound, hold for 15 to 20 minutes.

2. You can stop almost any bleeding with strong direct pressure and by elevating the wound above the heart to decrease the blood pressure on the cut. If it's your arm that's cut, hold it over your head. If it's your leg, lie down and put up your feet. When bloodflow stops, clotting starts. With pressure and elevation, you're giving the body time to do its work.

3. If there is significant bleeding or the wound is ½ inch deep or more (and so probably requires stitches), leave the cleaning to the experts. Apply direct pressure and a sterile gauze compress held in place by adhesive tape, elevate the area, and get to an emergency room.

   If the wound is minor and probably does not require stitches, remove any dirt and debris with tweezers once the bleeding has stopped. Sterilize tweezers, such as those in a Swiss Army knife, by flaming them with a match or cleaning them with an alcohol swab. If bleeding starts up again, just apply direct pressure.

Once the debris is out, cleanse the wound with hydrogen peroxide, Phisohex soap (an antibacterial skin cleanser), a povidone-iodine solution (a topical antiseptic microbicide), or just plain soap and water, which works about as well as anything. Don't scrub just the wound but also the skin for 4 inches around the cut because germs can crawl across skin surfaces.

4. Rinse it. After you've scrubbed, flush the soap or cleanser out of the wound with clean water. Do not use water from a lake or running stream, no matter how clean it looks. Use only the cleanest of drinking water.

5. Let the skin surface dry thoroughly, and, if you have it, apply a small bead of triple antibiotic ointment (bacitracin, neomycin, and polymyxin B) such as Neosporin or Mycitracin Plus to the cut. For shallow wounds, cover with a commercial bandage strip. If the wound gapes but isn't deep enough for stitches, use adhesive tape or butterfly bandages to pull it closed from each side.

6. Once the wound is clean and bandaged, you should check it every 2 days and reapply a clean bandage. Check the wound sooner if there are any signs of infection. If the bandage gets wet from showering, replace it. To prevent it from getting wet, tape plastic wrap over the bandage before showering—or take a bath.

Poisoning

1. If the victim has swallowed a poisonous substance, have him drink a half-glass (4 ounces) of milk or water. The drink will flush the chemicals out of his mouth and esophagus, where they can do the most damage, and send them to his stomach. But don't give him much more than a half-glass. If you flood the stomach with too much liquid, it will distend, exposing an even larger surface area to the poison. Once the victim has downed the milk or water, call the Poison Control Center immediately.

2. If the problem is a chemical that the victim has come in contact with, you need to get it off his body or out of his eyes as soon as possible. If it is a dry chemical, brush if off before getting wet. If you have quick access to a shower, put him in and have him stay under lukewarm water for 15 to 20 minutes. It's easier and more effective to wash off the substance in the shower than at a sink or with a cloth.

If you are near a hose or a sprinkler, you can use water from those instead. If the chemical is in the victim's eye, have him look straight into the shower head and blink his eyes under the water for 15 to 20 minutes as well.

3. The victim should shed every piece of clothing he has on if he has come in contact with a poisonous chemical, even if he doesn't think all of his clothing was contaminated. Wash the clothes immediately and don't mix them with other clothes.

4. Inhaling poisonous fumes can be just as dangerous as ingesting a chemical. If the victim has inhaled fumes, get him to fresh air immediately.

5. Do not force vomiting. Many people mistakenly believe that they have to force themselves to vomit if they've ingested poison. *Always* contact your Poison Control Center first for treatment recommendations. If certain substances get into the stomach in a small amount, it's not that bad. But if they go down the wrong pipe and get into the airways, they can be dangerous. Making the victim throw up increases the likelihood that the substance will go down the wrong pipe.

6. As soon as you have taken these immediate measures—to dilute the poison, rinse the skin or eyes, or get fresh air—call your local Poison Control Center. You can find the number on the inside cover or first page of the phone book. When you call, have the container of the poisonous substance on hand. They will either tell you how to handle the situation at home or advise you to call the proper authorities if you need medical attention. Then they will alert the facility where you are going and let them know that you are on the way and what the nature of the problem is. They'll also advise you whether you should induce vomiting.

7. Be prepared. When you call the Poison Control Center, you may be instructed to use either syrup of ipecac or activated charcoal. So it's a good idea to keep them on hand in case of emergency. Use them only as instructed.

Seizures

1. If you are around someone who's having a seizure, quickly move any furniture, sharp objects, or other potentially harmful items out of the way. Move anything nearby that could cause injuries.

2. Put a pillow or something else soft under the head of the person going into a seizure. The cushion will protect him from head injuries during the seizure.

3. A man's wallet is a perfect-size tool to keep a seizure victim from biting or swallowing his tongue. If you're around a person who's about to go into a seizure, insert the wallet—take the change out first—between his teeth and have him chomp down on it. If you don't have a wallet, use something that's not sharp and is too big for the person to swallow. Take care not to obstruct the airways: Put the wallet in the side of the mouth—don't stuff the whole thing into the mouth. Remove dentures if applicable. But if a person's in the midst of a full-blown seizure, don't try to force anything into his mouth. You could hurt him and yourself.

4. Leave him alone. Seizures can seem like they last forever. In reality, they usually last anywhere from 30 seconds to 5 minutes. During that time, be patient and don't panic. People who try to hold the victim down usually only end up hurting themselves and the person having the seizure. Don't try to shake him or wake him up. Let the seizure resolve itself.

5. During the seizure, put the person in the left-side recovery position if you can do this without injuring him. If not, wait until after the seizure is over to do this. Check to make sure that he is breathing and has a pulse. If not, call 911 and give rescue breathing or cardiopulmonary resuscitation as needed. Otherwise, monitor him until he fully recovers. (For step-by-step information on the recovery position, rescue breathing, and cardiopulmonary resuscitation, see Basic Lifesaving Techniques, beginning on page 481.)

6. Don't be alarmed. After a seizure, the victim may appear dazed, disoriented, even combative. Don't worry, this is normal, and it lasts from a few seconds to a few minutes. Just stay with him until he recovers.

Severed Appendages

First of all, call 911 immediately. The victim can bleed to death in 5 minutes if a cut has severed a major artery. Even less severe amputations like the tip of the finger can cause complications and be very painful. The quicker you get him to a hospital, the more likely that doctors will be able to reattach his severed body part.

While you are waiting for emergency assistance, do these things in this order.

1. Apply direct pressure to the wound using the cleanest object around, such as a shirt or a towel. Keep direct pressure on the stump until you get the person to the hospital. This will help stop the bleeding without the use of tourniquets and clamps, which often do more damage and are unnecessary if medical help is on the way.

2. If you can, elevate the injured appendage above heart level. Blood flows down with the help of gravity. By raising the body part above heart level, you'll slow down the blood loss.

3. If the appendage is hanging off or is only partly amputated, leave it alone. Removing a hanging piece of tissue will do more damage and make it harder to reattach. Apply direct pressure to the stump and support the other piece as best you can.

4. Soak sterile gauze with saline solution—the kind regularly used for contact lenses—and wrap the detached body part. It keeps the tissue moist and healthier. Saline is the best choice because it has the same salt content as human tissue, so it keeps the proper balance between salt and water in the cells. If you don't have saline solution, place the detached body part on dry, sterile gauze and cover it with the gauze. Try to avoid contact with regular water since it could be absorbed by the tissue, causing swelling and complications.

5. Once you've wrapped the severed part in sterile gauze soaked in saline solution, place it in a watertight container. Put the part in a cooler filled with ice. You want to keep it cool, but don't freeze it. Ice could damage the tissue. Also, don't allow water to get into the container. Soaking the appendage in water could also damage tissue and make it harder to reattach.

6. Even if you think that it is impossible to reattach, take the severed part to the hospital. You'd rather take something that can't be attached than not take something that could be.

7. If the victim feels light-headed, have him lie down with the stump elevated and wait for the ambulance.

Index

Underscored page references indicate boxed text. **Boldface** references indicate illustrations.

A

Abdominal crunches, 162–63
Abdominal fat, in men
    health risks from, 161
    reducing, with
        dietary changes, 162, 164
        exercise, 162–64
Abortion, teen pregnancy and,
        68–69
Absorbent products, for incontinence,
        297
Acarosan, for dust mite control,
        101–2
Accutane, for acne, 27
Acetaminophen
    for home medicine cabinet, 4
    mobility problems from, 322
    for treating
        fever, 54–55, 87–88
        muscle soreness, 328–29
        stomachache, 137
Acetic acid, for home medicine
        cabinet, 3
Acetyl-carnitine, for preventing
        memory problems, 316
Acidophilus suppositories, for yeast
        infections, 477
Acne
    cause of, 23–24
    cover-ups for, 25
    home treatments for, 24–27
    medical treatment for, 27

Actifed, poor concentration from, 373
Activated charcoal, for first-aid kit, 5,
        514
Activity, increasing, for mobility
        problems, 320–21
Acupressure, for menstrual discomfort,
        442
Addictions
    nicotine (see Smoking)
    sports
        dealing with, 250–52
        effects of, 249–50
        reasons for, 249
    TV
        negative effects of, 150
        overcoming, 150, 152–53
ADHD. See Attention
        deficit/hyperactivity disorder
Adoption, teen pregnancy and, 69
Agrimony, for incontinence,
        294–95
Alanine, for prostate enlargement,
        235–36
Alcohol, rubbing
    avoiding, as fever treatment, 89
    for first-aid kit, 5
Alcohol abuse, by teens, 72, 145
Alcoholic beverages
    effects of
        impotence, 214
        mobility problems, 322
    for preventing heart disease,
        193–94

Alcohol restriction
  in caregivers, 398
  for preventing
    cancer, 391–92
    migraines, 457
    snoring, 245
  for reducing abdominal fat, 164
  during smoking cessation, 240
  for treating
    gout, 192
    heart palpitations, 287
    incontinence, 296
    infertility, 432–33
    insomnia, 303
    sinusitis, 405
    urinary tract infections, 460
Allergies
  asthma and, 31–32
  causes of, 99
  chronic fatigue and, 407
  to dust mites, 101–3
  to foods, ulcer symptoms and, 264
  incontinence and, 297
  to mold, 103
  nettle for, 245–46
  to pets, 103–4
  to pollen, 99, 104–5
  snoring from, 243
  when to see the doctor about, 100
Allergy shots, 100
Allersearch ADS, for dust mite
    control, 101
Allicin potential, in garlic capsules,
    205
Aloe
  for hemorrhoids, 201
  for home medicine cabinet, 6
Alpha hydroxy products, for home
    medicine cabinet, 3
Alzheimer's disease. *See also* Dementia
  videos for, benefits of, 399
Amitriptyline, night vision problems
    from, 340
Amla, for baldness, 172–73
Amputations, first aid for, 515–16

Anemia
  causes of, 379
  treating, with
    diet, 380–81, 382–83
    herbs, 382–84
    iron supplements, 381–82
  when to see the doctor about, 380
Aniseed, for flatulence, 186, 187
Anorexia nervosa, 82, 85. *See also*
    Eating disorders
Antacids
  for home medicine cabinet, 3
  for ulcers, 264
Antibacterial soap, for home medicine
    cabinet, 3
Antibiotic ointment, for first-aid kit, 5
Antibiotics, for treating
  pneumonia, 368
  urinary tract infections, 459
Antidepressants
  side effects of
    insomnia, 302
    night vision problems, 340
    poor concentration, 373
  smoking cessation and, 238, 239–40
  for treating premature ejaculation,
    228–29
Antihistamines
  for allergies, 100
  avoiding, with colds, 56
  for home medicine cabinet, 3
  side effects of
    mobility problems, 322
    night vision problems, 340
    poor concentration, 373
Antioxidants. *See also* Beta-carotene;
    Vitamin C; Vitamin E
  for preventing dementia, 278–79
  for treating Parkinson's disease,
    357
Anxiety, poor concentration from,
    372
Apis, for treating
  gout, 191
  vaginitis, 465

Apnea, sleep, 244, <u>244</u>, 245
Appendicitis, symptoms of, <u>135</u>
Appetite loss, in older people, 344–45
Arginine, for intermittent claudication, 306
Arguments, sibling rivalry and, 131–34
Arnica
  for home medicine cabinet, 6
  for treating
    broken nose, 504
    bursitis and tendinitis, 175–76
    phlebitis, 364
    sprains, 256
Aromatherapy, for treating
  menstrual discomfort, 442
  poor concentration, <u>374</u>
  tension headaches, 453
Arsenicum album, for ulcers, 265
Arthritis
  causes of, 271
  hip pain from, 288
  nutrition for, 347
  treating, 271–75
  when to see the doctor about, <u>272</u>
Art therapy, for emotional and psychological problems, 9
Ashwaganda, for treating
  baldness, 172–73
  poor concentration, 373–74
Asian ginseng
  for increasing male fertility, 432
  for treating impotence, 215
Aspartame, avoiding, for blood pressure control, 204–5
Aspirin
  gout from, 192
  for home medicine cabinet, 4
  ulcers from, 267
Asthma
  symptoms of, 28
  treating, 28, 30–33
  when to see the doctor about, <u>29</u>
Astragalus, for colds and flu, 410
Atarax, poor concentration from, <u>373</u>

Attention deficit/hyperactivity disorder
  alienation due to, 110
  bad grades and, 34
  symptoms of, <u>36–37</u>

B

Baby bottle syndrome, 48
Baby powder, for home medicine cabinet, 3
Back pain
  causes of, 165
  treating, 165–69, <u>168</u>
  when to see the doctor about, <u>166</u>
Bacterial vaginosis, 462–63
Bad grades
  overcoming
    in adolescence, 39–40
    in grades 1 to 3, 34–36
    in grades 3 to 9, 36–39
    with school help, 40
  reasons for, 34
Baldness
  causes of, 170
  treating, 170–73
Bananas, as home remedy, 7
Bandages
  butterfly, for first-aid kit, 5
  elastic, for home medicine cabinet, 4
B-complex vitamins. *See also* Folic acid; Vitamin B_6; Vitamin B_{12}
  for preventing menstrual discomfort, 444
  for treating
    depression, 421–22
    menopausal problems, 436–37
Beano, for preventing gas, 185–86
Beans
  for chronic fatigue, 403
  preventing gas from, 185–86
Beclomethasone, night vision problems from, <u>340</u>
Beef, iron in, 380
Beer, for preventing heart disease, 193–94

Benadryl, side effects of
mobility problems, <u>322</u>
night vision problems, <u>340</u>
poor concentration, <u>373</u>
Benign prostatic hyperplasia (BPH)
preventing, 231–36
symptoms of, <u>230</u>, 232
treating, with
natural supplements, 232–36
prescription medication, 232
surgery, 232
Benzodiazepines, side effects of
mobility problems, <u>322</u>
poor concentration, <u>373</u>
Benzoyl peroxide, for acne, 26
Bergamot, for back pain, <u>168</u>
Beta-adrenergic blocking agents (beta-
blockers), side effects of
insomnia, <u>302</u>
night vision problems, <u>340</u>
Beta-carotene, for treating
Parkinson's disease, 357
vaginitis, 465
Betagan, night vision problems from,
<u>340</u>
Bilberry, for treating
diabetes, 183
night vision problems, 339
varicose veins, 469
Binge-eating disorder, 82. *See also*
Eating disorders
Bioflavonoids, for varicose veins,
469–70
Birth control, for teens, 126–28
Bitter melon, for diabetes, 182
Black cherry juice, for gout, 191
Black cohosh, for menopausal
problems, 438
Black currant oil, for preventing
menstrual discomfort, 443
Black haw, for treating menstrual
discomfort, 441–42
Blackheads, 24
Bladder control problems. *See*
Incontinence

Bladder drills, for incontinence, 294
Bladderwrack, for weight loss, 449
Bleeding
abnormal, <u>380</u>
in children, first aid for, 487–88
from open wounds, 512
from severed appendages, 515,
516
Blisters, from burns, 488, 489
Blood clots, varicose veins and, <u>468</u>
Blood pressure, high. *See* High blood
pressure
Blood sugar regulation. *See* Diabetes
Blue cohosh, for increasing fertility,
430
BMI, for determining overweight in
children, 119
Body clock, resetting, to overcome
insomnia, 298–99
Body mass index (BMI), for
determining overweight in
children, 119
Bones, broken. *See* Fractures
Boric acid suppositories, for yeast
infections, 476–77
Boron, for preventing osteoporosis,
351
Boswellia, for treating
arthritis, 274
bursitis and tendinitis, 175
BPH. *See* Benign prostatic
hyperplasia
Brahmi, for poor concentration,
372–73
Bras, for relieving
breast discomfort, 387
neck pain, 336
Breakfast
for chronic fatigue, 403
for weight loss, 447
Breast cancer
from estrogen replacement therapy,
280
flaxseed for preventing, 435
weight gain and, 389, 392

Breast discomfort
  causes of, 384–85
  treating, with
    dietary changes, 387–89
    home remedies, 385–87
    long-term strategies, 389
  when to see the doctor about,
    385
Breastfeeding, for preventing colds in
    infants, 53
Breathe Right, for preventing snoring,
    245
Breathing exercises
  for preventing premature
    ejaculation, 227
  for treating
    asthma, 32
    cigarette cravings, 242
    heart palpitations, 286
    memory problems, 319
    stress, 259
Breathing problems, in children, first
    aid for, 488
Broken bones. *See* Fractures
Broken nose, in adults, first aid for,
    503–4
Bromelain
  for preventing phlebitis, 365
  for treating
    bursitis and tendinitis, 176
    gout, 190
    intermittent claudication,
      307
    muscle soreness, 330–31
Bulimia, 82, 85. *See also* Eating
    disorders
Bullying
  grades affected by, 39
  helping child deal with, 42–44
  physical, 44–46
  prevalence of, 41
  seeking outside help with, 46–47
  signs of, 42
Bupropion, for smoking cessation, 238,
    239–40

Burns, first aid for
  in adults, 504–5, **504**
  in children, 488–89
Bursitis and tendinitis
  causes of, 174
  chronic, 177–78
  hip pain from, 288
  home remedies for, 175–77
  symptoms of, 173–74
  when to see the doctor about, <u>174</u>
Butazolidin, for arthritis, 274
Butcher's broom, for varicose veins,
    469
Butterfly bandages, for first-aid kit, 5

C

Cabbage juice, for ulcers, 264–65
Caffeine
  avoiding
    with breast discomfort, 388–89
    by caregivers, 398
    with depression, 423
    to increase fertility, 430
    to prevent kidney stones, 224
    with urinary tract infections, 460
  side effects of
    calcium loss, 353
    heart palpitations, 287
    incontinence, <u>295</u>, 296
    insomnia, 303
  for treating migraines, 456
Caladium, for vaginitis, <u>464</u>
Calamine lotion, for home medicine
    cabinet, 3
Calcium
  loss of, osteoporosis and, 353
  needs, of older people, 343–44
  for preventing
    kidney stones, 222
    menstrual discomfort, 443–44
    osteoporosis, 346, 348–50
  sources of, 6
  supplements, iron absorption and,
    381

Calendula
  for home medicine cabinet, 7
  for phlebitis, 364
Calorie needs, of older people, 343
Cancer
  breast
    from estrogen replacement
      therapy, 280
    flaxseed for preventing, 435
    weight gain and, 389, 392
  cervical, from human
      papillomavirus, 128
  preventing, with
    diet, 393–94
    lifestyle strategies, 390–93
  prostate
    preventing, 230–31
    symptoms of, 230
  stomach, 263
  symptoms of, when to see the doctor
      about, 391
Candy, hard, as home remedy, 8
Capsaicin cream, for arthritis, 272
Capsules, in herbal medicine, 13
Caraway seeds, for flatulence, 186
Carbonated drinks, flatulence from,
    187
Cardiopulmonary resuscitation (CPR)
  classes for, 481
  how to perform, 484, **485**
Caregivers
  planning by, 396–98
  problems affecting, 395–96
  profile of, 395
  stress in, when to see the doctor
      about, 396
  support groups for, 284
  ways of conserving energy for,
      398–400, 399
Carotene soup, for preventing
    pneumonia, 369
Carotenoids, for preventing cancer,
    393
Carotid pulse, checking for, 484, **484**
Cascara sagrada, for constipation,
    415–16

Castor oil, for treating
  breast discomfort, 386
  constipation, 416
Cataracts, night vision and, 338
Catnip, for colds, 58
Cat's claw, for ulcers, 265
Cavities, 47–52
  preventing, with
    eating habits, 50, 52
    tooth care, 48, 50, 51
Cayenne pepper
  cream, for back pain, 167–68
  as home remedy, 7
  for weight loss, 448
Celery seed, for gout, 192
Cervical cancer, from human
      papillomavirus, 128
Chamomile
  for home medicine cabinet, 7
  for treating
    bursitis and tendinitis, 177
    flatulence, 186
    insomnia, 301
    stress, 260
    ulcers, 266–67
Charcoal, activated, for first-aid kit, 5
Chasteberry
  for increasing fertility, 430
  for menopausal problems,
      438–39
Chemical exposure
  eye injuries from, 495–96
  poisoning from, 513–14
Chewing gum
  flatulence from, 187
  as home remedy, 7
  sugarless, for cavity prevention, 52
Chicken soup, as home remedy, 8
Chlamydia, 128, 458
Chlordiazepoxide, poor concentration
    from, 373
Chloroquine retinopathy, 312
Chlorpheniramine, night vision
    problems from, 340
Chlor-Trimeton, night vision problems
    from, 340

Choking, first aid for
in adults, 505–7, **506, 507**
in children, 490–92, **490, 491, 492**
Cholesterol
high (*see* High cholesterol)
types of, 207
Cholesterol-lowering medication,
208
Chromium, for controlling diabetes,
182
Chronic fatigue
with allergies, 407
sinusitis and, <u>404–5</u>
symptoms of, 401
treating, with
exercise, 401–3
herbs, 406–7
nutrition, 403, 406
when to see the doctor about, <u>401</u>
Cigarette cravings. *See* Smoking;
Smoking cessation
Cinnamon, for diabetes, 183
Citrus juices
avoiding, with urinary tract
infections, 460
for smoking cessation, 242
Cleansers, skin, for acne, 24, 26
Cloves, for macular degeneration, 311
Club drugs, abuse of, 73–74
Cocaine abuse, 73
Codeine, avoiding, with stomachache,
137–38
Coenzyme Q$_{10}$, for treating
chronic fatigue, 406
Parkinson's disease, 358
Colchicum, for gout, 190–91
Colds
pneumonia and, 367
preventing, 53, 55, 56, 408, 412–13
transmission of, 408
treating, 54–58, 409–12
when to see the doctor about, <u>54</u>,
<u>409</u>
Colic, massage for, <u>136</u>, <u>137</u>
Colloidal oatmeal bath, for home
medicine cabinet, 3

Comfrey, for treating
hemorrhoids, 201
sprains, 254–56
vaginitis, 466–67
Compresses
in herbal medicine, 14
for treating
back pain, <u>168</u>
gout, 190
Compression stockings
for preventing varicose veins,
471–72
for treating phlebitis, 362
Concealer, for hiding pimples, <u>25</u>
Concentration problems
with aging, 370–71
dealing with, 371–75, <u>374</u>
medications causing, <u>373</u>
when to see the doctor about, <u>371</u>
Condoms, 127
for preventing
premature ejaculation, 227
sexually transmitted diseases, 127,
129
urinary tract infections from, 462
yeast infections from, 476
Conflict
family, bad grades and, 40
resolution, for handling depression,
<u>420–21</u>
Congestion, in infants, 55
Constipation
in babies and children, 60–64, <u>61</u>
causes of, 59
regularity vs., 59
when to see the doctor about, <u>60</u>
effects of
hemorrhoids, 199, 200, 201
stomachache, 135, <u>136</u>, 138
varicose veins, 472
in women
avoiding laxatives for, 413
causes of, 414–15
preventing, 417
treating, 415–17, <u>416</u>
when to see the doctor about, <u>414</u>

Constriction bands, for preventing
  premature ejaculation, 227
Continuous positive airway pressure
  (CPAP), for snoring, 248
Contraception, for teens, 126–28
Convulsions. *See also* Seizures
  feverish, <u>90</u>
  without fever, first aid for,
    492–93
Corn silk, for treating
  incontinence, 294–95
  kidney stones, 222–23
Cortisone cream, for hemorrhoids,
    199–200
Cosmetics, acne from, 26–27
Cotton swabs and cotton balls, for
    home medicine cabinet, 4
Coughing
  in children, 55–56
  to stop heart palpitations, 285
  incontinence and, 297
Cough medicine, for home medicine
    cabinet, 4
CPAP, for snoring, 248
CPR
  classes for, 481
  how to perform, 484, **485**
Cramp bark
  for increasing fertility, 430
  for menstrual discomfort, 441–42
Cramps, menstrual. *See* Menstrual
    discomfort
Cranberry capsules, for urinary tract
    infections, 460
Cranberry juice
  for preventing kidney stones, 223
  for treating urinary tract infections,
    459–60, 461
Crunches, abdominal, 162–63
Curcumin, for treating
  arthritis, 274
  back pain, 169
  bursitis and tendinitis, 177
Curfews, 130, 148
Cyberdating, cautions about, 70

D

Dairy products
  avoiding
    with hemorrhoids, 201
    to prevent menstrual discomfort,
      443
  for controlling high blood pressure,
    204
  gas from, 184, 185, 187
Damiana, for treating
  inhibited sexual desire, 219
  menopausal problems, 438–39
Dandelion
  for liver protection, 212
  for treating
    anemia, 383–84
    constipation, 417
    kidney stones, 222
  for weight loss, 449
Dantrium, incontinence from, <u>295</u>
Dantrolene, incontinence from, <u>295</u>
Date book, for changing bad habits, 9
Date rape, 67
Date-rape drugs, 67
Dating
  dangers of, 67, 70–71
  establishing rules for, 64–67
  sex and, 129–30
  teen pregnancy and, <u>68–69</u>
Decoctions, herbal, 11
Decongestants
  for home medicine cabinet, 4
  for treating
    allergies, <u>100</u>
    broken nose, 503
    colds, 56
    sinusitis, <u>405</u>
Deep-vein thrombosis (DVT), 361
Deglycyrrhizinated licorice (DGL)
    lozenges, for ulcers, 267
Dehydration
  in older people, 296–97, 344
  from vomiting, 154, <u>156</u>, 157
Deltasone, insomnia from, <u>302</u>

Dementia. *See also* Memory problems
cause of, 276
dealing with, 281–84
preventing, 278–81, 279
signs of, 276, 277
when to see the doctor about, 277
Dental flossing, in children, 50
Dental phobia, avoiding, 49
Depo-Provera, for contraception, 127
Depression
bad grades and, 40
in caregivers, 396, 396
causes of, 418
memory loss and, 317
self-care for, 419–23
symptoms of
in children, 106
in women, 418, 419
visualization for overcoming,
420–21
when to see the doctor about, 419
Desensitization cream, for preventing
premature ejaculation,
227–28
Desyrel, night vision problems from,
340
DEXA, for identifying osteoporosis,
349
DGL lozenges, for ulcers, 267
Diabetes
causes of, 179–80
in children and teens, 119
controlling, with
chromium, 182
diet, 181
exercise, 180–81
herbs, 182–83
effects of, 180
impotence, 214, 214
intermittent claudication, 303
night vision problems, 338
yeast infections, 474
types of, 178–79
when to see the doctor about, 179
Diabetic retinopathy, 183

Diaphragm, urinary tract infections
from, 462
Diazepam, poor concentration from,
373
Diet(ing)
for diabetes, 181
low-fat
for heart disease, 196–97
for intermittent claudication, 308
for prostate cancer, 231
for reducing abdominal fat, 162, 164
weight-loss, 446–48
Digital/rectal exam, for prostate cancer
screening, 230
Diphenhydramine, side effects of
mobility problems, 322
night vision problems, 340
poor concentration, 373
Diuretics, insomnia from, 302
DMAE, for preventing memory
problems, 316
Doctors, herbal medicine, 16–17
Dong quai, for menopausal problems,
438, 439
Dopamine agonists, for Parkinson's
disease, 355, 356
Douching, for yeast infections, 476
Doxylamine, night vision problems
from, 340
Driving, night vision problems and,
340–41
Drowning
in children, first aid for, 493–94
saving someone else from, 509
saving yourself from, 508
Drug abuse
bad grades and, 39–40
dating and, 70
help for, 78–79
learning about, 71–72
parenting strategies for preventing,
74, 76–78
signs of, 75
substances involved in, 72–74
by teens, 145

Dust mite allergies, 101–3
DVT, 361
Dyslexia, 38

E

Eating disorders
    causes of, 82–83
    diagnosis of, 82
    symptoms of, 81–82
    treating, 83–85
    types of, 80–81
Echinacea
    for home medicine cabinet, 7
    for preventing yeast infections,
        477
    for treating
        colds and flu, 57, 58, 410
        phlebitis, 364
Ecstasy, abuse of, 73
Ejaculation
    premature
        causes of, 225
        preventing, 226–29
    for preventing prostate problems,
        231
Elastic bandages, for home medicine
    cabinet, 4
Elavil, night vision problems from,
    340
Eldepryl, for memory loss, 317
Elder flowers, for colds, 58
Electric shock
    in children, first aid for, 494
    saving someone else from, 510–11
    saving yourself from, 509–10
Emergency contraception, 128
Emergency medical services, how to
    contact, 481
Emetrol, for vomiting, 158
EPA, for gout, 190
Erectile dysfunction. See Impotence
Ergoloid mesylates, for memory loss,
    317
ERT. See Estrogen replacement
    therapy

Essential fatty acids
    for preventing memory problems, 316
    for treating prostate enlargement,
        235
Essential oils, in herbal medicine, 13
Estrogen replacement therapy (ERT).
        See also Hormone-replacement
        therapy (HRT)
    breast discomfort from, 385
    calcium requirement with, 348–49
    for preventing dementia, 280
Eucalyptus oil, for bursitis and
        tendinitis, 177
Evening primrose oil
    for preventing menstrual discomfort,
        443
    for treating
        arthritis, 273
        breast discomfort, 386
Exercise(s)
    beginning, 424–25
    breathing (see Breathing exercises)
    creating routine for, 425–27
    keeping fun in, 427
    Kegel
        for controlling incontinence,
            292–93, 297
        for preventing premature
            ejaculation, 227
    mental
        for poor concentration, 375
        for preserving memory, 315
    for preventing
        cancer, 392
        caregiver stress, 400
        heart disease, 195–96
        hemorrhoids, 200
        inactivity, 424–27
        memory problems, 315
        osteoporosis, 351–52
        phlebitis, 362–63
        pneumonia, 370
        prostate problems, 231
        snoring, 246–48
        sprains, 256
        varicose veins, 471

for reducing abdominal fat, 162–64
stretching (*see* Stretching)
for treating
  arthritis, 271–72, 273
  breast discomfort, 389
  chronic fatigue, 401–3
  cigarette cravings, 242
  dementia, 282
  depression, 423
  diabetes, 180–81
  high blood pressure, 203
  high cholesterol, 210
  impotence, 214
  inhibited sexual desire, 219
  insomnia, 302–3
  menopausal problems, 439
  Parkinson's disease, 359
  stress, 261–62
walking (*see* Walking)
for weight control, 121–22
for weight loss, 449–50
Eye injuries, first aid for, 494
  from chemical exposure, 495–96,
    513–14
  from foreign body, 495

F

Face mask, for first-aid kit, 5, 482
Falls
  first aid for
    in adults, 511–12
    in children, 496
  preventing
    from osteoporosis, 353
    from Parkinson's disease, 359–60
False unicorn root, for increasing
    fertility, 429–30
Family conflict, bad grades and, 40
Fat, abdominal. *See* Abdominal fat
Fat, body, breast discomfort and, 389
Fat, dietary
  as cause of
    heart disease, 196–97, 346–47
    intermittent claudication, 308
    prostate cancer, 231

Parkinson's disease and, 356–57
restricting
  for cancer prevention, 394
  for lowering cholesterol, 211
  for menstrual discomfort, 443
Fatigue
  chronic (*see* Chronic fatigue)
  poor concentration from, 372
Fatty acids. *See* Essential fatty acids;
    Omega-3 fatty acids
Fennel, for treating
  flatulence, 186–87
  menopausal problems, 436
Ferrous sulfate, for anemia, 381
Fever
  causes of, 85–86
  convulsions with, **90**
  roseola with, **88**
  taking temperature to determine,
    87
  treating, 54–55, 87–89, 91
  when to see the doctor about, **86**
Feverfew, for migraines, 453–54
Fiber
  needs, of older people, 344
  for preventing
    constipation, 62–63, 417
    varicose veins, 472
  for treating
    breast discomfort, 388
    constipation, 415
    hemorrhoids, 200
    high cholesterol, 209–10
  for weight loss, 447
Fiber supplement, for home medicine
    cabinet, 4
Finasteride
  for baldness, 170–71
  cautions about, 171
  for prostate enlargement, 232
Finger injuries, in children, first aid
    for, 496–97
First aid
  for adults
    broken bones, 501–3, **502**
    broken nose, 503–4

First aid *(cont.)*
  for adults *(cont.)*
    burns, 504–5, **504**
    choking, 505–7, **506, 507**
    drowning, 508–9
    electric shock, 509–11
    falls, 511–12
    open wounds, 512–13
    poisoning, 513–14
    seizures, 514–15
    severed appendages, 515–16
  basic lifesaving techniques
    checking for carotid pulse, 484, **484**
    CPR, 484, **485**
    recovery position, 486, **486**
    rescue breathing, 482, **483**
    shock position, 486, **486**
  for children
    bleeding, 487–88
    breathing problems and suffocation, 488
    burns, 488–89
    choking, 490–92, **490, 491, 492**
    convulsions without fever, 492–93
    drowning, 493–94
    electric shock injuries, 494
    eye injuries, 494–96
    falls, 496
    finger or toe injuries, 496–97
    frostbite, 497–98
    head injuries, 498–99
    poisoning, 500
First-aid kit
  for performing lifesaving techniques, 482
  supplies for, 5
Fish
  benefits of, 8
  for preventing
    cancer, 394
    heart disease, 8, 195
    menstrual discomfort, 443
  for treating rheumatoid arthritis, 8, 273
Fish oil, for treating
  arthritis, 273
  prostate enlargement, 235
5-HTP, for depression, 422
Flatulence
  causes of, 184
  preventing, 187
  treating, 185–87, <u>186</u>
  when to see the doctor about, <u>185</u>
Flaxseed, for treating
  constipation, 415
  menopausal problems, 435
Flaxseed oil
  for preventing memory problems, 316
  for treating
    arthritis, 273
    constipation, 8
    prostate enlargement, 235
    skin problems, 8
Flossing, dental, in children, 50
Flu
  preventing, 408, 412–13
  transmission of, 408
  treating, 409–12
  when to see the doctor about, <u>409</u>
Fluid(s)
  for colds and flu, 409
  needs, of older people, 344
Flunitrazepam, as date-rape drug, 67, 74
Fluoxetine
  insomnia from, <u>302</u>
  for premature ejaculation, 228–29
Folate, for preventing heart disease, 197
Folic acid
  for increasing fertility, 429
  for preventing
    cancer, 394
    phlebitis, 363
  for treating depression, 422
Food allergies, ulcer symptoms and, 264
Food record, for assessing constipation, 62

Fractures
    first aid for
        in adults, 501–3, **502**
        in children, 496
    from osteoporosis, 348
    preventing, 353
Frostbite, in children, first aid for,
        497–98
Fruit cocktail, antiulcer, <u>266</u>
Fruit juices, for preventing kidney
        stones, 222
Fruits
    for preventing heart disease, 194–95
    for treating
        chronic fatigue, 403
        constipation, 415
        heart disease, 346
        high blood pressure, 204
        macular degeneration, 310

G

Gangs
    help in leaving, 97–98
    preventing involvement in, 94–97
    reasons for joining, 91–94
    signs of membership in, <u>92–93</u>
Garlic
    benefits of, 8
    for preventing
        cancer, 394
        pneumonia, 369
        yeast infections, 477
    soup, for colds, <u>411</u>
    for treating
        high blood pressure, 205
        high cholesterol, 208–9
        intermittent claudication, 306
        ulcers, 265–66
Gas pain. *See* Flatulence; Stomachache
Gastroesophageal reflux, insomnia
        from, 301
Gauze, sterile, for first-aid kit, 5
Ginger
    for home medicine cabinet, 7
    soup, for colds, <u>411</u>

for treating
    arthritis, 275
    bursitis and tendinitis, 177
    colds and flu, 410
    gout, 190
    intermittent claudication, 307
    menstrual discomfort, 442
    muscle soreness, 331
    snoring, <u>247</u>
    stomachache, 139–40
Ginkgo
    for home medicine cabinet, 7
    for mental functioning, <u>279</u>, 318
    for treating
        back pain, 169
        high blood pressure, 206–7
        impotence, 215
        intermittent claudication, 306
        macular degeneration, 310–11
        migraines, 455–56
        Parkinson's disease, 357–58
Ginseng
    for home medicine cabinet, 7
    for increasing male fertility, 432
    for treating
        chronic fatigue, 406–7
        diabetes, 182
        poor concentration, 372
        stress, 260
Glasses, for night vision problems,
        341–42
Glucosamine sulfate, for arthritis,
        273–74
Glutamic acid, for prostate
        enlargement, 235–36
Glycine, for prostate enlargement,
        235–36
Glycolic acid, for acne, 26
Goldenrod, for treating
    kidney stones, 222
    urinary tract infections, 460
Goldenseal
    for home medicine cabinet, 7
    for preventing yeast infections,
        477
    for treating colds and flu, 410

Gotu kola
  for preventing varicose veins, 472
  for treating
    broken nose, 503–4
    chronic fatigue, 406
    poor concentration, 374–75
Gout
  cause of, 188
  diagnosis of, 189
  preventing, 192
  treating, 189–92
  when to see the doctor about, <u>189</u>
Grains, for chronic fatigue, 403
Grape juice, for preventing heart
    disease, 194
Grape seed extract, for treating
  bursitis and tendinitis, 178
  macular degeneration, 311
  varicose veins, 470
Green tea, for weight loss, 448
Grievous Bodily Harm, abuse of, 73
Guaiacum, for rheumatoid arthritis,
    275
Guggul
  for lowering cholesterol, 211–12
  for weight loss, 449
Gum, chewing
  for cavity prevention, 52
  flatulence from, 187
  as home remedy, 7
Gums, cleaning, in babies, 48
Gurmar, for diabetes, 182–83
Gymnema sylvestre, for diabetes,
    182–83

H

Hair loss
  causes of, 170
  treating, 170–73
Hairpieces, 172
Hair products, acne from, 26–27
Haldol, poor concentration from, <u>373</u>
Haloperidol, poor concentration from,
    <u>373</u>

Hawthorn, for treating
  high blood pressure, 205–6, 207
  high cholesterol, 212
  incontinence, 295–96
Hay fever, 99, 104–5, 243
Hazardous substances, preventing
    cancer from, 392–93
HDL cholesterol, 207, 210
Headaches. *See also* Migraines
  preventing, 456–57
  tension
    causes of, 451
    herbal remedies for, 452–53
  triggers of, 456
  when to see the doctor about, <u>452</u>
Head injuries, in children, first aid for,
    498–99
Heart attack
  cause of, 193
  intermittent claudication and, <u>304</u>
  from nicotine patch, <u>237</u>
  reducing risk of, <u>209</u>
  symptoms of, <u>194</u>
Heartburn, insomnia from, 301
Heart disease
  causes of, 193
  nutrition for, 346–47
  preventing, 193–97
  when to see the doctor about, <u>194</u>
Heart palpitations, 285–87
  when to see the doctor about, <u>285</u>
Heat, for treating
  back pain, 168–69
  hip pain, 288
  neck pain, 335
  phlebitis, 362
  stomachache, 135–36
Heating pad, for healing and pain
    relief, 9
Height and weight charts, for
    determining overweight in
    children, 118
Heimlich maneuver, performed on
  adults, 505–7, **506**
  babies, 490–91, **490, 491**

children over 1 year old, 491–92,
491, 492
self, 507, **507**
Helicobacter pylori, ulcers from, 262–63
Hemorrhoids
causes of, 198, 199
treating, 199–201
types of, 198
when to see the doctor about, <u>199</u>
Herbalists, finding, <u>17</u>
Herbal medicine
finding practitioner of, <u>16–17</u>
forms of
capsules and tablets, 13
compresses, 14
essential oils, 13
poultices, 14
salves, 13–14
solid extracts, 13
teas, 11–12
tinctures, 12
general guidelines for, 20
Herbal teas. *See* Teas, herbal
Herbs
buying, in bulk, 15, 18
for children, 56–57, 139
for home medicine cabinet, 6–7
for increasing appetite, 345
shopping for, 14–15
standardization of, 18–19
High blood pressure
in children and teens, 119
in men
causes of, 202
controlling, 203–7
readings of, 202–3
when to see the doctor about, <u>203</u>
in older people
dementia and, 280–81
diuretics for, <u>302</u>
intermittent claudication from, 303
High cholesterol
in children and teens, 119
in men

causes of, 207–8
health risks from, 208, <u>209</u>
reducing, 208–12
in older people, intermittent claudication from, 303
Hip pain
causes of, 288
treating, 288–91
when to see the doctor about, <u>289</u>
HIV, in teens, 128, 129
Holistic physicians, herbal medicine and, <u>17</u>
Homeopathic remedies, for treating
gout, 191
vaginitis, <u>464–65</u>
yeast infections, <u>475</u>
Honey, as home remedy, 8
Hormonal tests, for evaluating memory loss, <u>317</u>
Hormone-replacement therapy (HRT). *See also* Estrogen replacement therapy (ERT)
for menopausal problems, <u>436–37</u>
migraines with, 452
Horse chestnut, for treating
phlebitis, 363–64
varicose veins, 469
Horseradish, as home remedy, 8
Horsetail, for treating
gout, 191
incontinence, 293–94
Hot flashes, 438–39
Hot-pepper sauce, for weight loss, 448
HPV, 128
Human immunodeficiency virus (HIV), in teens, 128, 129
Human papillomavirus (HPV), 128
Humidifier, for relieving dryness, 9
Hydergine, for memory loss, <u>317</u>
Hydrocortisone cream, for home medicine cabinet, 4
Hydrogen peroxide, for first-aid kit, 5
Hydroxyzine, poor concentration from, <u>373</u>
Hypertension. *See* High blood pressure

I

Ibuprofen
    for home medicine cabinet, 4
    for treating
        bursitis and tendinitis, 175
        gout, 189
        hip pain, 289–90
        menstrual discomfort,
            440–41
        phlebitis, 362
Ice packs
    for first-aid kit, 5
    for treating
        arthritis, 275
        breast discomfort, 386
        hip pain, 288–89
        migraines, 456
        muscle soreness, 328
        neck pain, 335
        sprains, 253–54
Imipramine, side effects of
    night vision problems, 340
    poor concentration, 373
Impotence
    causes of, 213
    incidence of, 213
    psychological impact of, 213–14
    treating, 214–16
    when to see the doctor about,
        214
Inactivity, 424–27
Incontinence
    incidence of, 292
    from medications, 295
    treating, 292–97
    when to see the doctor about,
        293
Inderal, insomnia from, 302
Indigestion, insomnia from, 301
Infections
    sinus, 54, 404–5
    urinary tract (see Urinary tract
        infections)
    yeast (see Yeast infections)

Infertility
    avoiding
        general tips for, 432–33
        in men, 431–32
        in women, 429–31
    causes of, 428
    when to see the doctor about, 429
Infusions, herbal, 11
Inhalants, abuse of, 73
Inhalers, asthma, 28, 30–33
Inhibited sexual desire
    causes of, 216–17
    treating, 217–19
Insomnia
    causes of, 297–98
    medications causing, 302, 356
    treating, 298–303
    when to see the doctor about, 298
Insulin resistance, from aspartame
    abuse, 204–5
Intermittent claudication
    causes of, 303–4
    treating, 304–8
    when to see the doctor about,
        304
Ipecac syrup, for first-aid kit, 5, 500,
    514
Iron
    dietary sources of, 380–81,
        382–83
    excess, in men, 5–6
    loss of, anemia from, 379
Iron supplements
    for anemia, 381
    side effects of, 381–82
Isoflavones, for menopausal problems,
    434–35
Isopto Carpine, night vision problems
    from, 340
Isotretinoin, for acne, 27

J

Juniper oil, for bursitis and tendinitis,
    177

K

Karate, for protection from bullying, 45
Karo syrup, for constipation in babies, 62
Kava
 for home medicine cabinet, 7
 for treating
  incontinence, 296
  insomnia, 301
  stress, 261
Kegel exercises
 for controlling incontinence, 292–93, 297
 for preventing premature ejaculation, 227
Ketamine, abuse of, 74
Kidney stones, 220–21
 foods promoting, 224
 preventing, 221–25
 when to see the doctor about, 221
Kreosotum, for treating
 vaginitis, 465
 yeast infections, 475

L

Lactaid, for lactose intolerance, 185
Lactinex, for lactose intolerance, 185
Lactobacillus acidophilus, for lactose intolerance, 185
Lactose intolerance, gas from, 184, 185, 187
Latex gloves, for first-aid kit, 5
Lavender, for treating
 back pain, 168
 inhibited sexual desire, 218
 tension headaches, 453
Laxatives, avoiding, with constipation, 62, 413
LDL cholesterol
 heart disease and, 193, 197, 207
 lowering, with
  exercise, 210
  medication, 208

Learning disabilities
 bad grades and, 34
 symptoms of, 38
Leg pain. *See* Intermittent claudication
Leg stretches, for back pain, 166–67
Lemon, as home remedy, 8
Lemon balm, for tension headaches, 453
Lemon juice, for constipation, 416
Librium, poor concentration from, 373
Licorice
 for smoking cessation, 241–42
 for treating
  chronic fatigue, 406
  colds, 58
  constipation, 417
  ulcers, 267
Lifesaving techniques
 avoiding disease transmission from, 482
 checking for carotid pulse, 484, **484**
 CPR, 484, **485**
 learning to perform, 481–82
 recovery position, 486, **486**
 rescue breathing, 482, **483**
 shock position, 486, **486**
Lighting, for night vision problems, 337–39
Liver function
 breast discomfort and, 386–87
 high cholesterol and, 212
 Parkinson's disease and, 358
Lobelia, for smoking cessation, 241–42
Loneliness
 depression and, 106
 help for
  all children, 107–9
  teens, 110–12
  young children, 109–10
 recognizing, 105, 107
 as suicide risk factor, 110, 111
Low-fat diet
 for preventing
  heart disease, 196–97
  prostate cancer, 231

Low-fat diet *(cont.)*
  for reducing abdominal fat, 164
  for treating intermittent
    claudication, 308

M

Macular degeneration
  causes of, 308–9
  chloroquine retinopathy vs., <u>312</u>
  dealing with, 309–13
  night vision problems with, <u>338</u>
  when to see the doctor about, <u>309</u>
Magnesium
  deficiency of, 403
  for preventing
    menstrual discomfort, 443–44,
      <u>455</u>
    osteoporosis, 350
  sources of, 6
  for treating
    caregiver stress, 399–400
    intermittent claudication, 306
Male bonding, sports and, 249
Malic acid, for chronic fatigue, 406
Manganese, for bursitis, 176–77
Marijuana, abuse of, 72
Marshmallow root, for treating
  kidney stones, 222–23
  urinary tract infections, 460, 461
Massage, for treating
  bursitis and tendinitis, 175
  muscle soreness, 330
  stomachache, <u>136–37</u>
Masturbation, for preventing
    premature ejaculation, 226
Meat
  avoiding
    with gout, 192
    to prevent menstrual discomfort,
      443
  cured, migraines from, 456
  red, cancer risk from, 394
Medications. *See also specific medications*
  dementia and, 281
  for home medicine cabinet, 3–4

side effects of
  incontinence, <u>295</u>
  insomnia, <u>302</u>
  mobility problems, <u>322</u>
  night vision problems, <u>340</u>
Meditation, for poor concentration, 375
Memory problems. *See also* Dementia
  dealing with, 315–16, 318–19
  myths about, 313–14
  from nutritional deficiencies,
    345–46
  what to ask the doctor about, <u>317</u>
  when to see the doctor about, <u>314</u>
Menopausal problems
  hormone-replacement therapy for,
    <u>436–37</u>
  natural help for, 434–40
  symptoms of, 434
  vaginitis after, 463, 473
  when to see the doctor about, <u>435</u>
Menstrual discomfort
  migraines, 452
    preventing, <u>454–55</u>
  preventing, 443–44
  treating, 441–43
  types of, 440
  when to see the doctor about, <u>441</u>
Menstruation
  irregular, when to see the doctor
    about, <u>435</u>
  vaginitis before, 463, 473
Mercurius solubilis, for vaginitis, <u>465</u>
Mercurius vivus, for vaginitis, <u>465</u>
Migraines
  menstrual, 452
    preventing, <u>454–55</u>
  preventing, 456–57
  symptoms of, 451–52
  treating, 453–56
  triggers of, 456
Milk
  avoiding, with
    sinusitis, <u>405</u>
    ulcers, 264
  gas from, 184, 185, 187
  as home remedy, 8

Milk thistle, for liver protection, 358
Mineral oil, for constipation in
    children, 62
Minoxidil, for baldness, 171
Mobility problems
    dealing with, 320–24
    medications aggravating, 322
    stretching routine for, 324,
        324–27
    when to see the doctor about, 321
Mold allergies, 103
Motherwort, for treating
    high blood pressure, 206
    stress, 259–60
Mouthpieces, for preventing snoring,
    248
Muira puama, for treating
    impotence, 216
    inhibited sexual desire, 219
Multivitamin/mineral supplements,
    5–6
    for preventing
        cancer, 394
        memory problems, 315–16
        menstrual migraines, 455
    for treating
        caregiver stress, 398–99
        chronic fatigue, 406
Muscle soreness
    causes of, 328, 427
    treating, 328–33
    when to see the doctor about, 329

N

Naproxen sodium, for gout, 189–90
Nasal dilators, for preventing snoring,
    245
Nasal sprays
    avoiding, with allergies, 100
    for home medicine cabinet, 4
    for preventing snoring, 246
    for treating
        broken nose, 503
        sinusitis, 405
Naturopaths, 17

Neck pain
    causes of, 333–34
    treating, 334–36
    when to see the doctor about, 334
Nettle
    for treating
        prostate enlargement, 233
        snoring, 245–46
    for weight loss, 449
Nicotine addiction, 236. See also
        Smoking
Nicotine gum, for smoking cessation,
    239, 242
Nicotine patch, for smoking cessation,
    239
    heart attack from, 237
Nightmares
    dealing with, 116–17
    identifying, 114
Night sweats, in menopause, 439
Night terrors
    dealing with, 114, 116
    identifying, 113–14
Night vision problems
    causes of, 337
    dealing with, 337–42
    medications causing, 340
    when to see the doctor about, 338
Nootropyl, for memory loss, 317
Nose
    broken, first aid for, 503–4
    sore, from cold, 55
Nutrition
    basic nutrients for, 342–44
    for common health problems,
        345–47
    for lack of appetite, 344–45
Nyquil, night vision problems from,
    340
Nytol, poor concentration from, 373

O

Oak bark, for preventing snoring, 246
Oatmeal bath, for home medicine
    cabinet, 3

Oatstraw
  for smoking cessation, 241–42
  for stress relief, 259
Obesity. *See* Overweight
Ointment, antibiotic, for first-aid kit, 5
Olive oil, for heart health, 8
Omega-3 fatty acids
  for preventing cancer, 394
  for treating
    prostate enlargement, 235
    rheumatoid arthritis, 273
Onions, for preventing pneumonia, 369
Oral contraceptives, 127, <u>385</u>
Orange juice
  as home remedy, 8
  for iron absorption, 381
  for smoking cessation, 242
Oregon grape root
  for preventing snoring, 246
  for treating colds, 58
Orgasms, 225–26, 228, 431
Osteoarthritis. *See* Arthritis
Osteoporosis
  effects of, 348
  preventing, 346, 348–53
  when to see the doctor about, <u>349</u>
Overweight. *See also* Weight control; Weight loss
  in children
    dealing with (*see* Weight loss, strategies, in children)
    health risks from, 118
    methods of determining, 118–19
  effects of
    impotence, 214–15
    infertility, 433
  in women
    breast cancer and, 389, 392
    dealing with (*see* Weight loss, in women)
    when to see the doctor about, <u>446</u>
Ovulation, determining time of, 433

P

Pain
  back
    causes of, 165
    treating, 165–69, <u>168</u>
    when to see the doctor about, <u>166</u>
  gas (*see* Flatulence; Stomachache)
  hip
    causes of, 288
    treating, 288–91
    when to see the doctor about, <u>289</u>
  leg (*see* Intermittent claudication)
  neck
    causes of, 333–34
    treating, 334–36
    when to see the doctor about, <u>334</u>
Pain medicine. *See also specific pain medicines*
  for home medicine cabinet, 4
Palpitations, heart, 285–87
  when to see the doctor about, <u>286</u>
Papaya tablets, for flatulence, 186
Parkinson's disease
  effects of, 354
  lifestyle strategies with, 359–60
  medications for, 354–55
    reducing side effects of, 355–57
  supplements for, 357–58
  when to see the doctor about, <u>355</u>
Partridgeberry, for increasing fertility, 430
Passionflower, for treating
  insomnia, 299, 301
  stress, 260
Peanut butter, for preventing heart disease, 197
Pepper
  cayenne (*see* Cayenne pepper)
  for lowering cholesterol, 210
Peppermint
  for counteracting garlic and onion odor, 369–70
  for treating
    back pain, <u>168</u>
    colds, 58

flatulence, <u>186</u>
stomachache, 140
tension headaches, 453
Pepto-Bismol, for home medicine
cabinet, 4
Periods, irregular, when to see the
doctor about, <u>435</u>
Periwinkle, for preventing memory
loss, 318
Personal trainers, 427
Petroleum jelly, for home medicine
cabinet, 4
Pets, allergies to, 103–4
Phenothiazines, mobility problems
from, <u>322</u>
Phenylbutazone, for arthritis, 274
Phlebitis
causes of, 360–61
treating, 362–65
types of, 361
when to see the doctor about, <u>361</u>
Phobia, dental, <u>49</u>
Phospholipids, for preventing memory
problems, 316
Pillows
herbal, for insomnia, <u>300</u>
for neck pain, 336
Pilocar, night vision problems from,
<u>340</u>
Pilocarpine, night vision problems
from, <u>340</u>
Pimples. See Acne
Pine bark extract, for bursitis and
tendinitis, 178
Pipsissewa, for urinary tract infections,
460
Piracetam, for memory loss, <u>317</u>
Pitressin, for memory loss, <u>317</u>
Plaquenil, chloroquine retinopathy
from, <u>312</u>
Pneumococcal vaccine, for preventing
pneumonia, 367–68
Pneumonia
antibiotics for, <u>368</u>
causes of, 366–67
preventing, 367–70

symptoms of, 365–66, <u>366</u>
when to see the doctor about, <u>366</u>
Poisoning, first aid for
in adults, 513–14
in children, 500
Pollen
grass, for prostate enlargement, 234
hay fever from, 99, 104–5
Poor concentration. See Concentration
problems
Posture, for relieving neck pain, 335
Potassium supplements, for controlling
high blood pressure, 204
Poultices, in herbal medicine, 14
Prednisone, insomnia from, <u>302</u>
Pregnancy
obstacles to (see Infertility)
preventing varicose veins from,
471–72
teen, <u>68–69</u>
contraception for preventing,
126–28
myths about preventing, <u>125</u>
vaginitis during, 463, 473
Premature ejaculation
causes of, 225
preventing, 226–29
Pressyn, for memory loss, <u>317</u>
Propecia, for baldness, 170–71
Propoxyphene, mobility problems
from, <u>322</u>
Propranolol, insomnia from, <u>302</u>
Proscar, for prostate enlargement,
232
Prostate cancer
preventing, 230–31
symptoms of, <u>230</u>
Prostate enlargement
incidence of, 231–32
symptoms of, <u>230</u>, 232
treating, with
natural supplements, 232–36
prescription medication, 232
surgery, 232
Prostate gland, function of, 229
Prostatitis, symptoms of, <u>230</u>

Protein
needs, of older people, 343
for preventing osteoporosis, 352–53
Prozac
insomnia from, 302
for premature ejaculation, 228–29
PSA test
finasteride affecting, 171
for prostate cancer screening, 230
Psyllium, for constipation, 415
Pumpkin seeds, for treating
chronic fatigue, 403
prostate enlargement, 233–34
Punishments, for teen rebellion,
148–49
Pycnogenol, for varicose veins, 470
Pygeum
for increasing male fertility, 432
for prostate enlargement, 233

Q

Quercetin, for gout, 190

R

Rape
date, 67
statutory, 70
Rebellion, teen. *See* Teen rebellion
Recovery position, 486, **486**
Reishi, for high blood pressure, 206
Relaxation, for treating
heart palpitations, 285, 286–87
memory problems, 319
stress, 259, 261
Rescue breathing
classes for, 481
how to perform, 482, **483**
Respbid, insomnia from, 302
Retinitis pigmentosa, night vision
problems with, 338
Retinoids, for acne, 27
Rheumatoid arthritis. *See* Arthritis
Riboflavin, for preventing menstrual
migraines, 454

Risperdal, poor concentration from,
373
Risperidone, poor concentration from,
373
Rogaine, for baldness, 171
Rohypnol, as date-rape drug, 67, 74
Rosemary oil, for bursitis and
tendinitis, 177
Roseola, 88

S

Sage, for treating
baldness, 172
colds and flu, 58, 410–11
night sweats, 439
St. John's wort
for home medicine cabinet, 7
for smoking cessation, 240
for treating
bursitis and tendinitis, 177
depression, 420–21
Salicylic acid, for acne, 26
Saline solution, for first-aid kit, 5
Salt restriction
for preventing
calcium loss, 353
kidney stones, 224–25
for treating
breast discomfort, 388
high blood pressure, 204
Salves, in herbal medicine, 13–14
Sarsaparilla, for bursitis and tendinitis,
177
Saw palmetto
for home medicine cabinet, 7
for treating
baldness, 171–72
impotence, 216
kidney stones, 223
prostate enlargement, 232–33
Schisandra berry, for weight loss, 449
School problems
bad grades (*see* Bad grades)
bullying (*see* Bullying)
stomachache and, 138–39

Seafood. *See* Fish
Sea salt, for yeast infections, 475
Seizures. *See also* Convulsions
  in adults, first aid for, 514–15
Selegiline HCl, for memory loss, 317
Selenium, for increasing male fertility, 431
Senility. *See* Dementia
Severed appendages, first aid for, 515–16
Sex
  for conception, 430–31, 433
  frequency of, statistics on, 218
  oral, HIV from, 129
  for preventing prostate problems, 231
  teen
    forestalling, 129–30
    pressure to have, 67, 70
Sex drive, low. *See* Inhibited sexual desire
Sex education
  basics of, 66, 123–24, 126
  on pregnancy and contraception, 126–28
  on pregnancy myths, 125
  on sexually transmitted diseases, 128–29
Sexually transmitted diseases (STDs)
  educating teens about, 128–29
  teen incidence of, 145
Sexual problems. *See* Impotence; Inhibited sexual desire; Premature ejaculation
Shampoo, for baldness, 172
Shock, electric
  in children, first aid for, 494
  saving someone else from, 510–11
  saving yourself from, 509–10
Shock position, 486, **486**
Siberian ginseng, for smoking cessation, 241–42
Sibling rivalry, 131–34
Sinemet, for Parkinson's disease, 354–55, 356

Sinusitis
  in children, 54
  chronic fatigue and, 404–5
Skinfold measurements, for determining overweight in children, 119
Skullcap, for stress, 260
Sleep, for preventing memory problems, 315
Sleep apnea, 244, 244, 245
Sleeplessness. *See* Insomnia
Sleepwalking, 115
Smells, for inhibited sexual desire, 218
Smoking
  as addiction, 236
  as asthma trigger, 32
  avoiding, while using nicotine patch, 237
  effects of
    colds and flu, 413
    intermittent claudication, 303
    snoring, 245
  health risks from, 237–38
  quitting (*see* Smoking cessation)
Smoking cessation
  for preventing
    cancer, 391
    ulcers, 267
  strategies for, 238–42
  for treating
    heart palpitations, 287
    impotence, 214
    infertility, 432
    intermittent claudication, 307–8
    macular degeneration, 313
Smooth Move, for constipation, 416
Snacks
  for cavity prevention, 52
  for weight loss, 447
Snoring
  apneas with, 244, 244, 245
  causes of, 243
  preventing, 245–48, 247
  when to see the doctor about, 244
Soap, antibacterial, for home medicine cabinet, 3

Solid extracts, in herbal medicine, 13
Soreness, muscle. *See* Muscle
    soreness
Sore throat, in children, 55
Soups
    carotene, for preventing pneumonia,
      369
    chicken, as home remedy, 8
    for chronic fatigue, 403
    ginger-garlic, for colds, 411
Soy foods
    for lowering cholesterol, 210
    for menopausal problems, 434–35
Sperm problems
    infertility from, 431
    supplements for, 431–32
    from underweight and overweight,
      433
Spices, for increasing appetite, 345
Spinach, for macular degeneration,
    310
Spirometer, for asthma, 28, 30
Spitting up, in babies, 155
Splint, for broken bones, 501–2,
    502
Sponge bath, for treating fever, 89
Sports addiction
    dealing with, 250–52
    effects of, 249–50
    reasons for, 249
Sports drinks, as home remedy, 8
Sprains
    categories of, 253
    preventing, 256–57
    treating, 253–56, 255
    when to see the doctor about,
      254
Squats, for abdominal toning,
    163–64
Stalking, 71
Standardization, in herbal medicine,
    18–19
STDs. *See* Sexually transmitted
    diseases
Stinging nettle. *See* Nettle

Stockings, compression
    for preventing varicose veins,
      471–72
    for treating phlebitis, 362
Stomachache
    causes of, 134–35, 138–39
    treating, with
      herbs, 139–40
      home remedies, 135–39
      massage, 136–37
    when to see the doctor about, 135
Stomach cancer, 263
Strength training
    for treating
      menopausal problems, 439–40
      mobility problems, 320, 323–24
    for weight loss, 450
Stress
    caregivers and, 395–400
    dealing with, 195, 258–62
    effects of, 258
      colds, 56
      heart palpitations, 286
      impotence, 215
      nightmares, 117
      stomachache, 138
      tension headaches, 451
      ulcers, 264
      vaginitis, 467
    reasons for, 257
    when to see the doctor about, 258
Stretching
    for preventing
      muscle soreness, 331–33
      sprains, 257
      varicose veins, 471
    for treating
      hip pain, 290–91
      mobility problems, 324,
      324–27
      neck pain, 335
      tendinitis, 176
Strokes, intermittent claudication and,
    304
Stuttering, 140–44, 143

Suffocation, in children, first aid for, 488
Sugar avoidance, for preventing
    caregiver stress, 398
    depression, 423
    yeast infections, 478
Suicide, by teens, 110, <u>111</u>
Sunflower seeds, for chronic fatigue, 403
Sunlight, avoiding, with macular
    degeneration, 309–10
Supplements. *See also specific supplements*
    evaluating, with memory loss, <u>317</u>
Support groups
    for caregivers, 284
    for preventing teen loneliness, 110
Suppositories, for treating
    constipation in babies, 60–61
    yeast infections, 476–77

T

Tablets, in herbal medicine, 13
Teas
    green, for weight loss, 448
    herbal, for treating
        breast discomfort, 387
        bursitis and tendinitis, 177
        colds, 57, 58
        constipation, <u>416</u>
        flatulence, <u>186</u>, 187
        tension headaches, 453
    in herbal medicine, 11–12
    for preventing heart disease, 196
Teasing. *See* Bullying
Teen rebellion, 144–45
    dealing with, 146–49
    preparing for, 145–46
    risks associated with, 145
    serious, signs of, <u>147</u>
Television, positive uses of, <u>151</u>
Temperature, how to take, 87
Tendinitis. *See* Bursitis and tendinitis
Theophylline, insomnia from, <u>302</u>

Thermometer
    for constipation in babies, 61–62
    for home medicine cabinet, 4
    rectal vs. oral, 87
Thorazine, mobility problems from, <u>322</u>
Tinctures, in herbal medicine, 12
Tobacco, abuse of, 72
Toe injuries, in children, first aid for, 496–97
Tofranil, side effects of
    night vision problems, <u>340</u>
    poor concentration, <u>373</u>
Toilet training, constipation and, 63
Tomatoes, for preventing cancer, 393
Tooth care, in children
    for cavity prevention, 48, 50
    supervising, <u>51</u>
Toothpaste, for children, 48, 50, <u>51</u>
Toxic substances, preventing cancer
    from, 392–93
Trazodone, night vision problems
    from, <u>340</u>
Tribulus terrestris, for inhibited sexual
    desire, 218–19
Trichomoniasis, 462, 463
Tryptophan, for insomnia, 301–2
Turmeric, for arthritis, 274
TV addiction
    negative effects of, 150
    overcoming, 150, 152–53
Tweezers, for first-aid kit, 5

U

Ulcers
    causes of, 262–63
    preventing, 267
    symptoms of, 263
    treating, 263–67, <u>266</u>
    when to see the doctor about, <u>263</u>
Underweight, infertility from, 433
Unisom, poor concentration from, <u>373</u>
Urinary tract infections (UTIs)
    causes of, 457–59
    preventing, 461–62

Urinary tract infections *(cont.)*
 treating, 459–61
 when to see the doctor about, <u>458</u>
Urination problems. *See* Incontinence;
 Prostate problems
UTIs. *See* Urinary tract infections
Uva-ursi, for urinary tract infections,
 460

V

Vaccine, pneumonia, 367–68
Vacuum cleaner bags, for dust mite
 control, 102
Vaginal dryness, in menopause,
 438
Vaginitis
 causes of, 462–63
 diagnosing, <u>458</u>
 treating, 464–67, <u>464–65</u>
 when to see the doctor about,
 <u>463</u>
Valerian, for treating
 back pain, 167
 flatulence, <u>186</u>
 insomnia, 299
 stress, 260
Valium, side effects of
 mobility problems, <u>322</u>
 poor concentration, <u>373</u>
Valsalva's maneuver, for heart
 palpitations, 286
Vancenase, night vision problems
 from, <u>340</u>
Varicose veins
 cause of, 468
 preventing, 471–72
 treating, 469–70
 when to see the doctor about,
 <u>468</u>
Vasopressin, for memory loss, <u>317</u>
Vegetables
 for preventing
 cancer, 393, 394
 heart disease, 194–95

for treating
 constipation, 415
 heart disease, 346
 high blood pressure, 204
 macular degeneration, 310
Vegetarians, iron sources for,
 380–81
Vinca major, for preventing memory
 loss, 318
Vinegar, as home remedy, 8
Visine, for concealing pimples, <u>25</u>
Vision problems, bad grades and, 36
Vistaril, poor concentration from,
 <u>373</u>
Visualization
 with asthma inhaler use, 31
 for night vision problems, 339
Vitamin A
 for preventing
 menstrual discomfort, 444
 prostate cancer, 231
 for treating
 arthritis, 347
 colds and flu, 412
 vaginitis, 464–65
Vitamin B$_6$, for preventing
 heart disease, 197
 menstrual migraines, <u>454–55</u>
 phlebitis, 363
Vitamin B$_{12}$
 deficiency of, memory problems
 from, 346
 for preventing
 heart disease, 197
 phlebitis, 363
Vitamin C
 for increasing male fertility,
 431–32
 for preventing
 cancer, 394
 dementia, 279
 pneumonia, 368–69
 prostate cancer, 231
 varicose veins, 472
 sources of, 6

for treating
  arthritis, 347
  colds and flu, 412
  depression, 422
  intermittent claudication, 307
  menopausal problems, 436–37
  muscle soreness, 331
  Parkinson's disease, 357
  urinary tract infections, 459
  vaginitis, 465–66
Vitamin D
  for preventing
    dementia, 280
    osteoporosis, 346, 349, 350–51
  for treating arthritis, 347
Vitamin E
  for preventing
    cancer, 394
    dementia, 278
    heart disease, 197
    male infertility, 431
    menstrual discomfort, 444
    menstrual migraines, 455
    phlebitis, 363
    prostate cancer, 231
  sources of, 6
  for treating
    arthritis, 347
    breast discomfort, 387–88
    impotence, 215
    intermittent claudication, 307
    menopausal symptoms, 437–38,
      466
    Parkinson's disease, 357
    vaginitis, 466
Vitamin K, for preventing
  osteoporosis, 351
Vitamins and minerals. *See also specific*
  vitamins and minerals
  needs, of older people, 343–44
  recommended, 5–6
Vomiting
  in babies, 155
  treating, 154, 156–58
  when to see the doctor about, 156–57

W

Walking
  with Parkinson's disease, 359
  for preventing
    constipation, 417
    pneumonia, 370
  for treating
    arthritis, 273
    intermittent claudication,
      305–6
    menstrual discomfort, 443
    mobility problems, 323
Wandering, with dementia, 282
Warts, genital, from human
  papillomavirus, 128
Water, drinking
  for preventing
    breast discomfort, 388
    constipation, 417
    kidney stones, 221–22
  for treating
    menstrual discomfort, 443
    urinary tract infections, 459
Weight, ideal, determining, 445
Weight control
  for preventing
    breast cancer, 389, 392
    breast discomfort, 389
    varicose veins, 471
  for treating infertility, 433
Weight loss
  strategies, in children
    exercise, 121–22
    healthy eating, 120–21
    support, 122–23
  for treating
    arthritis, 272–73
    gout, 192
    high blood pressure, 203
    hip pain, 290
    snoring, 247, 248
  in women
    best time to begin, 446
    eating plan for, 446–48

Weight loss *(cont.)*
   in women *(cont.)*
      exercise for, 449–50
      realistic goals for, 445
Wheat, avoiding, with sinusitis, 405
Wheat germ, as home remedy, 8–9
White oak bark, for phlebitis, 364–65
Whole foods, for treating heart
      disease, 346
Wild yam, for snoring, 247
Witch hazel, for treating
   hemorrhoids, 200–201
   varicose veins, 469
Wounds, open, first aid for, 512–13

X

Xanax, mobility problems from, 322

Y

Yarrow, for treating
   colds, 58
   phlebitis, 364
Yeast infections, 462
   causes of, 473
   preventing, 476–78
   treating, 474–76, 475
   when to see the doctor about,
      474
Yellow dock, for anemia, 384
Yogurt
   as home remedy, 9
   for treating
      lactose intolerance, 9, 185
      yeast infections, 474–75
Y-Snore Anti-snoring Nose Drops,
   247

Z

Zinc
   for increasing male fertility, 432
   for preventing
      dementia, 280
      pneumonia, 369
   sources of, 6
   for treating
      burns, 505
      colds and flu, 412
      prostate enlargement, 234–35
      vaginitis, 466
Zyban, for smoking cessation, 238,
   239–40